SUPERFOODS TO SUPERHEALTH

Intelligent and sustainable food choices

for the next generation

Dr Johanna Ward

Disclaimer: Although the author and publisher have made every effort to ensure that the information in this book was correct at time of press, the author and publisher do not assume and hereby disclaim any liability to any party for any loss, damage, or disruption caused by errors or omissions, whether such errors or omissions result from negligence, accident, or any other cause.

This book is not intended as a substitute for the medical advice of physicians. The reader should regularly consult a physician in matters relating to his/her health and particularly with respect to any symptoms that may require diagnosis or medical attention.

First printing: 2019

ISBN-13: 978-1-9161087-0-7

Published by ZENii Ltd

British Cataloguing Publication Data:
A catalogue record of this book is available from The British Library.

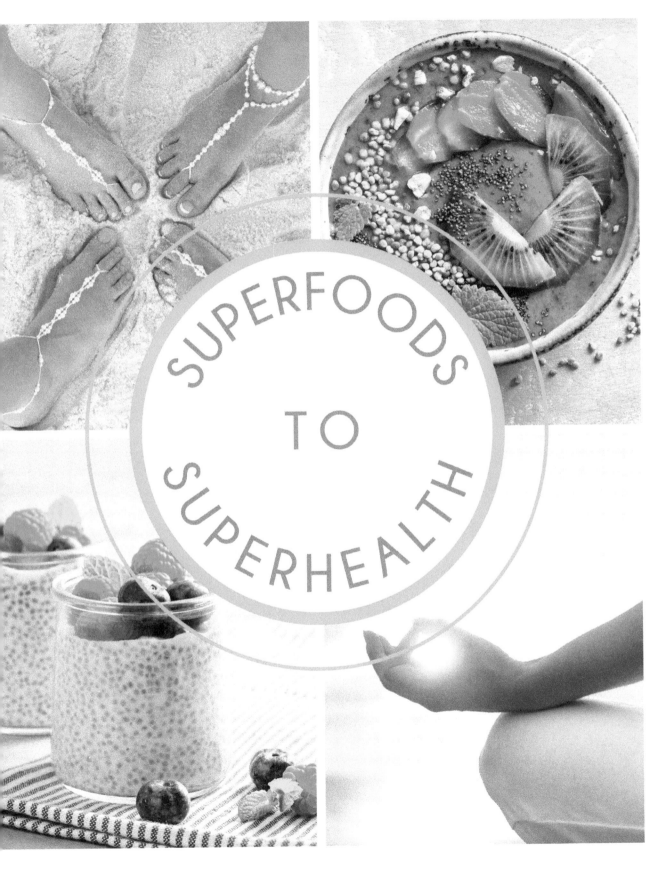

SUPERFOODS TO SUPERHEALTH

To our future generations

Thank you

This book is dedicated to my husband, my children and my family, all of whom have supported me in this project and in my every endeavour.

To my husband Craig - Without you I would be nothing and life would have been a totally lesser experience. Thank you for your unending love, support and inspiration and for helping me find soul deep joy.

To my beautiful children - It is for you that I write this book, to help protect your perfect bodies and beautiful souls from the perils of modern life. It is here for you to one day use to teach your own precious children how to live long, happy and healthy lives. You are my *raison d'être*, my joy, my love, my life.

To my mother and father - The education, love and life you have given me has been incredible - I consider myself truly blessed. You taught me to value people and not possessions and to live the life that I wanted to live. This was your gift to me.

Dad - Thank you for the inspiration to become a doctor. Your life has been spent serving others and you are nothing short of a total inspiration to me. Our health-related chats helped shape these words and these chapters and helped me realise that I needed to put my learning down to benefit others. If I am half the doctor you are, I will be happy.

Mum - Thank you for everything, big and small, that you do to support and love me and my family. Your warmth, gentleness and kindness of spirit will always be with me.

To my brothers Ville and David and my sisters Rebecca and Rachel - You all know how precious you are to me. This book is for your children and for all the future generations yet to come.

To my dearest friend Sally, who lost her mother at the age of 17 to cancer and whose young life showed me the great sadness and loss that cancer causes. I am so glad you finally found your Ray of Light. No one deserves it more than you.

To my friend Debbie and to my Auntie Aija - who are both currently battling breast cancer - this is for you because I know you both wanted and needed this information during your difficult journeys. Infinite love and prayers to you both.

To Dr Hilary Jones - Thank you for inspiring me and for teaching me the positive power of medical education via the media. Your friendship and mentoring are deeply valued.

To Dee Jones - My yogi, personal trainer and all-round muse - Thank you for sharing your infectious love of life and exercise with me. You truly have a gift.

To Charlotte Kjaer - Your cooking is simply divine. Thank you for creating with me the most wonderful and delicious recipes that grace this book. Hopefully together we can inspire the next generations to eat clean and green.

To Sam Burton - Thank you for years of wonderful friendship and mental support and for helping me to discover the joys of yoga, mindfulness, meditation and ashrams!

To Laurie Noble - Thank you for your unending patience and vision in bringing our recipes alive in your photos. Life is colour and beauty.

To Andy Hughes – You are a star. Thank you for everything and all the last-minute extras that I always throw upon you! I can't thank you or repay you enough.

CONTENTS

ABOUT THE AUTHOR

Dr Johanna Ward
BA Hons MBBS DRCOG MRCGP Dip Clin Derm

Dr Johanna Ward is a GP with a special interest in dermatology and nutrition. She studied English Literature at Oxford University and then went on to study postgraduate medicine at Guys, Kings & St Thomas' Hospital in London. Her postgraduate training was in family health, women's health, clinical dermatology and nutrition.

Dr Ward lives with her husband and children in Kent. She lectures nationally and internationally on the importance of lifestyle and nutrition in health and is frequently asked to comment in the media on all aspects of health, wellness and ageing. Dr Ward has won numerous awards for her health-promoting work, most notably 'Rising Star' (2011) and 'Best Blogger/Journalist' (2016). She is currently *Women's Health* magazine's resident doctor.

Most importantly, Dr Ward has dedicated her professional life to her patients and helps them on a daily basis to achieve better balance, health and happiness in their lives. She is a firm advocate of the power of preventative and nutritional medicine and wrote this book to set down some of her survival tips for the modern age.

FOREWORD BY DR HILARY JONES
GP, TV Presenter and Author

If you only buy one book devoted to health and wellbeing this year, *Superfoods to Superhealth* should be it. Irrefutably.

Dr Johanna Ward is a highly experienced doctor with dual qualifications in both science and arts, who manages to combine robust medical research with a compassionate, caring and holistic approach to everything she does and everyone she treats. She is passionate about the need for all of us to take greater responsibility for our own health in a world that is facing a number of increasingly urgent social, environmental and health-related crises.

Superfoods to Superhealth addresses head-on the great individual and public health challenges of our time: the conditions we all fear most, such as cancer, dementia, obesity, diabetes, heart disease, stress and autoimmune disease. It questions our naive over-reliance on pharmaceuticals, our unrealistic expectations of 'a pill for every ill' and the over-medicalisation of normal human responses to unhealthy lifestyles, stress, unhappiness and premature ageing.

For many people, both young and old, healthcare and modern medicine as we know it is failing us. We have somehow lost touch with the fundamentals of feeling and being totally well.

This book is the perfect and timely prescription and remedy. In it, Dr Ward explains clearly and precisely - with many a wise quotation to support her views - how small yet simple adjustments to the way we live our lives can pay unbelievable dividends in terms of our quality and quantity of life. Illustrated in colour with mouth-watering and healthy recipes along with easy-to-practice yoga and Pilates stretches, the book embraces state-of-the-art knowledge about the importance of good gut health and the benefits of a largely plant-based diet and explains how sound nutrition, a relaxed mindset and energy-generating physical exercise and mobility can transform us in mind, body and soul. Reading it will be seriously good for your health.

Dr Hilary Jones

WHY YOU NEED THIS BOOK

"If you think wellness is expensive, try illness."

Writing this book has been an incredible educational journey for me and I only hope that you enjoy the read as much as I enjoyed the research and writing of it.

I have always had an interest in health and wellbeing; it's no doubt the reason I chose to study medicine all those years ago. I had a desire to help and to contribute to the greater good of mankind. It has only been in recent years that I finally understood where I could make my contribution most impactful. My father is a surgeon and cancer specialist and he has inspired me enormously. He has worked like a trojan for the NHS over the years and his devotion to his patients is nothing short of incredible. His esteemed surgical career has inspired a generation of doctors and he taught me to enjoy the art and skill of medicine. It is thanks to him that I realised I needed to put my learnings down on paper for the benefit of others.

I am a GP with a special interest in preventative, nutritional and lifestyle medicine. I have devoted my professional career to the science and study of ageing and how we can preserve and optimise cellular health. In this book I have tried to examine how modern, industrialised living influences our genes and our overall health and I have put together a diet and lifestyle plan to help reduce disease risk. This diet and lifestyle plan is sustainable and has a low environmental impact. We now have enough scientific evidence to show a clear link between modern Western diets and lifestyles and the great medical problems of our age - obesity, diabetes, cancer, dementia, heart disease and stroke.

We have enormous power over the current health crisis that we face in the West. Many of the diseases we suffer and die from are dietary in their cause and are therefore preventable. We can positively influence our disease risk through the food and lifestyle choices we make each and every day. We have the power to preserve our lives or destroy them. And we have to be accountable for this and learn to become our own health advocates.

The world around us has changed immeasurably in the last hundred years. The food we eat, the lives we lead, the jobs we choose, the stress we endure - these all impact on our longevity and our health span. Our modern lives throw us into conflict with our traditional lives and serve as a source of disconnect between us and the natural world. We live in a modern, urban, global age. An age of 24/7. We are swamped by overflowing inboxes and endless technology. We work more than ever. We struggle to switch off. We eat fast, convenient, ultra-processed foods. We are overweight but undernourished. We live in an age of growing environmental pollution and planetary concern. An age of inadvertent chemical and toxin exposure. An age of cancer, dementia and cardiovascular disease. An age of spiritual anaemia and disconnect.

This book is my exploration of the impact of these changes on human life, happiness, cellular function, cancer risk, immunity and even the state of the planet. In essence, it is an essay on the perils of modern Western living and how we need to act now to reclaim our health. This book is a survival guide for the modern urban age. A preventative blueprint to help empower and navigate you back to health.

In order to live a long and healthy life there are many basic things we need to satisfy. To enjoy optimum health, we need to get the full range of micronutrients. This includes a daily intake of 21 essential minerals, 13 vitamins, 9 essential amino acids and 2 essential fatty acids. But most of us don't even know how to go about this, even if we are health motivated. We also need to have an effective detoxification system, an effective metabolism, an effective immune system and a balanced microbiome, to name just a few. In addition, science tells us more and more that those who stave off disease best and enjoy optimum health have fulfilment and love in their lives, positive support networks, regular relaxation and enjoy great mental health. So, there is a lot we need to optimise in order to survive, let alone thrive. Even the most educated and motivated person might have somehow missed out on this vital information and might not know how to connect the dots. I will show you how to reclaim and prioritise your health and escape the medical statistics.

More so than ever, humans are exposed to innumerable toxins, chemicals and radiation. We need to learn how to live a life that combats these pollutants on a daily basis and helps restore cellular heath and harmony. Too many people have become the victims of modern western living. Many have given up and resigned themselves to suffering the pain of chronic disease, to brain fog, toxic headaches, fatigue, poor mental health and the inevitable burdens of getting old. But it doesn't have to be this way. These are all compounded by the choices we make each and every day and made worse by toxin overload and nutrient deficiency. This book will help you to survive the toxic insults of daily life and will teach you how to take charge of your own health, reduce inflammation and live a long, healthy life. It also contains vital up to date scientific information on how to live a life that minimises the risk of cancer, heart disease and a whole host of other illnesses that are generally a result of our westernised lives. Throughout the book I have put together practical tips and health hacks to help you incorporate positive change into your daily routine. The good news is there is an enormous amount you can do yourself to improve your disease risk and to successfully age. You just need to know how - and you need to start now.

Our diets need to be rich in nutrients and not devised in labs. We need to eat real food that is in its natural state, whole and filling, rich in vitamins, minerals and the ever-important antioxidants. It's actually easier than you think to eat a well-balanced diet: you just have to make mindful food choices every day and hold tight against the temptations of high sugar, high GI foods that populate the food aisles of most supermarkets. A return to fresh, local, organic whole foods is the best way to guarantee achieving nutritional wellness.

We are the first generation predicted to live in excess of 100 years if we take care of ourselves. But what is the point if we are immobilised by chronic pain, or staggering around a nursing home with dementia so entrenched that we longer know who we or our loved ones are? The thought of living a long life only really appeals if we are blessed with the good health to enjoy it. What we do today and the choices we make each and every day become even more important if we want to maximise our potential lifespan and healthspan. The good news is that it's never too late to make positive changes to your diet and lifestyle that will profoundly improve your health. The body responds quickly to healthful choices and nurturing and has an incredible regenerative and reparative capability. Even if you are chronically ill or suffering from cancer it's never too late - so this book is for you.

Now IS the time to embrace dietary and lifestyle changes, to overhaul the toxic load and begin anew. Science already shows us that 80-90% of cancers are caused by the lifestyle and food choices we make, and we already know that once we have cancer there are many things we can do to extend remission and slow cancerous cells through our lifestyle and diet. So now absolutely IS the time to act. Do not put it off any longer. The benefits you will reap will ripple down through to your friends and family and you can teach them how to live well and long through simple daily changes.

Big pharmaceutical biotech companies have invested insane amounts of money trying to find a 'cure' for cellular ageing and disease. They have literally spent billions trying to find a cure for cancer, dementia and cardiovascular disease. But the truth is there really is no single pharmaceutical agent that can defeat or combat cellular ageing. And right now, there is no single chemical agent that can fight cancer or cardiovascular disease fully either. The truth is that pharmaceutics aren't the answer. Diseases that are caused by a lifetime of poor dietary and lifestyle choices can only be reversed through dietary and lifestyle improvement. There is no lazy option. No shortcut to health. No magic bullet or pill. It is something you have to choose to embrace every day for the rest of your life. And yes, it does take effort initially - a lot of effort and a lot of willpower! And yes, it's much easier not to bother. But once you rewire your brain into healthy mode it quickly becomes ingrained in your subconscious and healthful and positive choices will come with ease. You will automatically choose foods that nourish your body over junk foods. You will want to eat superfoods as part of every meal. You will want to cut out sugar when you realise how toxic it is. You will automatically choose to move and make exercise a daily ritual without really knowing it and most certainly without resenting it. In fact, days when you don't exercise you will miss it. Renewed energy, mental clarity and improved health will be your rewards. Everyone can benefit from healthful living and can reverse cellular damage and become biologically younger. And if you fall off the healthy bandwagon (which we all do occasionally!) you simply get back on and start again. What you do every day has far more impact than what you do every once in a while.

Obesity is on the rise - we have become overweight but undernourished. Our collective health is in decline. Obesity is the second biggest preventable cause of cancer after smoking. It is a big deal.

Our children, teenagers and young adults are at risk because they know no other world than processed foods, supermarkets, Subway, Starbucks, and the big chains that sell high-sugar, nutrient-depleted convenience foods. We need to help young people deal with the temptations they face every day. High-sugar and fast foods are highly addictive and have become entrenched in their way of thinking. The continual consumption of processed and unhealthy foods dumps on society in high healthcare costs, high disability and premature death. Recent studies have shown that teenagers in the UK eat less than one portion of fruit or vegetables a day (WHO 2014). This is highly worrying given that they more than anyone else need to have nutrient-dense food for growth, maturation and sound mental health.

Remember this - cheap food isn't cheap. It has a cost somewhere even if it's not at the checkout. Young bodies and minds are being polluted by this inner deluge of highly addictive junk foods with little intake of fruit and vegetables. Add to this their love of technology and phones, which makes them more sedentary than previous generations, and it's not hard to see how we have ended up with nearly a quarter of our youth obese. So we need to teach the next generation how to make healthy and positive lifestyle and dietary choices. We need to teach them how to cook and eat whole foods, show them how to enjoy movement and get off the couch. We need to lead by example in order for the generation that follows us to enjoy long and healthy lives. We also need to teach them how to make sustainable food choices, because the foods they choose to eat will determine the future of this precious planet.

This is no longer 'alternative' or peripheral medicine. A huge number of healthcare professionals are starting to realise that nutritional, preventative and lifestyle medicine is evidence-based medicine and progressive. It is the medicine of the future. Any doctor who ignores the power of nutrition and lifestyle is doing his or her patients a huge disservice. If that describes your doctor, get yourself a new doctor. The only way to change an epidemic of diet and lifestyle related diseases is to change the diet and lifestyle! It sounds obvious - and it is. It is time we change what is on our plate, what we put into our mouths and what we do with our spare time. Doing so will change the future of our planet and the future of our collective health.

The realisation and will to change comes to us all at different times. For me, my call to action was having my three children and realising that I had a duty to them to nourish and protect them as much as I possibly could in my lifetime. Before then, my commitment to my health was significantly less than it is now. For some of you, a cancer or diabetes diagnosis may be the wake-up call. For others, a life event like losing a loved one or divorce may trigger the desire to reprogram and prioritise.

The current state of the NHS makes access to preventative medicine much harder. Resources are limited and many doctors simply don't have the time in a 7-10 minute consultation to cover the vast topic of nutrition and lifestyle. Worse still, our current medical system works on payments for prescriptions and pills and doesn't always reward us for actual health improvements. Too many doctors prescribe symptom-suppressing, 'quick-fix' medicines instead of actually looking at the root cause of illness. And Big Pharma benefits from us being sick, not healthy.

In short, no one profits from lifestyle and preventative medicine except YOU. And unfortunately, mainstream medicine has become like a business with pharmaceutics and symptom-suppressing drugs top of the board. We have forgotten to treat the actual root cause of illness and instead practise a kind of fire-fighting medicine. What this means is that we can no longer be complacent and expect others to look after our best interests. We can't expect our doctors or the government to do it for us. Health and wellness needs to be self-served and self-motivated. We need to be accountable. It's time we invest in ourselves and learn how to be our own health protectors before the whistle blows.

The great news is that there is one diet that helps reduce ALL the diseases of western affluence and unhealthy behaviour. And there is one lifestyle that triumphs over ALL. That diet is a whole foods diet and that lifestyle is an active one. Westerners have been eating the wrong foods for the last hundred years and we have paid a heavy price. There are many healthy diets but the modern western diet is not one of them. I will show you in this book how eating the right foods can simultaneously save your life and save our planet. You don't need to rely on drugs and pharmaceutics to buy you extra time - diet alone can reverse disease, restore health and add up to 20 quality years to your life. Combine a healthy diet with daily exercise, mindful living, plentiful sleep and not smoking and you will cut your risk of heart disease by 80%, halve your risk of stroke, slash your risk of dementia and cut your risk of cancer in half. Not many drugs can do that!

With the world's population set to reach 9.6 billion by 2050 the question of WHICH diet takes on a fierce importance. For the sake of future generations, it is a matter of urgency that we realign our dietary choices with sustainability to save the planet from ecological ruin. Because there is no Planet B.

Our dietary choices need to be low impact whilst nutritionally dense, affordable and highly available. We have to puncture the twentieth century myth that humans can eat whatever they want, whenever they want, in whatever quantities they want. It's simply not sustainable. Food's role in environmental degradation is beyond dispute. In Europe, food is the European consumer's biggest source of greenhouse gases and meat and dairy account for over 20% of these greenhouse emissions.[1]

We must learn to live within our environmental limits, in harmony with nature and our surroundings. The Western dream of unlimited consumption is unsustainable and ultimately selfish. Americans eat an average of three hamburgers a week, or 156 hamburgers per person per year. With a population of over 310 million they eat over 48 billion hamburgers ever year, creating over 158 billion tonnes of greenhouse hamburger gases. This is simply insane. A $4 hamburger takes over 2,400 litres of water to make, which is more than 10 times the amount required for beans and grains and creates significant greenhouse gas emissions. What we don't pay for at the checkout we pay for in environmental damage and climate change. The real cost of that hamburger is much much more than $4. We use eight times as much land for feeding animals as we do for feeding humans. Land has been cleared globally on a huge scale to make space for livestock at the expense of forests that sequester greenhouse gases like carbon dioxide. Add to this the methane and nitric oxide gases caused by livestock rearing and it's soon obvious that if we want to save our planet we all need to cut back on our mass produced meat consumption for the sake of the greater good.

It's time we unite our food choices with planetary sustainability. Never has it been more important for us to try and live in harmony with our surroundings. Humans will pay the ultimate price if we keep chasing the western 'unlimited consumption' dream. The western world is now one of over-nutrition, where over one third of all foods are wasted despite huge issues with malnutrition in the developing world. We live in a modern, gluttonous world where there are vastly more overweight people (1.5 billion) than there are hungry people (0.9 billion). What a sad state we are in.

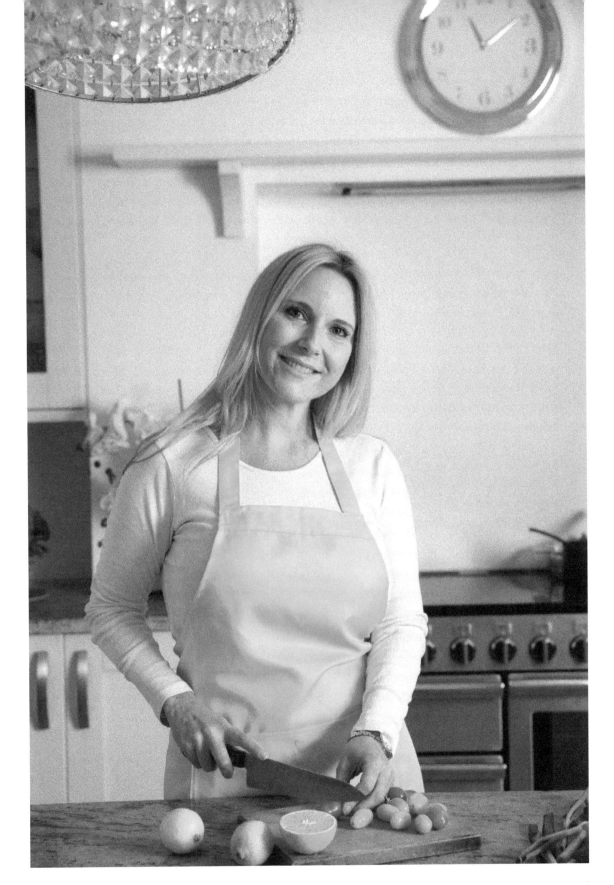

The educational website ForksOverKnives puts the issue of livestock, world hunger and sustainable living eloquently: "We are producing enough grain globally to feed two times as many people as there are on Earth. In 2011, there was a record harvest of grain in the world, with over 2.5 billion tons, but half of that was fed to animals in the meat and dairy industries. 77 percent of all coarse grains (corn, oats, sorghum, barley) and over 90 percent of all soy grown in the world was fed to livestock. Add to that the 30 percent food waste from farm to table, and we see clearly that the difficulty is not how to produce enough food to feed the hungry but rather where all the food we produce is going."[2]

Enough said. It's time to make some radical changes - if not for your own health, for the survival of future generations and for the survival of the planet. This book will help you do exactly that.

I would like to thank all my patients who have shared their health journeys with me over the years and who have asked so many intelligent questions. You all made me delve deeper and now I share what I have learnt. I have written this book in my head many times over so I am thankful for the time out of my clinical work to put it together and I am thankful that I can now finally share it with you all.

Thank you to all the scientists, biochemists, doctors, nutritionists and wellness advocates who have written up their findings in journals, books, and articles. No scientific or medical book can be written without the huge volume of work that goes before it by many others. This book is heavily indebted to you all and rests heavily on your shoulders.

Lastly, thanks to all the healthcare workers who devote their professional lives (and exhaust themselves daily) to serve the greater good of mankind. Without people like you, we would all be in much worse states of health. You have saved my life several times over already. For this you have my deepest and humblest thanks.

Finally, I hope this book inspires you, the reader, to become your own health advocate and to prioritise and take charge of your own health and wellbeing. Nothing matters more than your health. The real aim is to live to a great old age but to feel young and well when you get there!

Dr Johanna Ward, London, 2019

PREFACE

This book draws heavily on all the latest research and science. It is guided by an exhaustive number of research articles and studies. I have indexed all the journals, research papers and books that I mention for anyone who wants to delve deeper.

I have tried to make this book an educational guide and inspiration that will start a lifelong journey of health and wellness. It cannot and does not include everything but will hopefully begin a process of learning and education for you and your loved ones. Health is a lifelong commitment. Along the way I want to inspire you, motivate you, help you and, most importantly, make it so easy that you cannot help but embrace what I am saying and put it into use in your daily life. I have sought to make this book more visual and digestible in the hope that you stick with me for the entirety of the journey through to the very end, where you will find some fabulous life-enhancing recipes to start your precious journey.

I have tried to present the best science and the most up to date evidence in this book for your benefit. Establishing absolute proof in medicine, in particular in nutritional and lifestyle medicine, is an impossible task. There exists a complex interplay between genetics, lifestyle, food and health behaviours and it can be difficult to untangle one from the other. Furthermore, scientific studies are never perfect and are all limited by external factors - by the number of participants, by the study design, by time factors and by finances. The studies I cite in this book represent the best evidence that we have right now. Of course, more studies could always be done but the exciting thing is that more studies ARE being done all the time and more and more studies ARE showing us that improving our diets and lifestyles can be hugely positive and impactful.

The studies cited in the Superfoods section are of course less extensive and robust because very few companies are interested in investing their money into proving that foods like broccoli, berries and mushrooms have health benefits. Big Pharma can't patent and sell that. They are important nonetheless because they show us that our food choices can be healing and beneficial.

With a book like this there will always be people who insist that the evidence isn't truly reflective or that a study cites results that are insufficient. And there will always be those who cherry pick what I say, remove it from its context and criticise it. Scientific studies aren't perfect and will never give absolute proof but we can't wait for absolute proof; it will never come and in the meantime we will miss our chance to optimise health in the best way we know how.

As I write this I am reminded of the words of Albert Einstein, who once wrote: 'The truth of a theory can never be proven, for one never knows if future experience will contradict its conclusion.' It's the nature of the beast that our understanding of science is dynamic and continuously changing. At some point today's science becomes out of date as new understanding replaces and surpasses what we currently know.

Working in medicine, we all take the Hippocratic Oath that states 'Do no harm'. As doctors, scientists, researchers we are all trying to minimise risk and harm for our patients whilst also trying to push forward boundaries. Sometimes these two don't go hand in hand particularly well. We live in an age of litigation and defensive practice and it's important that we don't discourage risk taking and narrow our viewpoint so much that we stop pushing the boundaries and we stop trying to figure out the solutions. Trial and error is the way we have made significant progress over previous generations. We probably won't ever solve the problem of death and dying but (because most of us want to live forever!) I doubt humanity will ever give up trying… This is my small contribution.

I will show you how to improve your potential lifespan but it is always sensible to involve your own physician in your healthcare decisions. They will know things about you that I don't. Please reach out to them and start what may become a very powerful long-term dialogue and relationship between you and your physician.

This book has no corporate sponsorship or motive. I have no dietary agenda other than focusing on health and sustainability. As a mum of three, I want to do what I can in my lifetime to make the world that my children inherit safe, healthy and beautiful.

I hope this book will empower you, the individual - you don't have to wait for your own doctor to tell you to address your diet and lifestyle. You don't need a prescription. The changes I talk about in this book are things we can all do today, right now. And we can do them with our family, friends and loved ones to bring about better, healthier and happier lives for us all.

In recent years our numbers and statistics may 'look' better but actually we have just become better at living with chronic disease. I want to change that. The journey begins with you...

PART ONE
Our world in crisis

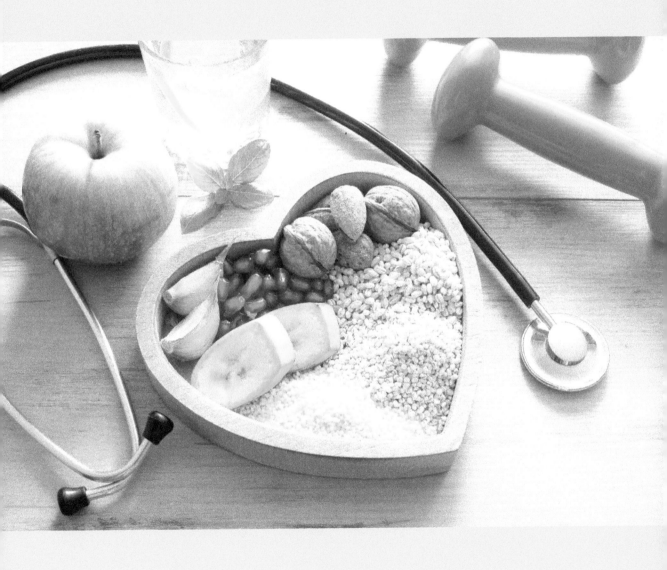

CHAPTER 1: Our World in Crisis

Mankind is on the edge of a healthcare crisis. Current trends suggest that one in two of us will get cancer and 75% of us will die from heart disease or stroke. Despite recent advances in science and medicine plus the billions spent on disease research and pharmaceutical development, millions of us are succumbing to preventable diseases every year. What on earth is happening and why is it happening?

There is compelling evidence now to suggest that it is our diets and lifestyles that are responsible for this crisis. Our current public health problems stem from over-eating industrially processed, junk foods and doing little physical movement to counteract the excess. It's called 'over-nutrition'. Eating too much, and eating too much of the wrong thing, spells disaster for a community. What we notice from the study of food in society is that any society that moves away from its traditional diet and embraces an industrialised, westernised, processed diet generally sees the same pattern of chronic disease follow - first obesity; then diabetes, heart disease, stroke and cancer. These are called 'western' diseases because they are really only seen in places that have adopted westernised, ultra-processed diets alongside lack of exercise and sedentary behaviour.

Cancer, heart disease and stroke are our biggest killers. They are increasing because of the lives we are living, the foods we are eating and the toxins we are exposed to. They are also increasing because of the things we are failing to do - the foods we fail to eat, the exercise we fail to do, the self-care we fail to practise. Disease levels go up when countries adopt more westernised living patterns. Our modern health crisis is a culmination of all the problems that modern, western living has brought - ultra-processed foods, inflammatory lifestyles, pharmaceutical overuse, chronic stress, environmental pollutants and a general breakdown in sense of purpose and wellbeing that I call 'spiritual anaemia'. The truth is that the last hundred years of human history have not served us well. Advancements in agriculture and technology have inadvertently brought us pollution, toxins and more chemicals in our food chain than we can even count or pronounce.

We need to actively engage in the protection and promotion of our own health. It is within our power to reduce the impending crisis and to improve our chances of surviving by changing the way we live. We are by no means powerless and the sooner we understand how our daily choices influence disease risk, the sooner we will be able to fight the crisis on our hands. If you focus on eating a more plant-centred, whole foods diet and exercising and relaxing more you can make a huge and positive impact to your overall health. These changes will create an inhospitable environment for cancer cells, they will reverse heart disease and stroke risk and will be better able to sustain you in your future life. Your risk for cancer, heart disease, diabetes and stroke will all come down if you embrace healthful eating and healthful living. And of course, all of this can exist alongside your conventional medical treatment plan until one day you may find that you don't need your cholesterol, blood pressure or diabetic pills anymore.

Medical anthropologists have described our current era as the Age of Degenerative and Man-Made Diseases.[3] We now survive the infective diseases of the previous century, like tuberculosis and smallpox, only to succumb to diseases caused by our global abuse and overuse of food. Our collective mentality seems to be to eat whatever the hell we want and then erase the consequences with pills. Global spending on prescription drugs is estimated to surpass $1.5 trillion by the end of 2020, with Big Pharma sales larger than the GDP of more than 15 developing countries combined. Blood pressure and cholesterol-lowering medications are the most prescribed drugs in the UK, with an estimated one in seven of us on statins to control cholesterol. They have an incredible list of side effects and can cause everything from muscle damage, insomnia, dizziness, memory loss and confusion to liver toxicity, and in rare instances even death. What a risk to take when our cholesterol and blood pressure respond so easily to simple lifestyle measures.

Is it that we are too lazy to do it ourselves or could it be that the public have been kept in the dark about the power of nutritional and lifestyle medicine? I strongly feel it is the latter. The problem is that lifestyle and nutritional measures feature very little in our consultation and hospital processes - so little that they get forgotten. We stick a band aid on most medical problems by prescribing drugs and carrying on until the problem presents itself again. Modern medicine is rather like crisis management. If we hurt our bodies every day with our food and lifestyle choices, we are going to find it really hard to live long and healthy lives.

The last hundred years have given rise to the most radical change in the way we humans eat. Wherever we see traditional diets dropped in favour of westernised patterns of eating we see obesity, diabetes, high blood pressure, stroke and heart disease. The pattern is so well recognised that early researchers such as Dennis Burkitt in Africa and Weston Price in Peru called these diseases 'western diseases'.

The main features of a westernised diet are processed foods, processed meats, damaged fats, super-added sugars, soft drinks, alcohol - an abundance of everything, basically, except fruits, vegetables, beans, legumes, nuts, seeds and whole foods. Rarely in traditional, native populations did they see any of the medical problems that we face nowadays. Rarely did they see heart disease, cancer, diabetes, obesity, diverticulitis, appendicitis, dental decay, haemorrhoids, inflammatory bowel disease and so on. This all points to the fact that what we eat and what we don't eat has a direct impact on our health.

Studies have shown that the average time doctors spend talking about diet and lifestyle with their patients is less than one minute. In fact, an interesting study of 4454 patients found that their GPs spent less than 10 seconds talking about the importance of diet.[4] It follows then that patients don't understand the worth of dietary and lifestyle changes because doctors pay no importance to them in their consultation. I now consider it a huge disservice to my patients if I don't include dialogue about lifestyle and diet in my consultations.

Looking back, I realise that our ignorance about the power of preventative medicine comes from medical school, where we spend very little time learning about nutrition and a disproportionate amount of time studying copious pharmaceutical agents and their interactions, side effects and contraindications. Crazy, isn't it? Part of the wider solution has to be the re-education of healthcare professionals so they understand the power of nutritional, preventative and functional medicine. The other part of the solution is to educate the public and to empower individuals to make their own positive health choices. As I write this book a huge positive has been announced in the state of California - plant-based meals have been agreed for every hospital. This represents a huge step away from the general junk food found in hospitals. Schools next! Then the world...

There is another major problem - the public are confused. There is so much conflicting advice about what to eat that no one really knows what to believe or what to eat anymore. Many doctors, nutritionists and healthcare workers are spilt into different political and dietary camps. Some advocate a 'keto' diet (high fat, low carb), others a high protein diet, whilst others still preach the benefits of Paleo eating (caveman, meat-based diets). Are they all aiming for the same goal - better long-term health and a reduction in disease risk? Some diets are focused on short-term weight loss that can come at the expense of long-term health. Through all of this we have left the general public utterly confused. Are eggs healthy or not? Is milk good or bad for you? Is red meat to be avoided? Does fat make you fat? The water is so muddied and the message so confused that even the most intelligent person can get it wrong (including doctors!). Countless diet fads, diet books and food industry propaganda exist that are designed to utterly confuse you and make a fortune out of that very confusion! Confusion is an actual tactic used by the food industry - the more confusion they create the more likely you will give up and just eat whatever ends up in your lap.

In truth, there are many healthy diets. But the modern western or Standard American Diet (aptly abbreviated SAD) isn't one of them. There is an old saying, 'The whiter your bread, the sooner you're dead.' This certainly rings true for the modern western diet, which has become characterised by incredible amounts of refined carbohydrates, processed foods and super-added sugar.

I don't believe in diets and I am certainly not here to give you a step by step 'diet' plan. Many diets focus on short-term gain but sabotage long-term health. My 'diet' is probably best called the disease prevention diet. I am more concerned with the numbers on your blood tests than I am the numbers on your bathroom scales. The ultimate objective of food is to provide nourishing fuel for your body, reducing your disease risk and adding years to your life. If at the same time we can eat foods that have a positive impact on the state of the planet and prevent ecological ruin, then that is a sure win-win.

Many diets focus on the macronutrients (fat, protein, carbohydrates) but forget to improve the micronutrients. In reality, few people in the West are deficient in protein, fats or carbs (the macronutrients) but many are deficient in micronutrients. Micronutrients are the small units of vitamins, minerals, antioxidants, phytonutrients etc. that you get from foods. If you aim to eat plentiful micronutrients each day this crowds out the junk food, nourishes your cells, floods your body with antioxidants and generally provides low calorie foods that fill and nourish you simultaneously. It is these very micronutrients that are your powerful anti-cancer allies and are the key to long-term health. In order to achieve high micronutrient intake, you need to focus on increasing your intake and diversity of plant-based foods. Plant-based foods are all rich in micronutrients. Eating for good micronutrient intake will automatically push junk foods and excess refined carbs off your plate and make space for more nutritious and healthful food choices. Long-term health should never be mortgaged for short-term gain and the best diet is the one that aligns with disease prevention and health and is one that you can sustain.

Dean Ornish MD and Colin Campbell - both giants in terms of their contribution to the study of nutritional medicine - have done incredible work to show that whole food diets with a high intake of plant-based foods can reduce so much of modern, western, chronic disease. Both have spent their professional lives showing how poor diet is the single most significant contributor to our current state of ill health, from heart disease to cancer, stroke and diabetes. Despite their valiant research efforts, the message hasn't really rippled through yet and we still find ourselves in an era of food inertia where we would rather rely on quick fix pharmaceuticals than change what's on our plate.

Dr Dean Ornish has done studies to show that our number one killer - heart disease - can be prevented and indeed reversed with simple dietary changes. His research found that whole food, plant-based diets alongside active living can reverse even the most advanced and refractory heart disease. But what has mainstream medicine done with that information? Turned a blind eye.

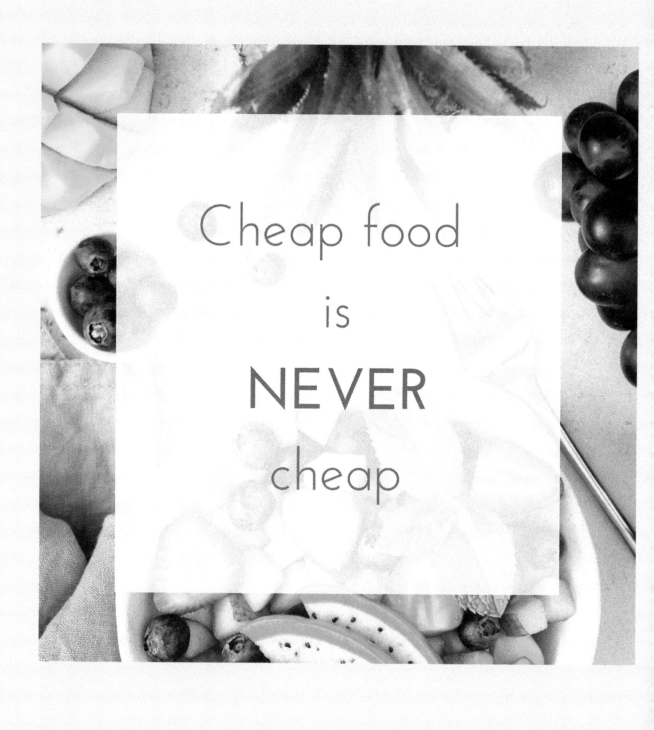

Cheap food

is

NEVER

cheap

85% of us will die from heart disease or stroke - largely preventable and reversible diseases - but we choose rather to continue eating inflammatory, artery clogging fast foods and ignore the fact that the very answer to modern illness is already upon us. Changing what you eat for breakfast, lunch and dinner is surely worth it for your life?

We used to think that heart disease, stroke and cancer were just the consequences of old age, something inevitable that happened when the body tired, aged and wore down. But actually, they are not. The vast majority of heart disease is acquired through a lifetime of unhealthy choices that create sustained inflammation in the body, compounded every day by the repeated consumption of junk foods and the preference for sedentary behaviour. It's the same inflammatory process for most cancers and most strokes. They are generally not diseases of overuse and old age. Nor are they predominantly pre-programmed in our genes. They are simply the cumulative result of a generation of people eating the wrong foods for a long period of time and not taking enough exercise. In short, they are preventable and (thankfully) reversible. By making a few simple changes to what you eat and the way you live today you can drastically cut your chances of a premature death.

We are not totally to blame for what has happened to our health. It has happened to some extent without us even being conscious or complicit. Convenience and fast foods were created to help us in our busy lives. We didn't do a deal with our lazy selves to get to this place. What has happened for most people is an accidental slip into a toxic relationship with food and most people still don't realise the powerful negative consequences of our modern way of life. If you would struggle to eat a mainly whole foods, unprocessed diet - a diet centred around fresh fruits, vegetables, nuts, legumes and seeds - all that tells me is that you have drifted very far away from what is ideal for your health. It should indicate in no uncertain terms that you need to make the change sooner rather than later. The standard western or 'American' diet is slowly killing us all. And the sooner we realise this the sooner we can start the journey back to health. It reminds me of Anne Wigmore's powerful words: 'The foods you eat can be either the safest and most powerful form of medicine or the slowest form of poison.'

People often assume that what they die of is pre-programmed genetically and therefore they have a fatalistic view of chronic diseases like heart disease, diabetes and cancer. They think that if their parents had heart disease or diabetes then they too will get it, irrespective of their individual behaviours and choices. But the truth is that even if you have been dealt some poor genes you can totally trump and dwarf your genetic hand with a careful diet and an active, healthy lifestyle. Science shows that our genes are only responsible for about 5-10% of our disease risk. The rest is the way we choose to eat and live.

For example, rates of cancer and heart disease go up when people move from a low risk area to high risk area as they adopt the diet and lifestyle of their new surroundings. Migration studies show us it is not our genes that do this but the new lives we live when we move to new places. An interesting study of Japanese men relocating to Hawaii noticed that the study participants (8,006 in total) acquired the same heart disease risk as locals within a single generation because of their switch to the Standard American Diet.[5] Alzheimer's risk also went up.[6] This is not genetics or anything to do with ethnicity - this is simply a case of Japanese men changing their diet and lifestyle according to their new American surroundings. This is what happens when inflammation becomes the driving pathological force in the body. Similarly, we know that Nigerians have a low risk of Alzheimer's if they live in their native Nigeria but if they move and adopt a western pattern of eating and living their dementia risk increases fourfold.[7]

In fact, you don't even have to relocate anymore. Developing nations are fast embracing convenient, ultra-processed foods with an increase in processed foods, meat, dairy and egg consumption. Now that all kinds of foods are available globally the Japanese in Japan have started to consume triple the dairy they used to (uncommon in Asia) and six times the meat. It should then come as no surprise that their rates of heart disease, cancer and Alzheimer's have shot up over recent years. The same is happening in urbanised parts of India, China, Indonesia, Africa and all over Central and South America. Wherever people start eating the western diet they start acquiring an increased risk of western diseases. And they start dying of western diseases too.

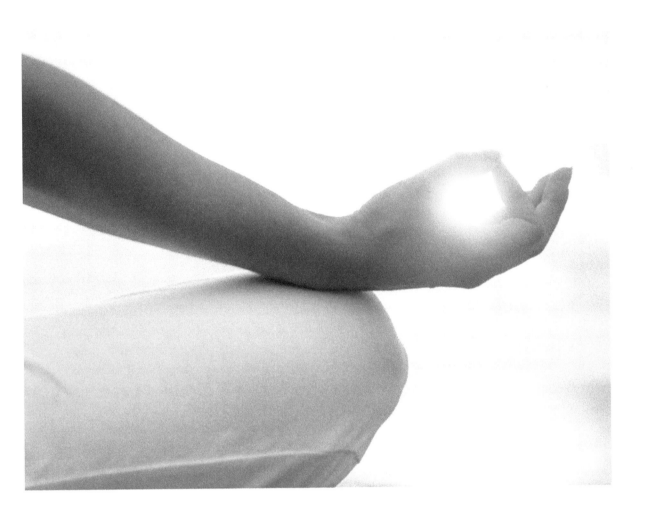

Lifestyle trumps genetics

There is a single point in history when modern western diseases took a stronghold and started to snowball. This point was the Industrial Revolution. Whilst it brought convenience and all the mod cons we enjoy today it also singlehandedly reversed the state of our health. The unfortunate price we paid for the revolution was toxic pollution. That pollution was external and internal and resulted in the sea of toxicity we are now all drowning in. Many of the production techniques used to make modern foods, toys, cosmetics, cleaning products, cars, planes, trains, fuels, electricity, computers, smartphones and everything else in between come with toxic by-products. It's almost impossible nowadays to separate all these different types of pollutants and to pinpoint the ones that might be responsible for disorder and disease. You only have to look at power plants to see how many toxic fumes are spewed into the air. You only have to look at food labels to see how many chemicals we have introduced into our food chain. And if you read the label of a domestic cleaning agent or personal care product you will see chemical after chemical listed as ingredients.

Whilst many of these chemicals have been approved for human use in small doses, what they don't do is account for synergistic or combined toxicity. Certain chemicals in isolation may be safe and approved in small doses but when you add them all together with regular or even daily use the cumulative and synergistic effect may be where the toxicity lies. An interesting study of common chemicals conducted by Brunel University in 2015 showed how over 50 common chemicals became toxic when combined. The main culprits identified were triclosan (antibacterial hand washes), titanium dioxide (mechanical sun blocks and cosmetics), acrylamide (fried foods such as french fries), BPA (from plastics), phthalates (from plastics) and dioxins (by-product of industrial processes) amongst numerous others. My point really is that we are sinking in a toxic swamp with risks that are impossible to quantify. The only way to reduce this is to systematically remove the main toxins and pollutants from our lives and to eat and live clean and green. The fact that this is no easy task is testament to the amount of toxins around us.

Remember also that toxins can come in the form of medicines. We have been conditioned to trust doctors and medicines and to think that they are always beneficial, but this is not always the case.

Many of the medicines released onto the market nowadays end up having intolerable side effects and just don't perform as well in real life, real people situations. Statins are a good example of this. We once thought statins (a type of cholesterol lowering drug) were the panacea to all ills and gave them out like sweeties to anyone with high cholesterol (regardless of the nuances). At one point they were the most widely prescribed drugs. However, we have since realised through our excessive use of statins that the side effects were grossly underestimated in clinical trials and the benefits generally exaggerated. Given all this, it's obvious where we ought to invest our energy. The safest thing to do is to optimise your diet and lifestyle first rather than rely on potent pharmaceutics to do the hard work for you. Most of the medical problems blighting the western world are due to chronic, systemic inflammation. Since they are not deficiency diseases, isn't it worth addressing the inflammation rather than relying on drugs and a chemical fix?

It's worth knowing that the third biggest cause of death in the USA after heart disease and cancer is a category called 'iatrogenic'. Iatrogenesis refers to disability and death caused by prescription medicines, doctor intervention, investigations or pharmaceutics. In the USA over 225,000 people die each year as a result of medical intervention[8] and over half of these (127,000) die as a result of taking a prescribed medicine at the right dose - in other words, death by prescription.[9] This must surely tell us that medicines aren't always the answer and that doctors can be dangerous people!

Adjusting your diet and lifestyle is a much safer option. With a few simple changes you can boost your health, improve your brain function, improve your skin health, boost your cardiovascular function and improve your chances of getting old. Who doesn't want that?!

Sadly, most westerners think they are 'healthy', but surveys have shown that less than 10% are considered to be living a 'healthy life' combining a heathy diet with ample exercise, minimal stress and good quality sleep. 50% of the food consumed in the UK is processed, putting us disgracefully top of the list for processed food consumption in Europe. It won't surprise you then that most people eat less than the recommended amount of fruit and vegetables each day. Only 11% of the average American diet is from plant-based calories[10] and 66% of Brits eat less than three portions of fruit and vegetables per day.[11]

Most worrying, however, is the news that British teenagers consume less than one piece of fruit or vegetable a day. It's not surprising then that one in four British children are overweight by the time they leave primary school (average age of 11). Once our children learn poor dietary habits it can be exceedingly difficult to reverse these behaviours. It requires total re-education. Obesity doesn't run in families because of genetics. There may be a genetic component to obesity, but most people aren't born 'fat' with no way of being healthy and slim. Obesity runs in families because *diets run in families,* eating habits run in families and sedentary behaviours run in families. Obesity is an incredibly complex behavioural and lifestyle/diet problem which affects how our genes are expressed. It is virtually inconceivable that anything solely genetic has occurred in our population in the space of 30-40 years on such a massive and global scale that it has caused the enormous epidemic of obesity. Behaviour trumps genetics.

Worldwide, the rate of obesity has doubled since 1980. In 2014 nearly 30% of the world's population (2.1 billion people) were overweight or obese.[12] Humans are the only species that manage to overeat themselves into a premature grave. You don't see overweight animals running around the Amazon or the Savannah. <u>Obesity is the western dream of unlimited consumption manifested</u>. The most overweight people routinely underestimate the extent of their obesity and undercount their food and calories. They also underestimate the extent of their food problem and underestimate the effect it might be having on their health. I call this 'food amnesia' and we all suffer from it from time to time. Being honest with yourself is hard but it's an incredibly important part of the Back to Health journey.

Sadly, BBC News recently broadcast the fact that millennials are predicted to be the fattest generation ever recorded in history by the time they reach 40.[13] And fat kills. Being fat increases your risk of virtually every disease, especially cancer. Obesity is responsible for about 40% of cancers and is second only to smoking as a preventable cause of cancer. It also increases the risk of insulin resistance, diabetes, hormone dysfunction, chronic inflammation, poor mental health and reduced immunity. Fat is directly related to what you put in your mouth and represents a warning sign that you need to cut back and get back in shape. Pronto.

We have to educate whole families, whole communities and virtually a whole generation about the changes that have occurred in our food behaviours over the last century.

We also need to reduce our portion sizes, which have significantly increased over the last fifty years. A 2002 US study found that portion sizes of hamburgers, french fries and sugary drinks have increased 2-5 times from the recommended portions.[14] This was mirrored by studies in the UK by the British Heart Foundation which found 53% increases in size of supermarket curries compared with curries in 1993 and foods like crumpets which are now 20-30% bigger. The only way to ensure we improve the health of our nation at the grassroots level is to educate people about the dangers of excess consumption. It's unsurprising that we have become a fat nation, with soaring rates of heart disease, cancer and diabetes, when the majority of our calories come from ultra-processed foods.

An interesting global meta-analysis of 95 studies performed by Imperial College London and the Norwegian Regional Health Authority looked at fruit and vegetable intake and health outcomes. Its findings were staggering and highlight our urgent need to increase fruit and (especially) vegetable consumption. The researchers looked at the relative risk of dying from heart disease, stroke, cardiovascular disease, cancer and all-cause deaths. They looked at outcomes for every 200g increase in fruit and veg consumption and showed that eating 800g a day gave the biggest all-cause risk reduction for all five categories of disease. Given that these diseases are our biggest killers, it's a good idea that we take note.

In real terms, this means we need to strive for at least 10 different plant-based foods a day, not the standard 'five a day' that the UK government recommends. Diversity and variety is the important message to take away. The researchers estimated that 5.6 million early deaths occurred in 2013 due to eating less than 500g of fruit and vegetables per day and that eating 10 portions of fruit and veg per day would prevent 7.8 million premature deaths globally.[15] These findings are huge and have far too much significance to ignore. Once again (and over and over again) you will see that increasing your superfoods consumption and reducing your processed foods consumption is the key to safeguarding and future-proofing your health.

The answer to most western diseases is actually quite simple. To paraphrase Michael Pollan:[16] Eat real, whole foods. Eat less rather than more. Eat from the bottom of the food chain - mainly plants. Sleep more. Move more. Relax more. That is nearly all it takes to reduce your all-round disease risk. And I promise you it's not that hard.

CHAPTER 2. The Heart Disease Crisis

"Surgeons can cut out everything except cause." Herbert Shelton

Heart disease is currently the single biggest killer across the globe and is thought to be largely preventable. Outside A&E and your doctor's office, optimising your food and lifestyle choices is the most powerful intervention that you can make to reduce your heart disease risk.

In the UK there are currently 2.3 million people affected by heart disease.[17] In the USA heart disease kills in excess of 633,000 people annually and 28.1 million Americans currently live with a diagnosis of heart disease.[18] Globally, heart disease is the number one cause of death and kills 17.7 million people annually.[19]

Heart disease is wiping us out in massive numbers. We need to stop it in its tracks, and we can - we just need to act now. Can you imagine if a war killed 17.7 million people annually? We would never just shrug our shoulders and allow it to happen. But day after day we let heart disease kill millions of people in the prime of their lives because we haven't yet connected the dots and made the profound realisation that heart disease is simply the manifestation of our unhealthy diets and lifestyles.

We know the cure for heart disease - it's a good diet, an active lifestyle and avoiding inflammation. For years we were going around in circles trying to find the cause of heart disease whilst ignoring the huge problem of inflammation. Inflammation is the elephant in the room in heart disease and connects virtually ALL modern western diseases. Heart disease is almost impossible to get if you avoid inflammation. Inflammation is caused by a number of mechanisms but things that cause it in the modern western diet and lifestyle are high sugar, high saturated fats, processed foods, high alcohol, smoking, lack of exercise and high stress conditions. To avoid heart disease, you need to eat a nutrient-dense, whole foods, low GI diet, give up smoking and move plentifully. Unless you have a rare genetic cardiac defect there really is no reason to get heart disease. Why? Because heart disease is almost entirely preventable in the majority of people.

It's amazing how reluctant people are to hear this and how reluctant they are to make the small changes necessary to prevent our biggest killer. Instead of curing ourselves with active changes to our diet and lifestyle (both of which are evidence-based), we'd rather rely on pills and risky surgical and interventional procedures to try to manage and control it. But wouldn't it make more sense if we prevented heart disease in the first place? All it requires is you adjusting what's on your plate, reducing your glycemic load, managing your stress better and moving a bit more. It's that simple.

For a long time, we thought that heart disease was just what happened when the heart tissue aged, got old and clogged up with plaque. We had a fatalistic view of heart disease, that it was somehow a natural and unavoidable consequence of ageing - like weight gain, joint stiffness and grey hair! Something inherited from your parents. But this is not the case. You can get heart disease in your 20s if you have widespread inflammation.

The heart pumps 115,000 times per day, 42 million times per year and literally billions of times during the average lifespan. Amazingly, it doesn't just tire out and stop. Heart disease is not caused by straightforward ageing and wear and tear. We know this because when we look at the ageing process in rural, traditional communities (those that do not indulge in the same inflammatory diets and sedentary lifestyles) we see that they suffer very little heart disease. In rural China, for example, and the world's 'Blue Zones', where people frequently live well into their hundreds, their hearts are healthy in old age. Colin Campbell's *The China Study* studied thousands of rural Chinese people eating a mainly plant-based diet and found that in a region of over 500,000 people heart disease was virtually non-existent.[20] The truth is that a very small number of heart disease cases are genetic (less than 10%) and the rest are a direct consequence of our unfortunate relationship with cheap, processed, sugary foods.

Heart disease occurs because of inflammation and mechanisms that drive chronic inflammation. We used to think it was a consequence of eating too much dietary cholesterol and that the vascular tubes simply got 'clogged up' with fatty, cholesterol-derived gunk. But this is not entirely the case. Inflammation is the driving force. Diet, lifestyle and stress all compound our dietary mistakes, creating the plaque build-up that can mean the end of life.

High sugar and unhealthy fats drive plaque formation through many different mechanisms that lead to build-up in the lining (endothelium) of our vessels. Interestingly, it is not the narrowing of vessels that causes most heart attacks; rather, it is when the inflammatory plaque ruptures and bursts (causing downstream issues) that most heart attacks occur. Up to 30% of heart attacks are fatal so it's important that you never get to this stage.

If we eat the standard western diet and do little in terms of movement, the process begins in childhood and accumulates over a lifetime. Studies and post mortems of young people who died from non-heart-related causes demonstrate that heart disease is evident already in our childhood, teens and early 20s.

Autopsies of young people who died in accidents have shown children as young as 10 to have what's known as 'fatty streaks' in their vessels - the first sign of inflammatory plaque build-up.[21] 300 autopsies on young US soldiers from the Korean War showed a whopping 77% rate of heart disease, with some having up to 90% coronary artery obstruction.[22] Given these were young, fit and supposedly healthy men this just goes to show how heart disease is not simply a consequence of increasing age. Something else is going on.

We know now that when you regularly consume a western diet it is impossible for it not to gradually destroy your vascular system. To keep it simple and spare you the heavy science, it is the excess sugar and unhealthy fats in the modern western diet that are driving our heart disease epidemic. They do this via an enormous number of inflammatory mechanisms. You find excess sugar and unhealthy fats in most processed and convenience foods, which is why we need to go back to eating whole, unprocessed foods. These two together are a dreadful and toxic combination for the vascular system and a driving factor in our heart disease epidemic.

Low omega 3 (DHA & EPA) combined with high omega 6 (from vegetable oils) also drives inflammation. Low levels of vitamin D, vitamin K2, vitamin C and magnesium compound the problem. Lack of good quality sleep also has a mechanistic action, driving arterial disease through the stress hormone pathways and cortisol. Lack of regular exercise and smoking also add significantly to the problem.

These are all the primary drivers of heart disease. Anyone who is overweight with a prominent belly or girth is likely to be well on the path to advanced internal inflammation and insulin resistance. We all need to change our relationship with processed foods in order to survive.

Our heart disease 'numbers' may look like they are going in the right direction, but we are only fooling ourselves. Every year in the UK over 75,000 coronary angioplasties are performed (where a balloon is passed into a blocked coronary artery that supplies the heart with blood to try and improve blood flow) and over 20,000 people have their chests cracked opened to receive life-saving heart bypass surgery. Yes, we have got better at 'treating' heart disease and yes, science and technology have advanced so our survival rates are higher. BUT the incidence of heart disease isn't decreasing so actually our numbers haven't improved; we are just better at treating heart disease once it's established.

The fact is that most of us have heart disease already and 30-50% of us will die because of its impact on our vessels. The other fact is that it is largely preventable.

Inflammatory plaque slowly obstructs the inner lining of the coronary vessels that carry blood to the heart. Plaque is a greasy, buttery textured layer of proteins, fats (including cholesterol), immune cells and other cellular debris. It builds up and accumulates slowly over years until it compromises the heart tissue downstream, causing either a drastic rupture of a plaque (likely to die) or a slow tissue death (may survive). It's a bit like a kink in a pipe. Every time the plaque builds up the muscle cells get less oxygen until a critical low level is reached where the tissue cannot survive. Oxygen deprivation begins the process of cell death that we commonly call a 'heart attack'.

When we put the numbers into perspective, that is 17.7 million needless premature deaths per year, globally. Unless we do something right now to improve the diet of a whole generation, we will continue in this epidemic of suffering and death - and so will our children.

Did you know…?

1 out of 3 people who have a heart attack will die.

Every 7 minutes someone in the UK has a heart attack.[23]

Every 3 minutes someone dies of a heart attack in the UK, which means we lose 180 people daily to heart disease.[24]

Every year we spend about £9 billion managing the symptoms of heart disease with a mass of pills, defibrillators, sutures and scalpels but these do not effect a cure. We are using drugs to camouflage our heart disease. These all just prolong the inevitable if a person continues to eat cheap, sugary, inflammatory foods and live a sedentary lifestyle.

As doctors, we absolutely have to tell our patients about the success of changing diet and lifestyle in the management of heart disease and we have to empower the people we serve. You can attack the problem from all angles and significantly reduce your risk of heart disease and virtually every other disease by simply cutting out unhealthy fats and sugar. Ask your doctor to help you establish your vascular risks. Chronic disease is now the main cause of death and disability in the western world and we need to respond as a medical profession to this changing landscape of disease pattern. It's not infections that are killing us off any more, but simple, preventable diseases mostly caused by widespread (systemic) inflammation. The change has to start in our hospitals and GP surgeries. Doctors have to educate the people they serve about the benefits of healthy diet and regular movement. This then has to ripple down to our schools, supermarkets, homes and kitchens if we want to cut these junk foods out.

"

It's no coincidence
that health contains
the word heal

"

According to WHO - the World Health Organisation - the eight key risk factors for heart disease are high blood glucose, high blood pressure, high body mass index, high alcohol use, tobacco use, high cholesterol, low fruit and vegetable intake and low physical activity. These account for as much as 61% of all cardiovascular deaths and over three quarters of all cardiovascular disease.[25] If you can manage to reduce all of these risk factors you can virtually 'heart attack proof' your body. If you look carefully you will see that all these risk factors are to do with (or are a consequence of) our diet and lifestyle.

These are the key things in your life that shape your health destiny. A least six of the eight WHO risk factors can be improved by cutting out processed foods and sugar and swapping it for low GI whole foods. Studies have shown that individuals who eat fried foods, fast foods and ultra-processed foods are ten times more likely to have a heart attack than someone who eats with health as the focus.[26]

We can reverse and prevent so much heart disease by reducing our consumption of foods that cause the inflammatory plaque to build up in the first place. This has to start by reducing sugar and refined carbs to reduce insulin resistance. Foods to avoid are ultra-processed foods, sugars and refined carbs PLUS anything with a label on, as it will generally fit into the inflammatory high vegetable oil category. The Harvard Health Professionals follow-up study showed that men and women who make time for healthier diets and lifestyles can reduce their risk of heart disease by 90 and 92% respectively.[27]

Whole food, low GI diets are incredibly effective in correcting and preventing heart disease. Heart-healthy foods should be minimally processed and in their natural and most nutritious state. An array of low GI plant-based foods that are rich in vitamins, minerals, antioxidants and phytonutrients will also help flood your cells with nutrients and help sequester cellular inflammation. They are like water to the flame.

8 key ways to reduce heart disease risk

Reduce your blood pressure

Reduce your blood sugar

Reduce your cholesterol

Reduce your body weight and waist circumference

Reduce alcohol

Increase your fruit & vegetable intake

Increase your physical activity

Stop smoking

Dr Dean Ornish and Caldwell Esselstyn (both US doctors) have been great and vocal advocates for the preventative power of dietary change in heart disease. Both doctors have conducted comprehensive studies on low GI plant-based diets in people with significant heart disease and have shown how heart disease can be treated and even reversed with improved diets and simple lifestyle interventions such as stress management, cessation of smoking and daily movement.

In the Lifestyle Heart Trial, Dr Ornish took a group of patients with severe heart disease and placed them on a low GI vegetarian diet, made them exercise five times per week, asked them to stop smoking and helped them manage their stress levels. He demonstrated that even established coronary heart disease can be halted and reversed with simple lifestyle measures.

Eating processed, nutrient-depleted fast foods is one of the worst things you can do for heart health. Fast foods are not just those sold at drive-throughs and fast food counters but also the same foods found in our refrigerators and cupboards, served up daily in our homes. Inadvertently and unintentionally, most of us eat fast foods every day and in every meal. The only way to avoid this is to cook all meals and foods from scratch.

As a general rule I classify processed food as anything with more than five ingredients on the label. As soon as a food has more than five ingredients I suspect that it has been processed, stabilised, modified, enhanced and manipulated for taste, longevity and shelf life. So processed foods actually include what many people would consider shopping staples such as white bread, pastries, cereals, commercial yoghurts, sauces, meats, cheeses, burgers, pizzas, ice creams, soft drinks, salad dressings and much much more. These are all junk foods and just as unhealthy as foods from McDonalds or Burger King but most people don't realise they are bad. This food ignorance is what keeps us buying the same things over and over again, week after week without realising the health consequences. These foods have been altered, manipulated and adulterated with chemicals, preservatives, salt, sugar, oils, whitening and a whole host of other toxins that are bad for us. These foods have seeped into every aspect of modern life and some people exist solely on these foods, all the while thinking they are fine.

What happens when we eat processed foods all the time is that our taste buds adjust and we no longer enjoy the taste of natural, wholesome, healthy foods. Worse still, these ultra-processed foods wreak havoc on our blood sugars, drive insulin resistance and undermine our health. 'Pack mentality' tells us that if everyone else is eating these foods, they must be okay. If the food manufacturers are allowed to make these foods, they must be okay? Following everyone else will lead you to a future of heart disease, diabetes and a whole host of other illnesses.

We have all fallen prey to the commercialisation and bastardisation of the foods in our food chain and we have all become addicted to 'fake' foods. On this one the government has failed to protect us, because the policy makers either don't realise what they are doing or they put capitalistic gain first. What we need to realise is that these foods are chemically incompatible with our genetic make-up and wreak havoc on us at a cellular level. They are damaging our hearts, damaging our brains, damaging our very DNA and making us addicted to the very things that will end our lives prematurely. Junk foods have no long-term benefits for us. We need to let them go.

You may not realise it but your choice of food each day is one of the most important decisions you make. If you make the same unhealthy choices every day you are creating the same inflammatory traumas for your body every day. Over weeks, months and years these add up and compound to big traumas and one day, before you know it, you may be faced with some serious health problems. As Dr Michael Greger puts it, why hit yourself over the head with a hammer every breakfast, lunch and dinner? That's what eating bad food does. It creates repeated, cumulative trauma for your body to have to repair.

Choosing a whole foods diet is a powerful way to align your food choices with health. Whole foods are rich in vitamins, minerals, antioxidants and phytochemicals - all of which are needed on a daily basis for every cell in your body to survive and thrive. Ultra-processed, fast foods are devoid of these nutrients and fill you up with calories but little else. In contrast, plant-based foods help support your body's production of something called nitric oxide, an amazingly protective molecule that prevents plaque build-up and cellular inflammation.

Esteemed biochemist Earl Stadtman once said: 'Ageing is a disease. The human lifespan simply reflects the level of free radical damage that accumulates in cells. When enough damage accumulates, cells can't survive properly and they just give up.'[28] Ultra-processed foods are consumed in such quantities now in the western world that they represent one of the biggest problems for humanity - they cause so much toxic and inflammatory damage to our cells over a sustained period of time that eating fast foods now kills more people prematurely than smoking cigarettes does.[29]

High Blood Pressure

High blood pressure has been identified as the number one risk factor for premature death from all causes.[30] In terms of heart disease it is the number one enemy alongside inflammation because it contributes to so many diseases (heart disease, stroke, kidney failure, vascular dementia and brain haemorrhage, to name just a few). It is a huge priority that you reduce your blood pressure if it is elevated because the consequences are so far-reaching in health terms.

When Colin Campbell conducted his ground-breaking *The China Study*, he found that the average blood pressure of someone in the second half of their life living in rural China was 110/70. That means that blood pressure in these people remains stable throughout the entirety of their adulthood, where they mainly exist on plant-based whole foods. In contrast, by the age of 60 in industrialised countries the average person has a blood pressure reading of 140/90, which is high. It's no surprise then that the death rate from heart disease in America is 17 times the death rate in rural China.[31] It's the same in rural Africa. It's the same for native Amazonians.[32] Blood pressure increases very little in adulthood in these native, rural populations.

Why is it then that one in three Americans and Brits have high blood pressure?[33] The simple answer is that it is primarily related to our diet and lifestyle. Westerners tend to eat far more processed foods, animal products, dairy, sugar and salt and they tend to exercise less than rural populations. The explosion in heart disease and stroke follows very closely with our increasing consumption of these kinds of foods coupled with an inactive lifestyle.

Interesting Facts

The death rate from heart disease in America is 17 times
the death rate in rural China.

20 million Brits have high blood pressure –
and up to one third don't even know they have it.

High blood pressure kills 9 million people worldwide each year
and contributes to millions more deaths.

Studies have estimated that eating too much salt
kills nearly 4 million people a year.

Salt reduction would save up to 90,000 heart attacks per year
in the USA alone.

Not eating enough fruit and vegetables kills an estimated 5 million a year.

A 2014 meta-analysis of vegetarian, plant-based diets found them
particularly effective at lowering blood pressure.

Vegetarians are observed to have the lowest blood pressures
in industrialised countries.

Simple dietary changes equate to millions of lives saved.

Studies have shown that we consume five to ten times more sodium (salt) nowadays than our bodies are designed to handle.[34] Your lifetime salt intake correlates to your lifetime risk of heart disease and stroke because excess salt systematically damages the human vascular system. A large prospective trial published in the well-respected *Lancet* medical journal showed a frighteningly strong correlation between high salt intake and all-cause mortality.[35]

Primitive man ate a low salt diet and for most of civilisation we have eaten little salt because we ate from the soil and existed largely on plant-based, raw diets with occasional fish and meat. That all changed when we discovered that you could preserve foods with salt. In other words, salt creates a convenient 'shelf life' for food. Unfortunately, this discovery has meant that we now add commercial levels of salt to huge numbers of foods. This is another damaging effect of processed foods - reducing your daily intake of salt is absolutely vital.

The average Brit consumes more than double the daily recommended salt intake and around three quarters of our salt intake is in ready-made foods, so you probably don't even know you are consuming an excess. For example, most people know that roasted peanuts and crisps are high in salt but so too are foods like bread, pizza, cheese, cakes, pies, cereal, meat, milk, soups, salad dressing, ketchup and other sauces. A small serving of commercial vegetable soup can contain over 1200mg of sodium despite being low in calories and full of vegetables.[36] That's almost an entire day's worth of salt in one small, supposedly 'healthy' meal... And only one slice of pizza can contain half your daily salt allowance. It's no wonder pizza is the number one source of dietary salt for American kids. Unsuspecting white bread is the number one source of dietary salt for the 20-40 age group, and chicken ranks number one in the over 50 age group.[37]

So you see, even if you aren't adding salt to your meals yourself, someone else is! And that's the problem. When we eat convenience foods, or any foods that aren't made from scratch in the home, we are delegating the responsibility to someone else. And that someone else is the food industry - and they want you to become a consumer for life. So they add salt. They add sugar. They add preservatives and a whole host of other chemicals that do not serve you in any healthful way but entice you to always want more. More food. More drink.

A typical intake of cereal for breakfast, sandwich for lunch and ready-made meal for dinner would easily get you twice over your daily salt intake and that's without counting any salt from snacks. If you simply cannot avoid processed foods in your day, then look for 'low salt' or 'no added salt' products. Better still, make your own foods each day so you know exactly what you are eating.

Taking back control and responsibility is what is needed. The earlier in life that you begin eating for health the greater the long-term benefits. Obesity and multi-organ disease are what happens when we allow the food industry to feed us. Delegating our nutrition to the food industry is simply insane. If they feed us, they will kill us.

A reduction in daily salt intake from 8g (current British daily average) to 6g (maximum daily recommended consumption) would prevent over 8,000 premature deaths each year in the UK and would save the NHS over £570 million annually in medical costs.[38] Staggering, isn't it?

So get used to reading food labels; it will certainly help you navigate the confusing issue of hidden salts in foods and may well help you reduce your blood pressure too. Better still, avoid foods with labels and eat whole foods - whole foods never come with labels and don't come with added salt! Food may taste a little bland and boring for the first few weeks when you reduce your salt but very rapidly your taste buds will adjust and foods that were once overly salty won't have the same appeal. Try flavouring your foods with vegetables and herbs instead - peppers, tomatoes, onions, garlic, paprika and oregano all make great healthful additions to most dishes.

"I have saved the lives of 150 people with heart transplantation. If I had focused on preventative medicine earlier, I would have saved the lives of 150 million."

Christiaan Barnard, Heart Transplant Surgeon

Salt facts

· ·

The DASH study showed that westerners consume
about 5 times as much salt as they should and that it raises
blood pressure significantly.

Salt and sodium are measured differently.

Maximum salt intake per day is 6g and maximum
sodium intake is 2.5g.

Most of your daily salt is hidden in processed foods.

One pizza slice can contain half your day's salt allowance.

Reducing salt from 8g to 6g per day would save the NHS
£570million annually.

Once you have cut down your salt intake it might be good to cut back on your meat. Reducing meat from the diet is associated with lowering blood pressure. Reduced animal product consumption and increased plant intake is thought to be the reason why high blood pressure is rarely seen in rural Africa, China and other remote parts of the world. In these countries they eat low salt diets and high amounts of plant-based whole foods, with little animal protein. We have known since the 1970s through epidemiology studies that diets that are low in animal products correlate with lower blood pressures. Strict vegetarians are observed to have the lowest blood pressures in industrialised countries.[39] Studies have shown that blood pressure can increase in a matter of days if a vegetarian switches to a high meat diet.[40]

In a large study of almost 90,000 Californians, those who cut out all animal products and ate a plant-based diet reduced their risk of high blood pressure by 75%.[41] This is remarkable and is testament to how much power we ourselves have to influence our health destiny. Too many times we reach for the pills when a simpler and safer option would be changing what we eat.

In addition to cutting out salt and increasing plant-based whole foods, regular movement and exercise can also help reduce blood pressure. As technology has advanced over the years our lives have become more sedentary. The manual labour that used to govern our lives has been replaced with technology. Humans were made to move and movement is fundamental to our health. It also feels great when we move more, and our brains are hardwired to enjoy the endorphin release that comes with movement.

In terms of blood pressure and heart disease, the British Heart Foundation estimates that around 20 million adults (or 39% of the UK population) are insufficiently active. 'This puts them at a significantly higher risk of heart and circulatory disease and premature death', which costs the taxpayer £1.2 billion a year.[42] BHF-funded research showed that middle-aged women could significantly lower their risk of heart disease and stroke by exercising even just two or three times a week. So adding regular movement into your day can have a profound impact, not just by reducing the risk of heart disease but reducing rates of cancer, dementia and stroke. If you don't already exercise for 30 minutes, 3-5 times a week, now is absolutely the time to start.

If your physician or doctor doesn't stress the importance of diet and exercise in the management of your heart disease then they are doing you a huge disservice. What you eat every day is what you eventually become. Superior nutrition coupled with regular exercise will not only help prevent insulin resistance and high blood pressure but will also prevent the myriad of diseases that they cause. There is no way around it - our food and lifestyle choices are killing us, and we need to put things right.

In the words of Dr Michael Greger from his book *How Not to Die*, the insidious consequences of heart disease 'may not be apparent until you are lifted into an ambulance or lowered into a grave'.[43] Harsh but true. **This is your wake-up call.** The good news is you don't need to die from heart disease or stroke - a few simple lifestyle changes now can swiftly reduce your risk and save you from that early grave.

Actions to Reduce Heart Disease

Avoid processed foods (anything in a packet)

Reduce vegetable oils and damaged fats

Reduce sugar and refined carbohydrates

Improve your Omega 3: Omega 6 ratio

Improve Vitamin D, C, K2 & magnesium status

Exercise daily for 30-40 minutes (housework and walking count!)

Reduce or cut out alcohol

Learn to manage your stress (meditation, yoga, Pilates, reading)

Prioritise sleep (aim for 8 hours every night)

Stop smoking

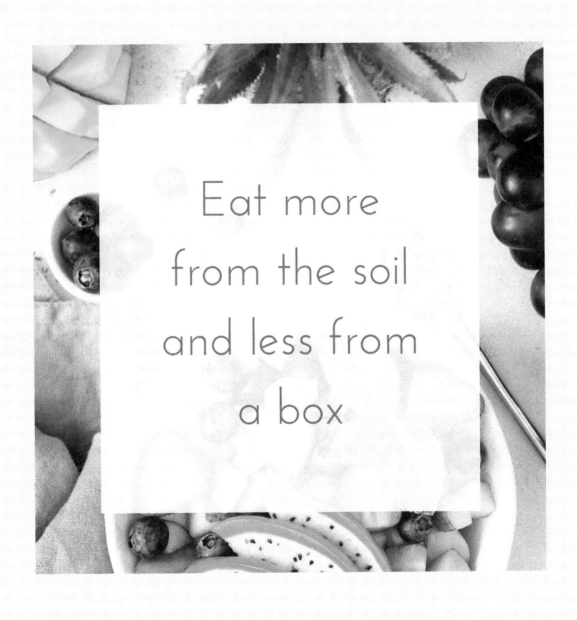

Eat more
from the soil
and less from
a box

CHAPTER 3. The Cancer Crisis

Cancer is the plague of our generation. Anyone born after 1960 in the UK now has a one in two risk of cancer in their lifetime (Cancer Research UK).

The Industrial Revolution represents the single most significant point in history where human cancer rates started to explode. Whilst the Industrial Revolution paved the way for the incredible modern conveniences that we now enjoy (from mass transportation to mass food production) the price we paid for progress and convenience was a deluge of toxic pollutants and chemicals. These are effectively a slow form of poison that compound every day. Now our food, water, air, land and soil are heavily polluted and one in five cancers are caused by environmental pollutants.[44]

It is thought that cancer will soon overtake heart disease as our leading killer. A cancer diagnosis is a terrifying thing. It is made significantly worse by the fact that we still don't entirely understand cancer. Cancer refers to a group of more than 200 different diseases, all of which are related to cell change and uncontrolled cell growth. Because there are so many different types of cancer there will never be one singular cure. Each type requires a different treatment because each type is unique.

Because of its biblical complexity cancer always has and continues to elude us. Like heart disease, our 'numbers' haven't really improved; it's just that we have got better at detecting cancers and living with cancer. To give you an idea of what is happening with cancer, between 1940 and 2005 cancer rates increased every single year. Despite the millions of pounds (and dollars) spent and the significant 'progress' we have made with cancer drugs and medical treatments, we have not improved the death rates for most cancers. Non-Hodgkin's, Hodgkins, testicular cancer and childhood leukaemia are the main exceptions. Survival rates for solid epithelial tumours (accounting for 80% of all cancers) have improved very little over the years.

What we do know is this - cancer exploded when we (humanity) made significant changes to how we eat, exist and live. Sadly, the truth is we probably did this to ourselves. The Industrial Revolution started a snowball that is getting bigger and faster and rolling out of control.

In December 1971, President Nixon declared a federal funded 'War on Cancer' and brought hope to millions suffering from cancer when he signed the National Cancer Act. But we were overconfident in our abilities to overcome cancer and have spent many billions trying to defeat it, only to find that it's one of the most complex and elusive diseases ever known. Cancer research to date has been a sophisticated wild goose chase. In the eloquent words of Travis Christofferson, 'we can split an atom, get man to the moon and map the human genome but sadly we still can't figure out cancer'.[45] Perhaps what we forgot to do is look at what we are putting inside our bodies and instead we blamed our genes.

For years the medical and pharmaceutical industries have ignored the mountain of evidence that shows that most cancers are caused by poor diet and lifestyle. Prevention and treatment therefore has to start with diet and lifestyle correction. The problem is the chemical cancer industry is booming. Big Pharma generates over $100 billion in revenue per year selling cancer treatments - so where is the incentive to start winning the war? Big Pharma can't patent healthy diets and lifestyles, but it can sell us chemotoxic drugs. The problem is that losing the war on cancer is lucrative and chronic disease such as cancer is where Big Pharma gets its massive payout.

In the UK, cancer rates have increased by 13% since the 1990s (Cancer Research UK), with 359,960 new cases diagnosed each year. Around the world cancer remains a leading cause of death with new cases predicted to increase by a whopping 70% in the next two decades alone.[46] To put it into context, in 2017 cancer took the lives of 8.8 million people globally. Four million of those cancer deaths are classified as a premature death, i.e. the person who died was aged 30-69.[47]

Given these staggering numbers and our lack of success so far, it's unlikely we will win the 'war' any time soon. The breakthroughs that we thought were on the horizon have never quite worked out.

Currently, the buzz word in oncology is immunotherapy and there are thousands of trials underway trying to determine if it will be successful. Most of those trials haven't seen a breakthrough and we need to start looking at other strategies.

Given that we haven't made the advances we thought we would, it's important that we learn how to defend ourselves against cancer and live lives that equip our immune cells with the power to fight a good fight. This is the only way we can escape the dreary one in two statistic. We have so much compelling evidence now that lifestyle factors can significantly reduce our cancer risk. Diet and lifestyle are the missing links in the existing cancer treatment model.

Ten years ago, the suggestion that diet, lifestyle and mental wellbeing might be linked to improved cancer survival rates would have been dismissed (or even laughed at) by the conservative medico-oncology fraternity. The standard of care was surgery, chemotherapy and radiotherapy and little else was considered. Nowadays, if you are not considering nutritional and lifestyle factors in addition to standard therapy you are missing a most powerful and legitimate part of a person's survival strategy.

Chances are that most of you reading this book have a number of mutant potential cancer cells already. I certainly have. I have been treated for pre-cancerous cells twice. That's not to be alarmist - it simply aligns with the fact that cancer can take anywhere from 5-25 years to become evident in the body as a tumour or a detectable mass. It also aligns with the fact that one in two of us now get cancer. Some of us get several types of cancer.

Most cancers have a latency period where exposure happens many years before the actual cancer is diagnosed. So there is almost always a delay and a period of slow but persistent growth. What this means is that we have the potential to influence the development of cancer in a positive way, before it becomes a tumour, a lump, something detectable, something fatal. With diet and lifestyle, we can interrupt it and change its course and direction.

Within the next 5-10 years it is very likely that we will all have access to blood biopsy technology. This kind of technology will allow us to detect cancers in the very early stages, long before they have become solid masses or detectable tumours. Whilst this technology is incredible, the problem will be that we will all realise we have microscopic cancer. What do we do then?

Well, diet and lifestyle have been shown to be incredibly effective at halting and preventing early stage cancers. This knowledge will force us out of our laziness and into some urgent and healthful habits. We then have to live lives that reduce cancer growth and proliferation. We will likely find that medicines combined with diet and lifestyle will be the magic bullet we have all been waiting for.

Cancer starts in a cell or a small group of cells. Our bodies contain 30 trillion cells (excluding microbial cells) - written out that's 30,000,000,000,000. It starts with mitochondrial and DNA damage and then the entire cell changes so much that it escapes the body's natural defence systems and proliferates. Every one of us has mutant cells already but what matters is whether these cells are given a hostile or receptive environment in which to grow. This is called 'cell proliferation'. Lifestyle and diet can hugely impact cell proliferation.

Many things have to happen for a cell to become cancerous and a threat to our existence. The following, as described by eminent scientist Robert Weinberg, are pivotal:

Mitochondrial damage

DNA coding mistakes

Uncontrolled growth

Evasion of cell death (apoptosis)

Replicative immortality

Ability to grow a new blood supply (angiogenesis)

Spread to distant site (metastasis)

It is actually not that easy for a cell to escape the body's natural and sophisticated defence systems - but it can and does happen. Cellular mistakes occur regularly. Each time a cell divides it copies billions of DNA 'letters' that make up its unique genetic code. This is an enormously intricate and demanding task. It doesn't always happen error free. But amazingly, the body has developed exquisitely robust safety mechanisms to prevent and repair any mutations. However, if we swamp our cells repeatedly with carcinogens such as tobacco, alcohol, chemicals, processed foods and other toxins, our cells will find it more difficult to do this task without mistakes. Despite the body's safety mechanisms, sometimes the system becomes overloaded.

The most important cellular events in this entire process are mitochondrial and DNA damage. The mitochondria is the cell's powerhouse. It's where energy is produced. Many things damage the cell's mitochondria - some avoidable, some not. Some things, like oxidation, are unavoidable. Oxygen is a double-edged sword for humans. Whilst we need it to live, the very process of using the oxygen that keeps us alive continuously damages our cells. The by-products of oxidation are called free radicals and they cause a constant biochemical 'rusting' or erosion of our mitochondria. So the irony is that whilst we need oxygen to sustain life, it also robs us of life too.

To combat this, the body has an elaborate system of free radical neutralising agents called antioxidants. Antioxidants shield us and neutralise the potential damage caused by these rogue free radicals. Antioxidants come in the form of co-enzyme Q10, glutathione, superoxide dismutase, vitamin C, vitamin E, lipoic acid, uric acid and other antioxidant enzymes. As we age, we become less able to neutralise these free radicals and if we pollute the body with huge amounts of toxins our antioxidants can't keep up and our mitochondria bear the brunt of this toxicity.

We cannot avoid the oxidation process because it is part and parcel of the cell's life cycle, but we can avoid smoking, alcohol, dietary toxins, environmental pollution, X-rays, CT scans and unnecessary medicines, all of which increase our risk. We can also actively increase our dietary antioxidant intake to try and fight the battle better.

Don't ever feel like you have no power against cancer. You absolutely do. In fact, your dietary and lifestyle choices matter so much that they far outweigh the genes you have been dealt. These avoidable factors involved in cancer formation are what you and I can influence in our lifetime. NEVER give up and think that nothing can be done.

On the scientific side, recent studies of cancer such as The Cancer Genome Atlas (TCGA) have told us that one of the main problems with cancer is the mutations and changes that happen in the mitochondria and DNA vary from person to person and are vastly different, sometimes incredibly random. What has become clear in the last few years of cancer research is that each person's cancer is unique, almost like a fingerprint or snowflake. Given that the mutations vary so much from person to person and are so random and unpredictable, pharmaceutical researchers have an almost impossible task trying to find a medicinal cure for such a complex target. As Larry Loeb, a cancer researcher from the University of Washington, says: 'The mutational complexity found in cancer is truly daunting.'

A more novel approach is to look at the way in which cancer cells metabolise and see if we can halt their proliferation. This kind of approach is now being hailed as the way forward. It looks at the metabolism of the cancer cells and how it differs from normal cells and then uses that information to outsmart the cancerous cells.

Genetics and genetic mutations are thought to cause only 5-10% of cancers. The constant focus on genetics has hidden the truth - that most cancers are caused by our lifestyle choices and by the things that influence our mitochondrial health. Yet most cancer programmes fail to include or even mention lifestyle and environment changes. The truth is that genetics isn't to blame for most cancers, and diet and lifestyle can trump bad genes. Understanding this allows us to understand that cancer is about primary prevention.

Every cell in our body uses sugar (glucose) for energy but cancer has a perverted appetite for sugar. Tumour cells can absorb glucose much faster than healthy cells and refined or processed sugars are like drinking through a fire hose and fuelling huge amounts of inflammation and stress through sugar. Cancer cells love cheap circulating, processed sugar and stuff themselves with excessive glucose. This is why PET scans, the most accurate way of scanning for active metabolising cancer, dramatically visualises cancer's perverted cellular metabolism and perverted appetite for sugar. Before a PET scan they give you radioactive sugar to drink and the scan lights up anywhere where the cancer is actively growing. I suspect the future of cancer will focus on the metabolic aspects so that even if all our cancer mutations are different and unique, the way cancer cells metabolise is the same. This is where we can affect and target renegade cancer cells. Avoiding refined and cheap sugars is a great place to start.

Leading research by Seyfried in 2000 showed that a ketogenic diet can effectively starve cancer cells of the glucose needed to grow and survive. It can potentially block off the ability of cancer cells to create their own new blood supply, a term named angiogenesis. Seyfried wrote in his book, 'all oncologists should know that dietary restriction is the nemesis of many cancers'.[48]

A lot more research needs to be done on the dietary aspect of cancer metabolism before we can really understand the potential of a ketogenic or calorie restricted diet in cancer prevention and treatment. What we do know so far is that simple calorie restriction shrinks tumours and avoidance of sugar metabolically restricts cancer cells and reduces their ability to survive. This kind of manipulation of the diet may hold therapeutic potential. Cancer most certainly has a sweet tooth.

Tumours need a blood supply to grow. We cannot grow large tumours unless the tumours themselves develop their own blood supply. This is a process called angiogenesis. The great news is that some of the most potent blockers of tumour angiogenesis are plant-based foods. Fruits and vegetables contain an abundance of phytonutrients that stop tumours developing their own blood supply.

Plant-based foods that are known to block angiogenesis (as well as having a whole host of other positive anti-cancer benefits!) include:

Parsley	Celery	Onions
Strawberries	Green tea	Ginseng
Blueberries	Blackberries	Cherries
Grapefruit	Turmeric	Nutmeg
Garlic	Dark chocolate	Lemons
Apples	Red grapes	Pumpkin

So you should focus on getting these anti-cancer foods into your diet The best all round anti-cancer plant-based foods were listed in a great study published in 2009. They showed garlic to be one of the most powerful anti-cancer foods that exists, capable of stopping seven different cancers in their tracks.[49] Here is a list of the best anti-cancer foods taken from that 2009 study listed from most effective down:

Garlic	Leek	Yellow onions
Red Onions	Broccoli	Brussels sprouts
Cauliflower	Kale	Red cabbage
Green beans	Spinach	Beetroot
Asparagus		

From this list it is clear that the allium family (garlic, onions, leeks) and the cruciferous vegetable family (broccoli, Brussels sprouts, cauliflower) are the anti-cancer superstars. You should pack fresh versions of these plants into your diet EVERY SINGLE DAY if possible. Supplements and extracts are not as effective as the real thing so dash out and buy fresh garlic, leeks, onions and kale and start dropping them into all your recipes. It will pay dividends in the long run. Unfortunately, in the west, the most commonly consumed vegetables are potatoes, carrots and lettuce and these aren't nearly as chemoprotective as the ones listed above. Dark green leafy and cruciferous vegetables account for only 1% of the current western diet so we need to start drastically upping our dose of these wonderful life-promoting plants.

The only way to deal with the huge epidemic that we are seeing worldwide is to start practising preventatively and to start exploring the role that nutrition and lifestyle play in preventing cancer. Modifying as many factors as we can and balancing our toxin exposure with natural antioxidants in foods is a low-cost way to try and remain cancer free. Comprehensive lifestyle and dietary changes remain a powerful antidote to cancer. For those currently with cancer, this needs to happen alongside targeting the abnormal cells with surgery, radiotherapy and chemotherapy. The best thing to do right now if you have cancer is to enlist the help of a specialist oncology nutritionist and work closely with them to tweak your diet in ways that can positively benefit your short- and long-term health.

Reducing your overall calories as well as reducing sugar, processed meats, dairy, trans fats, salt, chemicals, additives, pesticides and anything artificial in your food is a positive step in the right direction. Increasing your consumption of dietary vitamins, minerals, antioxidants, phytochemicals and fibre is also vital. This can only be done if you ensure a rich and diverse array of plant-based foods features in your diet. If you have been diagnosed recently, you should aim for at least 10 different plants in your diet every single day. The aim is to absolutely flood your cells with the healing nutrients found in plants on a regular basis throughout the day. Remember, plants are nature's superfoods. They contain an abundance of micronutrients. Superfoods bring superhealth. Your aim is to create a robust body with a robust immune system that can heal and repair, quell inflammation and better fight the cancer fight. Start eating to restore your cells, restore your health and restore your life.

"

Eating healthy can cost
you money.. Eating
unhealthy can cost you
your life
"

HOW TO PREVENT CANCER

Every day our bodies are dealing with mutant cells that are the start of cancer, so to speak. But an effective immune system knows how to detect these errant cells and annihilate their cellular material. Without an effective immune system, mutant cells might slip through the net.

Building immune resilience is tied in with all aspects of our lives. Modern western living holds us so firmly in its grip that most of us are not even aware of how far we have drifted away from true health. We all need to relearn the art of healthy eating and healthy living if we are to truly win the war on cancer.

We urgently need to reduce our sugar, refined carbohydrates, alcohol, damaged fat and toxin consumption. We need to eat more raw, organic and local plant foods free from pesticides and toxins. We need to get back in the kitchen and make changes that start in our supermarkets and end on our dining room table. We need to teach our children how to do the same - they are a generation of young people who think Subway and Starbucks are normal because it's all they have known. We need to eat more from the earth and less from a box. We need to learn the art of proper nutrition and feed the body wholesome, nourishing foods. We also need to prioritise deep, restorative sleep. Sleep is a critical immune-building reparative activity that is vital to healthfulness and wellbeing. I like to think of sleep as a super nutrient. It should not be compromised, interrupted and neglected because of a busy schedule. The body heals from the day's cellular insults at night and uninterrupted sleep is vital. Rediscovering the art of movement through an activity like yoga and meditation will help better align our physical and mental wellbeing. Physical movement is both therapeutic and anti-inflammatory. Studies have shown that those of us who work full time in office-based jobs are estimated to be sedentary for 21 out of 24 hours a day. This is not right. Humans were made to move. If we don't move, we risk ill health.

"It's time we understand there is a sweet spot where wellness and disease intersect."
Dr Lorenzo Cohen, author, Anti-Cancer Living

We live in a noisy, busy world so finding quiet time is key. Mental tranquility is vital for wellbeing. And positive mental wellbeing is linked to cancer prevention. Those individuals who choose to live well and decide they are going to beat cancer often do. Your choices and your mental approach are fundamental to your survival. All these things add up to rebuilding a pathway back to health and they are all integral to survival. It's only when we become accountable for our health that we see our health improve.

THE EVIDENCE

A 2016 study by a Harvard University research team reviewed 135,000 people's data over a 40-year period and found that not smoking, alcohol in moderation, exercising regularly and maintaining a healthy BMI could prevent 41% of cancer cases and 59% of cancer deaths in women and 66% of cancer deaths in men. Had the alcohol been zero, I think the rates would have been even more impressive.

Another study conducted in 2017 involving over 800,000 people categorically showed that eating a diet consisting of inflammatory foods caused increased risk of colorectal cancers. Colorectal cancer risk increased by 51% for men who ate pro-inflammatory foods and by 25% for women.[50] Similar smaller studies have been done where two very different types of population have switched foods for a number of weeks to observe the changes that take place.

In 2015, an interesting study was carried out by Professor Stephen O'Keefe at Pittsburgh School of Medicine, who switched the diets of 20 rural Africans with 20 African-Americans. He wanted to try and understand why the level of colon cancer in native Africans was so much lower than in Afro-Americans, who are known to have the highest levels of colon cancer of any race in the USA. The native African diet is plant-based, high in fibre and low in fat; when the African-Americans switched to this diet their microbiome and inflammatory markers improved within two weeks. When the native Africans ate the Standard American Diet, they were noted to experience an increase in inflammation and negative intestinal changes - risk factors for colorectal cancer.[51]

In 2005, Dr Dean Ornish conducted an interesting study to test the diet and lifestyle cancer hypothesis. He took a group of men with prostate cancer and divided them into a diet and lifestyle group and a control group. The men in the diet and lifestyle group were assigned a low sugar, plant-based diet, instructed to exercise for 30 minutes, six days a week, and reduce their stress with daily yoga and meditation. They were also given a weekly group support session. The diet and lifestyle group were found to have a 70% suppression in human prostate cancer cell growth compared to a 9% change in the control group. The study ended up showing that the greater the lifestyle changes a participant undertook, the greater the prostate cancer improvement, as measured by PSA blood levels.[52] PSA is an enzymatic marker used to measure cancer cell activity in prostate cancer. Increases in PSA correlate to increased activity of prostate cancer cells.

Whilst the idea that sugar 'feeds' cancer is a slight over-simplification we know there is a clear link between sugar and cancer. For example, studies have shown that post-menopausal women eating high levels of sugar have twice the risk of colon cancer[53] and Swedish researchers found that men who drank a 340ml can of sugary fizz each day increased their risk of prostate cancer by 40%.[54]

Obesity is also linked to over 13 types of cancer and accounts for one in five cancers globally.[55] [56] Sugar is hugely implicated in our global obesity problem and we know from Chapter One that excess glucose or sugar causes the dreaded insulin resistance, a precursor to many modern diseases. When you combine obesity with a sedentary lifestyle, cancer risks increase by more than 30%. Sugar is at the heart of many of these problems.

If you remain unconvinced about the link between cancer and sugar then how about this fact - excess sugar consumption causes type 2 diabetes, which affects more than one in ten adults globally. Type 2 diabetes is linked to double the risk of pancreatic cancer and double the risk of prostate cancer. The path to cancer through diabetes is very real and threatens the health of millions. Four hundred and fifty million, to be exact.

In terms of specific food groups, there is plenty of good evidence showing the anti-cancer benefits of specific foods. Researchers at Cornell University have tested the anti-cancer effects of many different fruit and vegetables. In one such study they extracted the juice of 11 common fruits and drizzled them in a lab over a petri dish with human liver cancer cells. What they found was exciting. Bananas and grapefruit performed wonderfully, cutting the liver cancer cell growth rate by 40%, but red grapes, apples and strawberries performed staggeringly well and were twice as potent as the bananas and grapefruit groups. Lemons and cranberries, however, came out top, cutting the liver cancer cell growth rates by a whopping 85%.[57]

Berries also have great anti-cancer properties. They contain immune-boosting and anti-cancer compounds like ellagic acid, caffeic acid and anthocyanins. One study showed that participants who ate two cups of blueberries a day for six weeks showed significant increases in their Natural Killer cells from two billion to four billion cells.[58] Natural Killer cells are part of your body's immune defence against cancer and low numbers equate with a low level of resilience against cancer.

We have literally thousands of studies showing that the micronutrients in plants are chemoprotective, but we seem to have chosen to ignore them. It is abundantly clear from studies (and from real life) that the daily choices we make about food, exercise, stress, sleep, work and play all have a profound effect on our health, wellness and in particular on our susceptibility to cancer.

It goes beyond the scope of this book to discuss every kind of cancer, but I want to briefly pay particular attention to breast cancer, colon cancer and prostate cancer - the Big Three. These cancers account for more than half of all cancer deaths in the UK.[59] We are clearly not winning the war on cancer, but our best hope now is to reduce the numerous co-factors that 'pull the trigger', metaphorically speaking.

BREAST CANCER

A woman's lifetime risk of developing breast cancer is currently one in eight, but many things can reduce this risk. Adjustments such as optimising diet, lifestyle, BMI, exercise and vitamin D levels can profoundly affect the trajectory and outcome of cancer. In fact, the more positive lifestyle changes we make, the more benefit each lifestyle adjustment has.[60]

87% of women diagnosed with breast cancer do not have a first degree relative with the disease so we can no longer hold firm to the idea that breast cancer is a pre-determined genetic condition. The identical twin sister of a woman with breast cancer has only a 20% chance of developing it - which is exactly the same risk as a non-identical sister. If DNA called all the shots this wouldn't be the case. So something in our environment is interacting with our genes to trigger the levels and rates of breast cancer we are now seeing. This is called epigenetics - how our environment interacts with our genes and suppresses them or excites them. A good example of epigenetics is the observation that Japanese women generally have a low incidence of breast cancer if they live in their native Japan. However, if they move to Hawaii their cancer risk significantly increases and if they move to mainland USA then their cancer risk increases even further. Studies like these show us that genetics cannot be blamed - some other factor (or factors) in our diet and lifestyle causes these changes. The following are all factors that can help reduce the incidence of cancer in addition to eating well.

Vitamin D and breast cancer

Vitamin D optimisation could save many breast cancer lives. Numerous studies have shown that optimising vitamin D levels should form part of any anti-cancer strategy. Research shows that most breast cancers occur in people with sub-optimal vitamin D levels (between 10-40ng/mL) and that if you can get your level above 60ng/mL then your breast cancer risk is reduced by more than 80%.[61] The 2016 PLOS One study mirrored these results and found that women aged 55 and older who had a vitamin D level of 40ng/mL or greater had a 67% reduced risk of breast cancer compared to those with suboptimal vitamin D levels (defined as < 20ng/mL). Overall, breast cancer patients were found to be 1.5 times more likely to be deficient in vitamin D.[62]

A recent Japanese study published in the *British Medical Journal* showed that higher vitamin D levels were associated with a 20% lower relative risk of internal cancers in both sexes, with no increased cancer risk in those with higher levels of vitamin D.[63] Another study published in 2011 looked at vitamin D and all invasive cancers and concluded that post-menopausal women who increased their vitamin D level to more than 38ng/mL lowered their risk of all invasive cancers, including breast cancer.[64]

Vitamin D has also been shown to increase your chances of survival if you do get breast cancer.[65] [66] In one study published in the *American Journal of Clinical Nutrition,* breast cancer survival rates were doubled in those with high vitamin D levels.[67]

It is abundantly clear from recent research on vitamin D that optimisation should form part of breast cancer awareness and survival programmes. Vitamin D works to boost and support the immune system, which is the first line of defence against cancer. Unfortunately, the protective benefits afforded by vitamin D have not been well publicised and have not yet trickled down to the very people who would benefit from it. More than one billion people are vitamin D deficient globally,[68] so small changes like vitamin D optimisation could have a huge impact on health and wellness.

According to one study, during the winter months 87% of the UK population have vitamin D levels below optimum.[69] Anyone who doesn't live near the equator should supplement vitamin D3 in the winter months. In the UK, Public Health England recommends that all Brits do this. Pass this information on to those you love. It could help keep them alive and well.

I tend to recommend anywhere from 1,000-4,000iu of vitamin D3 daily as a standard adult dose for supplementation. Ask your doctor to check your vitamin D levels with a simple 25(OH) blood test and make sure your levels are optimal.

Whilst there is no set optimum level, most experts agree that being on the higher side (rather than on the lower) has powerful health benefits. My family and I take vitamin D3 all year around to support our immune system.

Breastfeeding

Breastfeeding is known to be protective against the development of breast cancer. It shows its greatest benefits when mothers breastfeed for six months or more. Breastfeeding generally suppresses the menstrual cycle, which means fewer periods and, when added to the nine periods missed during pregnancy, this significantly decreases an individual's total lifetime oestrogen exposure. Women also tend to eat better, drink less alcohol and exercise better self-care when pregnant and when feeding a baby. Plus, at the cellular level, it is thought that breastfeeding makes the breast tissue and breast ducts less susceptible to carcinogens.

A 2015 study on breast cancer and breastfeeding published in the *Journal of the National Cancer Institute* in the USA found that a history of breastfeeding decreased the risk of breast cancer recurring by 30% overall. The researchers also found that breastfeeding was protective against the most commonly diagnosed breast cancers and that women who breastfed were 28% less likely to die from the disease.[70]

Did you know?

Most breast cancers are to do with our diet, lifestyle and cumulative toxin exposure, not genetics.

Breast cancer risk is related to lifetime oestrogen exposure. The higher the oestrogen exposure, the higher the risk of breast cancer.

Breast cancer risk increases if a girl has early periods.

Breastfeeding reduces the risk of breast cancer. Breastfeed if it is at all possible.

Avoid endocrine disruptors that act directly or indirectly to stimulate oestrogen. They are found in a wide variety of processed foods, plastics, pesticides, cosmetics, fragrances, cleaning products and even in unfiltered water.

Breast cancer risk increases in young girls who eat frequent portions of french fries, likely due to inflammation due to trans (damaged) fats.[71] Avoid all fast foods and reduce processed foods.

The more french fries a child eats between the ages of 3-5, the greater the risk of breast cancer in later life. Each additional serving of fries per week can increase breast cancer risk in later life by 27%.[72]

In a study of 23,963 women, those who ate little or no fish had half the breast cancer rate compared to those who ate it several times a week.[73] This is thought to be due to bio-accumulation of toxins in fish (mercury, dioxins etc.). Make sure you eat wild-caught fish and not farmed fish to reduce risk of toxin exposure. And choose small fish like sardines and anchovies that don't bioaccumulate as much.

Alcohol increases the risk of breast cancer. Studies have shown that for every 10g of alcohol (less than one drink), breast cancer rates increase by 7%-12%.[74] Avoid or reduce alcohol.

Physical activity of 30-60 minutes per day reduces breast cancer risk by 20-30%.[75] Get moving daily!

COLON CANCER

"If you step back and look at the data (on beef and cancer) the optimum amount of red meat you eat should be zero." Walter Willett MD, Chairman of the Nutrition Department, Harvard School of Public Health

Without doubt, the colon reflects the health of the food that passes through it every day and cancer of the colon is the cancer most strongly linked to our food choices.

We know the risk of cancer of the colon is 250% greater for women who eat red meat daily than it is for those who only eat it infrequently (< 1 per month)[76].

We also know that those eating poultry are not totally safe either. Risks of colon cancer in those eating poultry meats regularly (> 4 times per week) are 200-300% higher than in those who don't.[77] Even low levels of meat consumption are linked to 30-50% more colon cancer that those who enjoy a meat-free diet.[78] Studies show us that those who eat diets rich in lentils, beans and leafy greens at least twice per week enjoy a 50% lower colon cancer rate than those who don't.[79] And diets that are rich in B vitamins (found in abundance in leafy greens) are also significantly protective against colon cancer.[80] So it's not just what you eat, it's *what you fail to eat too* that determines your colon cancer risk. If your plate is piled high with processed foods and a lot of animal products then this pushes protective green, beans, legumes, nuts and seeds off your plate.

Processed meats are now classed as human carcinogens according to the WHO, alongside asbestos and smoking. This means that hot dogs, ham, corned beef, canned beef, party sausages and packaged hams and meats need to be avoided. These are the very foods widely available at supermarkets, in canteens, service stations, hospitals and at kids' play zones. Where did it go so wrong?

"Rates of colorectal cancer ... are strongly correlated with per capita consumption of red meat and animal fat and inversely associated with fibre consumption."

Peter Cheek, Professor of Animal Science at Oregon State University

Red meat accounts for about 58% of meat consumption in the USA[81] and consumption of red meats like beef is increasing in developed nations and developing nations alike.[82] [83] Numerous studies now show a link between red meat and colorectal cancer rates and also a link between red meat consumption and cancers of the kidney,[84] prostate[85], oesophagus[86], liver[87], lung[88] and pancreas (in men)[89]. In one large study involving 500,000 people, those eating the highest amounts of red meat also had the highest incidence of dying of cancer.[90]

The way we cook meat adds to our cancer risk. Cooking meat at high temperatures (especially grilling and BBQing over a naked flame) creates toxic heterocyclic amines (HCAs) and polycyclic aromatic hydrocarbons (PAHs) that are known to be highly carcinogenic.

Snacking and frequent eating have also been shown to increase colon cancer in men.[91]

Nitrites are also bad for human health. They are found in processed meats and are used as antibacterial agents to keep meats from going putrid and off. Nitrites are found in cured meats and smoked cheeses, often to keep out the dangerous *Clostridium Botulinum* toxic bacteria. The main issue is the formation of N-nitroso compounds (NOCs) which, when ingested, are classified as 'probable human carcinogens - 2A' by the International Agency for Research for Cancer.[92] Cured meats and processed hams are officially off the healthy list, I am afraid.

Red meat is also associated with increased intake of heme iron - a highly absorbable type of iron found in red meat, organ meat and shellfish. There is no heme iron in plant foods. In excess, heme iron causes oxidative stress and inflammation and is known to increase the risk of colorectal cancer as well as stomach and oesophageal cancer. If you want to eat meat it is best to eat smaller amounts (think of it as the side and not the main!) and choose grass-fed, pasture raised meats that are less likely to have been adulterated.

Another thing to be aware of is that heavy meat consumption increases your levels of an essential amino acid called methionine. Several cancers - including breast, ovarian, colorectal and melanomas - use the amino acid methionine for growth. Non-cancer cells can survive without methionine but many cancer cells cannot - they stop replicating and die without methionine. Methionine is found abundantly in animal protein especially red meat, chicken, fish, eggs and dairy. Plant foods generally have much lower levels. In animal studies, methionine restriction in mice and rats successfully improves lifespan and suppresses cancer. More studies need to be conducted on the effects of methionine and cancer but its worth being aware of if you already have a cancer diagnosis and are wanting to reduce your all round risk. Plant based diets are low in methionine so once again focusing on a good intake of plants and whole foods will help to prevent excessive methionine intake.

"If beef is your idea of real food for real people
then you'd better live real close to a really good hospital."
Neil Barnard MD, President of the Physicians Committee for Responsible Medicine

Things to Know

· · · · · · · · · · · · · · · · · · · ·

Colon cancer is the cancer most closely linked to diet.

Poor fibre intake is linked to increased colon cancer risk.

The average Brit eats only 18g of the recommended
30g of daily fibre.

Slow transit of food through the gut increases the risk of
colon cancer due to toxic accumulation. Food should ideally pass
through the gut in 24 hours.

Vegetarians have lower rates of colon cancer than red meat eaters.

Nitrates found in processed meats are classified as probable human
carcinogens and increase the risk of colon cancer.

BBQ'ing or cooking meat at high temperatures creates Heterocylic
amines (HCA's) and Polycyclic aromatic hydrocarbons (PAH's) which
are both carcinogenic.

In the USA meats frequently contain sex hormones because they haven't followed the 1995 EU ban of sex hormones in livestock. The EU has generally protected us from these hormone exposures but sex hormones progesterone, estradiol, 17 beta-oestradiol, testosterone and trebolone acetate have all been found in US tested meats. These are known to be human carcinogens so be cautious of meat from countries outside the EU. Even supposedly hormone-free US meat was found to contain unacceptable levels of hormones when spot checked.[93]

Slow passage of food through the gut due to constipation from low fibre intake is also a significant risk for colon cancer. One of the first people to study the importance of fibre in the diet was Weston Price who, in the 1930s, went to Africa and started examining native populations. He marvelled at why things like heart disease, diverticulitis, cancer, haemorrhoids, constipation and dental decay were virtually non-existent in rural Africa but widespread in the west. He was way ahead of his time when he proposed the theory that eating a largely westernised and processed diet 'breaks the rules of nature, severs us from our natural diets and disrupts the flow of food through our bodies'.

He wrote in his book: 'Western diets are so low on bulk and so dense in calories that our intestines just don't pass enough volume to remain healthy.'

Fibre is found in abundance in fruit and vegetables but many manmade foods are fibreless. A diet centred around low GI plants and whole foods will help reduce colorectal cancer rates by providing essential fibre. 30g of fibre a day is what is needed to keep the colon healthy, but Brits consume woeful amounts at about half the recommended daily amount. A diet low in fibre results in sluggish bowel movements because fibre bulks out stools and supports peristalsis, the rhythmic movements of the intestine that help push food through the digestive tract. In diets that are low in fibre these peristaltic movements occur less frequently, resulting in less frequent passage of stools. If waste foodstuff is allowed to sit around the colon for too long (as in the case of constipation) there is a risk of toxic accumulation and increased colon cancer risk. In an ideal world you should pass soft stools once a day, they should be passed whole (not in pellets), be light/medium brown in colour, not smell offensive and be passed without the need to strain. Any less and you have an increased risk of colon cancer. A simple, protective measure is to eat more dietary fibre. Plants are abundant in soluble and insoluble fibre, both of which are vital to good gut and colon health.

PROSTATE CANCER

The prostate is an organ about the size of a walnut tucked between the bladder and the penis. Prostate cancer accounts for 26% of all new male cancer cases in the UK and the incidence is set to rise 12% by 2035.

Genetic factors likely account for about 5-10% of prostate cancers (such as BRCA genes) but the majority of prostate cancer is due to increasing age combined with diet and lifestyle factors. We know that prostatitis or inflammation of the prostate increases prostate cancer risk. Obesity also increases prostate cancer risk, as does smoking. Men who eat a lot of red meat are known to have higher rates of prostate cancer too. These men tend to eat less fruit and vegetables so it's not quite clear which one is the causative factor - the high intake of red meat or the lack of protective fruit and vegetables. In some studies, high consumption of dairy products has been shown to increase prostate cancer by up to 70%.[94]

According to a study published in the *International Journal of Cancer*, researchers observed significant increases in prostate cancer levels with increases in dairy. They monitored the dairy intake of just under 1,000 men with prostate cancer as part of the Physicians Health Study over 10 years. Those men who consumed more than three servings of dairy per day had a 141% higher risk of death due to prostate cancer compared to those men who consumed less than one serving. Both high and low fat dairy had the same impact and mortality was likely due to increased inflammation caused by Insulin-like Growth Factor -1 (IGF-1). Cow's milk contains steroid hormones like estradiol and testosterone and peptide hormones like IGF-1.

We know that IGF-1 is an inflammatory growth factor hormone that increases with dairy exposure. What we don't know is its exact mechanism of action but there is some concern now that it is linked to higher rates of cancer and systemic inflammation. For anyone concerned about prostate cancer it would be wise to reduce milk and dairy intake from a dietary staple to a dietary 'occasional'. More studies need to be performed on potential dietary links with all kinds of cancer but anything that raises inflammation is worth reducing in the interim.

Things to know

Smoking, obesity and increasing age increase prostate cancer risk.

A diet rich in plant-based foods reduces the risk of prostate cancer.

Men who consume two or more servings of tomato sauce (because of the lycopene content) per week have 23% less risk of prostate cancer than those who have it less than once per month.[95]

Cruciferous vegetables (such as broccoli, cabbage, and Brussels sprouts) offer protection against prostate cancer.

Milk and dairy may increase the risk of prostate cancer due to increased Insulin-like Growth Factor 1(IGF-1).

TOBACCO

No chapter on cancer would be complete without the mention of tobacco. Smoking is the single largest risk for all-cause cancers. Obesity is the second. We know that tobacco is not just the cause of lung cancer but has now been linked to 14 other cancers[96] as well as accelerating the ageing and damage of all tissues and organs in the body. We also know it is a powerful and addictive toxin - a symbol of the destruction of the industrialised age. Anyone who doubts the impact that lifestyle factors have on cancer risks only needs to look at the lessons we learnt from the tobacco industry. Despite knowing the risks associated with cancer, 1.1 billion people worldwide still smoke, with disproportionate numbers of people smoking in poorer parts of the world. The World Health Organisation calls the tobacco epidemic 'the biggest public health threat' to man and has launched campaigns like 'Tobacco Breaks Hearts' to try and drive home the message.

Each year tobacco kills more than seven million people (WHO 2017), with six million of these deaths directly attributable to tobacco and almost one million due to the effects of second-hand smoke. Much of the world's smoking happens in low socioeconomic areas where standards of living are poor and education is limited.

The tobacco industry has been responsible for millions of deaths and suffering and yet still cigarettes are being sold. How crazy is this to an outsider looking in on our world?

Where tobacco is concerned there is no denying that lifestyle factors hugely affect our cancer risk. In the UK in 2016, in excess of 35,000 people died of lung cancer. Unfortunately, we have allowed the tobacco industry to reinvent itself and poison us in another way, through vaping. This brings with it a whole new list of chemicals and unknown toxins that will show their effect in 5-15 years' time. Vaping is simply another way to justify nicotine consumption and we have a whole young generation now addicted to vaping. Not cool. Remember that absence of evidence is not the same as absence of harm. There have been few studies on the long-term safety of e-cigarettes because they haven't been around long enough so I would strongly suggest that you stay well away from them. Anything that is inhaled introduces foreign matter into the lungs which can trigger inflammation and cell change. We urgently need action on vaping and e-cigarettes before the next generation suffers the impact of these unknowns.

OBESITY

Obesity is the second most significant and avoidable risk factor for cancer after smoking. It has been estimated that 20% of cancers are caused by being overweight.[97] Obesity has been linked to 13 different types of cancer, with The International Agency for Research into Cancer and the World Cancer Research Fund linking obesity to breast, endometrial, kidney, oesophageal, prostate and colorectal cancer. Given these links, it is vital that we all learn to control our diets and lifestyles to ensure we don't supersize either our physical bodies or our cancer risk. Being overweight or obese increases risk of cancer through a number of different clinically evidenced mechanisms.

Obesity increases levels of insulin and insulin-like growth factor 1 (IGF-1), which is thought to drive and stimulate cancer proliferation.

Obesity increases leptin (a hormone released by fat cells), which is linked to increased risk of breast, prostate and colorectal cancer.[98]

Obesity in its own right drives chronic inflammation, which is linked to increased cancer risk.

Oestrogen production increases when there is excess body fat and drives hormonally receptive cancers like breast and endometrial cancer.

Obesity interferes with signalling and growth suppressors via adipokines, which are proteins secreted by fat cells.

Obesity is correlated with low vitamin D levels, which is responsible for 20% of the cancer risk attributed to high body mass index.[99]

Obesity is linked to higher rates of oxidative stress that the body cannot always sequester or neutralise, leaving it vulnerable to renegade free radical activity.[100]

Did you know...?

Obesity is linked to twice the rate of liver and kidney cancer[124]

Being overweight increases thyroid cancer risk by 10%[125]

Obesity doubles the risk of oesophageal adenocarcinoma[126]

Risk of a slow-growing brain tumour called meningioma
is increased by 50% in obesity[127]

Obesity is linked to increased rates of breast cancer
in post-menopausal women

Obese women have four times the risk of endometrial cancer[128]

Obesity increases the risk of multiple myeloma[129]

Childhood obesity increase the risk of cancer in adulthood by 10%[130]

EXERCISE

Exercising 5-7 hours a week can lower cancer risk.

Exercise helps control blood sugars, reduces inflammation and reduces an IGF-1 which is implicated in many cancers.

In addition, maintaining a low body weight helps reduce certain cancer risks because fat cells make oestrogen and carrying excess body fat raises oestrogen production. In simple terms, this means the higher your BMI the higher your risk of breast cancer. So it is indeed Survival of the Fittest.

ALCOHOL

Research consistently shows that drinking alcohol increases the hormone-positive breast cancer risk. Alcohol creates a toxic breakdown product called acetaldehyde that is the culprit in increasing cancer risk. It also has no nutrient value and lots of calories and sugar. Even light drinking is linked to increased risk. Women who have only three alcoholic drinks per week have been shown to have a 15% higher risk of breast cancer than women who abstain. And a 2013 study estimated that nearly 5,000 breast cancer deaths could be attributed to light drinking.[101]

It's worth knowing that the WHO upgraded alcohol to a definitive human breast carcinogen in 2010.

Alcohol damages the DNA in cells, predisposing us to all kinds of cancer, not just hormonal cancers such as breast cancer. Keeping your body weight down, exercising regularly, eating an abundance of plant-based foods, avoiding excessive meat and dairy consumption, not smoking and minimal alcohol will all help you avoid the Big Three.

SLEEP

Sleep is a super nutrient equivalent. Getting enough sleep is vitally important if you want to ensure reduced cancer risk. At night time the body heals and recovers from the day's toxic insults. Your body needs that time to physically recover. Studies have shown that women who disrupt their sleep-wake cycles with shift work have an increased risk of breast cancer because of a decrease in melatonin. Melatonin is made in the pineal gland and peaks in the night time when it's dark. A good night's sleep ensures that your melatonin levels are balanced and protects you against cancer.[102]

LOVE AND SUPPORT

If you have been diagnosed with any kind of cancer, it's important you get your friends and family to rally around you and help support you. We know that support is a huge factor in cancer survival. Companionship in all walks of life helps us feel connected and loved but in cancer, connectedness takes on a new meaning as a wealth of studies now show that social connections help shield us from cancer growth and proliferation through reduced inflammatory pathways. It is also recognised that excess stress erodes our sense of wellbeing and promotes cancer growth and proliferation.

MAKE CHANGE TODAY

Things we do today can significantly affect our health destiny and can reduce the risk of a future cancer prognosis. Cancer is not pre-determined but is something you can take charge of and hopefully prevent. Remember we now have a mountain of evidence that shows that most cancers - probably somewhere in the region of 80-90% - are a direct consequence of our diets and lifestyles.

It's easy to think when we are young 'It won't happen to me' but the sad reality is it will. Cancer now affects half of us so even if it doesn't hit you, it will likely hit someone you love and may even take them away from you prematurely. Trust me when I tell you there is nothing more distressing than to see a young person die of cancer. Each year over 8 million people die from cancer. It is vital that we take action and learn how to prevent these cancers. Despite billions of dollars invested and despite our best efforts, we have failed to win the war on cancer.

Change what's on your plate by focusing on what your body needs rather than what you want. Try to remind yourself every day about the science that shows that eating well, sleeping well and living well expands and extends your lifespan. If the science alone doesn't motivate you, think of the people in your life you want to live for.

The way I see it is that any oncologist or doctor who doesn't connect diet, lifestyle and cancer is doing their patients a huge disservice and possibly even negatively impacting their chances of survival. The same goes for other chronic diseases such as cardiovascular disease and diabetes. What we choose to do each and every day has a direct impact on our disease risk. I encourage everyone to start correcting their diet and lifestyle today. Tomorrow may be too late.

"Fast food diets are even damaging our genetic code, which is passed on to future generations."
Joel Fuhrman MD

THE ANTI-CANCER DIET

The World Cancer Research Fund and the American Institute for Cancer Research systematically analysed more than 1,000 studies on cancer and diet and found that diets low in fibrous plant-based nutrients and higher in animal products were linked to cancer. As a result, they both recommend plant-based whole food diets for the prevention of cancer.[103] Vegans and vegetarians in general have lower risks of cancer and lower rates of type 2 diabetes than omnivores and they are also some of the longest living westerners in the world.[104] We also know that a high sugar diet is a disaster for those with cancer. An anti-cancer diet needs to remove added sugars, improve consumption of healthy fats and avoid all additives and chemicals.

The problem with the current westernised diet is that animal product consumption, processed food consumption and sugar consumption has skyrocketed whilst fibre, fruit and vegetable consumption has plummeted. It is estimated that only 10% of the calories in the modern western diet are derived from whole foods like fruits, vegetables, beans, nuts and seeds. In inner city 'food deserts', where access to fresh foods is low, these figures are much worse and sit at around 5%. The reason this is a cancer-promoting diet is that low consumption of vegetables, nuts, beans and seeds results in low levels of vitamins, minerals, antioxidants, phytochemicals and fibre - all of which are incredibly effective at preventing cancer. At the cellular level these micronutrients are needed daily to ensure mitochondrial and DNA protection, efficient cell renewal and repair, toxin neutralisation and waste removal. Without these key nutrients, cellular function can be compromised and toxic metabolites can accumulate.

It is extremely common to find poor antioxidant status in cancer patients. Poor antioxidant status is a major risk factor for cancer in the first place, which might be why we find poor status in these people. But it's also partly because the three main treatments for cancer (surgery, chemotherapy and radiotherapy) all act to deplete antioxidant levels through a massive increase in free radical load.

If you have cancer, it's incredibly important to have an abundance of antioxidants as these are one of the body's most important first line defence mechanisms. The main frontline antioxidants are co-enzyme Q10, glutathione peroxidase and superoxide dismutase. In my view these should be all measured in oncology patients and supplemented through dietary change as necessary. These three single-handedly mop up millions of excess unstable electrons and pass them back to the second line antioxidant defences, such as vitamins D, K, E, B, lipoic acid, melatonin and many others, which then recycle the electron back to the ultimate electron - ascorbic acid. Ascorbic acid is vitamin C and its role in cellular health cannot be underestimated. Make sure your daily diet contains abundant antioxidants.

Fortunately, many of these antioxidants can be topped up through the diet - the exact way Mother Nature intended - so it's incredibly important during cancer treatment (and for prevention) that you eat a diet rich in vegetables, nuts, seeds, berries (and fruit to a lesser extent because of the fructose) and avoid beige foods that are generally processed and refined. Plant foods are superfoods and are rich in vitamins, minerals, phytonutrients and life-saving antioxidants. They will be your anti-cancer allies. In order to make the most of this natural anti-cancer potential I suggest you enlist the help of a professional nutritionist if you have been diagnosed with cancer. Allow the professionals to design you an anti-cancer diet that is balanced, nutritious and full of antioxidants, one that will starve the cancer of its fuel source (sugar) and boost your antioxidant defence.

We need to connect the dots and realise that what we put into our bodies every day has an impact on our disease risk. The path to preserving health is one that limits toxin exposure and maximises intake of healthful nutrients. When pro-inflammatory diets and lifestyles are adjusted the body has incredible capacity to prevent, to heal and to renew.

"What is remarkable about the diet-cancer story is the consistency with which certain foods emerge as important in reducing risks across the range of cancers. Millions of cancer cases could be prevented each year if more individuals adopted diets low in meat and high in fruit and vegetables."[105]
J Cummings, British Medical Journal

CHAPTER 4: The Diabetes Crisis

Diabetes is a disease of pancreatic insufficiency or overload. It is the dreaded insulin resistance in full picture and massively increases your risk of everything from heart disease and cancer to dementia and stroke.

10% of all cases of diabetes are classified as Type 1 diabetes and are genetically determined, the other 90% are classified as Type 2 diabetes, meaning that it is acquired throughout a person's lifetime. Type 2 diabetes occurs as a direct consequence of excess glucose and recreational eating. It is overconsumption coupled with underactivity. If ever there was a disease that typifies the modern western diet it would be Type 2 diabetes. It develops as a consequence of a lifetime of excessive calorie consumption and sedentary behaviour.

Type 1 diabetes is a genetic condition where you get impairment of pancreatic function through immune destruction of the beta cells of the pancreas. This normally happens in infancy or childhood. The beta cells are responsible for insulin production. Insulin is a hormone that regulates and controls the sugar in our blood. In Type 1 diabetics, pancreatic function will always be impaired. Dietary and lifestyle choices don't cause it, but a healthy lifestyle and diet can certainly improve it and lessen its impact. Sadly, more than one third of all Type 1 diabetics die before the age of 50 because of the destructive impact of uncontrolled sugar on their vessels, tissues and organs. They often die of heart disease, stroke, cancer and infections.

Type 2 diabetes is an entirely different beast and is caused primarily by food. To be specific, it is caused by overconsumption of the wrong types of foods. In Type 2 diabetes the pancreas starts off entirely normal and healthy in youth but over time and with sustained exposure to excess glucose it stops being able to adequately respond to the insulin being produced. Modern western diets, high in sugar, refined carbohydrates and junk foods, cause this excess demand on the pancreas such that it slowly burns out. The UK's *Lancet* medical publication called it 'a public humiliation' that diabetes has become such a global epidemic given that it is diet related and caused by our own lack of self-control. Type 2 diabetes is nothing short of a public health and preventative health car crash. Eat too much of the wrong foods and Type 2 diabetes will be the consequence.

Type 2 diabetes is a diet-related problem and therefore requires a dietary solution. It occurs when too many unhealthy and sugary foods are consumed in too high a volume and when too little physical exercise is undertaken to control the excess. It starts in our youth with unhealthy food choices and compounds over and over again throughout our lives when we make these same poor food choices. As parents we have to teach our children to eat well, otherwise they will face a future of obesity, diabetes, heart disease and chronic suffering. Healthy behaviours start in our youth; some people argue that it is a form of neglect to fail to teach children the benefits of healthy eating. The best way to avoid a diagnosis of diabetes is to eat less, reduce weight and get fit.

Food and beverage companies spent over $1.7 billion in 2009 marketing junk to our children because they see them as lifelong consumers of junk foods. 72% of this was spent on marketing breakfast cereals, fast foods and sugary soft drinks.

Food availability and food choices have significantly increased our rates of diabetes. According to the WHO there are now 422 million people with diabetes compared to 108 million in 1980.[106] Diabetes now affects one in eleven of the world's adult population. This figure is expected to rise to 642 million people by 2040.

The global cost of diabetes is set to almost double to $2.5 trillion by 2030, according to research from King's College London. For a diet-induced condition this is diabolical and frankly frightening. We are literally eating ourselves to death. These figures only mention the financial cost of diabetes, but the human suffering and disability endured by diabetics is profound. In the UK alone, four million people have diabetes and it's estimated that almost another million have undiagnosed diabetes.[107]

"The reason for our massive explosion in diabetes is our expanding waistlines."

Dr Joel Fuhrman

Diabetes has become the accepted norm in western societies where being overweight or fat is very common. Unfortunately, medication has become the favoured treatment for diabetes but it never corrects the cause. Weight loss, healthy eating and regular exercise are all highly effective means of stabilising and indeed reversing Type 2 diabetes. But often people don't bother with this - or maybe their doctors don't emphasise the importance of lifestyle and dietary changes enough?

Either way, our population prefers the quick fix of a tablet or injection to the effort of changing their ways. The drugs insulin and metformin have revolutionised survival for diabetics. They help in the short term but bring their own problems in the long term (insulin, for example, is a growth promoter). Before insulin, diabetics were doomed to death and would last a few years at most once the condition was full blown. But the problem with medications (in Type 2 diabetes) is that they never actually address the root cause of the problem, which is excess consumption of sugar such that the pancreas cannot cope. In medicine, if we don't ever address the root cause of a problem then we don't ever effect a cure. It's that simple. If we use drugs to mask symptoms so we can carry on longer, the collateral damage is lessened but the problem is still there. If a person continues to eat the very diet that made them diabetic in the first place then the problem just continues. In short, if you don't ever institute dietary and lifestyle changes in diabetics then you never really stop the ravages and pathology of the disease.

Left unchecked, the excess sugar from diabetes will destroy virtually every organ in your body, age your tissues and shorten your lifespan. In its advanced stages diabetes leaves people with eye problems, nerve problems, vascular problems and kidney problems. In hospitals we actually have wards just for diabetics and they are full of people with advanced heart disease, amputated limbs (from peripheral nerve problems and ulcers), blindness (diabetic retinopathy) and vascular dementia (known as 'type 3' diabetes). Almost half of all diabetes deaths are premature deaths, meaning they affect people under the age of 70. It is absolutely imperative that we emphasise prevention of diabetes in public health campaigns, GP surgeries, in the community and in the media. It is also vital that we make the food industry take some responsibility and make significant efforts to reduce excess and hidden sugar in commercial foods and drink. Thirdly, we need to take some responsibility ourselves and stop our recreational and excessive overeating, particularly of sugar and refined carbs. We need to exercise portion control (and self-control) and eat foods with a low GI index. We need to eat a more healthful, beneficial, micronutrient-rich diet so as to avoid the disability and devastation that comes with a chronic disease like diabetes.

Diabetes was virtually non-existent in previous centuries when food wasn't so sugary, processed and readily available. In countries where being overweight is the new norm diabetes has exploded. This isn't just western countries; Type 2 diabetes is also skyrocketing in India, Asia, Central and South America. In all corners of the world diabetes is taking hold because the modern diet is totally unsuited to our DNA. Even slim people can get diabetes if they eat the wrong foods. If you have already been diagnosed with insulin resistance (pre-diabetes) or have diabetes, the best way to halt it is to adapt and adjust your lifestyle and diet. Whilst the modern western diet is dangerous for everyone, for diabetics it is incredibly dangerous and is, in fact, pathogenic.

Some blame has to fall with us doctors. Studies have found that only 33% of us educate our patients about the positive role of exercise and diet in diabetes management.[108]

As well as changing our diet we need to change the way we live. Sedentary behaviour is a key factor in Type 2 diabetes. The 2008 European Society of Cardiology congress study showed how important exercise is in beating and reducing Type 2 diabetes. It showed that diabetics who pursued physical fitness had a 65% reduced risk of death compared to those with low levels of physical fitness.[109] No diabetic medicine can produce these kinds of mortality improvements so it's very important that diabetics know the value of daily exercise for their overall health. All doctors need to remind their diabetic patients that daily physical exercise is an absolute must if they intend to reduce the deadly impact of their disease. If exercise could be prescribed for all, trust me, it would be.

DIABETES AND OBESITY GO HAND IN HAND

Diabetes is linked with obesity. In very simplistic terms, both diabetes and obesity are caused by overconsumption and 'super-sizing' of the modern western diet. A diet high in sugar, high in refined carbs (pre-sugar sugar), high in trans fats (bad fats) and high in portion size is the road to both obesity and diabetes. They are like two peas in a pod. In the USA, women are consuming 335 more calories per day and men are consuming 168 more calories daily than 30 years ago (Wright, 2004). They are not moving or exercising enough to compensate and mitigate for this increased calorie intake and therefore end up putting on weight. A US woman would need to walk an extra 75 minutes per day to burn off these extra calories!

Fast and convenience foods must take a lot of the blame. Studies have shown that people who eat take away or fast foods two or more times a week are 50% more likely to become overweight (Pereira, 2005). Lack of exercise is also to blame for the increasing levels of obesity in the modern world. We are largely a sedentary society now with the convenience of mass transport to take us from A to B and the world at our fingertips online. Most people sit at desks for extended parts of the day and fail to walk the minimum 10,000 steps a day. It is estimated that if you work a full-time job you are likely to be sedentary for 21 out of 24 hours in a day (including your 8 hours of sleep).

INTERESTING FACTS ABOUT DIABETES

By 2020 it is estimated that more than half of Americans will be pre-diabetic or diabetic, costing the US economy £3.35 trillion.[110]

Diabetes increases cancer risk. Diabetics are 30% more likely to develop colorectal cancer,[111] 20% more likely to get breast cancer and 82% more likely to develop cancer of the pancreas.[112]

Three quarters of all diabetics have high blood pressure - a risk factor for heart disease and stroke.

80% of diabetics die of heart disease and stroke - diabetes increases your risk of heart disease and stroke by more than three times.

Diabetes is the leading cause of kidney failure, limb amputations and adult onset blindness.

Insulin levels are a strong predictor of heart attack and shortened lifespan.

90% of diabetics are classified as ype 2, caused by poor food and lifestyle choices.

Diabetes has increased 700% in the last 50 years.[113]

Women with diabetes are more than 30% more likely to develop depression; women who take insulin are 53% more likely to develop depression.[114]

Diabetes is not just caused by excess sugar. The pathology is that microscopic particles of fat deposit in the muscle and liver cells cause the dysfunction of insulin. The fat stops insulin from being able to move from the blood stream into the cell. If you eat a lot of fatty junk foods and vegetable oils this can cause the blockage of the activity of insulin. So it's important to eat low sugar, low processed foods and vegetable oils if you suffer from diabetes or pre-diabetes and focus on low GI index whole foods with minimal processing. This kind of diet will help take the pressure off your pancreas and help shape a better, healthier future for you. NB: If you are diabetic please see your doctor before you change your diet. They may need to significantly reduce your diabetic medications so as not to over treat you. That's how effective it can be!

CHAPTER 5: The Brain Crisis

Our brains are our most fragile and complex organs. They are protected and encased in the hard and sturdy skull and protected internally by the exquisite blood brain barrier. Most of us take brain health for granted without realising the complex relationship that our brains have with the foods that we eat and the lives we live.

We are living longer than ever. Life is now an ultra-marathon with the ceiling for human existence constantly increasing. Genetics is thought to account for 25% of ageing but the rest is related to nutrition, lifestyle, environment and socio-economics. The 20th century has witnessed a boom in longevity with the average lifespan increasing from fifty to eighty years in industrialised countries. Most of this is due to better public health, better sanitation, clean water, widespread vaccines and better medicines. But when it comes to brain health, are we the victims of our own success? Our increase in lifespan does not necessarily come with clarity of mind or quality of life. The truth is that for many people these additional years come with poor mental health, cognitive dysfunction and a sense of despair. Much of this is due to brain deterioration, which happens slowly over the years. Given that it takes many years to get to a state of cognitive loss and full-blown dementia there is lots we can do ourselves to prevent and mitigate the damage and to gift ourselves a better old age.

As Dr Lisa Mosconi eloquently puts it, 'Of all the challenges to ageing in the 21st century nothing compares to the unprecedented scale of Alzheimer's.' The drastic explosion of dementia rates worldwide has brought widescale suffering for those it affects and for those who care and support those afflicted. The financial, emotional and human cost of our current epidemic of dementia is huge. There are currently an estimated 46 million people living with dementia worldwide and this is set to increase to 132 million by the year 2050. So, whilst we are all living longer, are we really living well? Is it really value added if we are staggering around a nursing home with dementia so entrenched that we no longer know who we, or our loved ones, are? It's not nice to feel lost and vulnerable, especially when we are elderly.

If we are all living longer then we all need to learn how to take care of our brains. They need to last eighty to a hundred years, not just sixty.

In the same way that heart disease and cancer are primarily caused by diet and lifestyle, dementia is much the same. A small number of people have genetic defects that code for dementia (<5%) but the vast majority do not. Instead it is a slow and gradual deterioration of brain function largely caused by repeated and cumulative brain insults influenced by a person's choices of food and how they live.

Taking care of your brain is a life-long commitment and, like most things, starts in our youth. Unlike other parts of the body that can regenerate (like the skin, the liver and red blood cells) the brain's capacity for regeneration is much more limited. This makes brain cells incredibly precious (and also vulnerable) because the vast majority of them are with us for life. Since they cannot easily be regrown, restored or replaced it is vital that we learn to live brain-friendly lives and learn how to protect and nourish our wonderful brains. Doctors call this neuro-nutrition - nourishing our brains with a lifetime of good food and lifestyle choices.

Blue Zones show us that dementia is not a consequence of old age and bad genes. Many people in these longevity hotspots live well into their 90s and 100s with good cognitive capacity. In the majority of people, dementia is not determined by genes but is driven by insulin resistance and inflammation caused by poor diets and sedentary lifestyles. It is possible to live well into your hundreds with a sharp and agile mind if you know how to feed and nourish your brain.

To show the impact that diet and lifestyle has on brain health, scientists have looked at brain imaging in the form of MRIs of people following differing diets and compared them. In one well-known study they compared MRI imaging of a 50-year-old who ate a typical Mediterranean diet for the entirety of her life and a second participant who ate a typical westernised diet characterised by high amounts of processed foods, sugar, salt, damaged fats and fizzy drinks. The difference in brain health between the two 50-year-olds was remarkable. The MRI from the person eating a western diet showed brain shrinkage (atrophy), neuronal loss, enlarged ventricles and accelerated ageing of the hippocampus, the memory centre of the brain. The MRI of the participant eating the Mediterranean diet showed much better brain preservation, better memory centres and healthy neuronal numbers. What studies like this show us is that there is a clear link between brain health and food health. Studies like these are visual, tangible proof that dietary management should be part of any anti-ageing and anti-dementia regime.

Our brains need a multitude of nutrients in order to survive and thrive. Because of this our brain is highly dependent on positive food and lifestyle choices. Excess sugars, chemicals, additives, toxins, hormones, pesticides, arsenic, heavy metals and GMOs found in poor quality foods are all accelerators of brain deterioration. Alzheimer's dementia has now been dubbed 'Type 3 Diabetes' because it is so clearly linked to a form of insulin resistance in the brain. All the same dietary and lifestyle changes that minimise your risk of heart disease and stroke as well as diabetes are the same changes that prevent dementia. Unsurprising really, since it's all linked.

Changing what you eat has profound health benefits. Cutting out ultra-processed and junk foods, reducing sugar and eating low GI index foods is a great place to start. But there are also some specific measures you can take to really power up your brain. Increasing your omega 3 intake, ensuring adequate intake of vitamins C, B and E and ensuring good protein intake are all essentials for brain health.

It is thought that increased omega fat consumption was one of the single most important factors in the development of the human brain in evolutionary terms. Historians think that when consumption of DHA doubled in the million years between Homo Erectus and Homo Sapiens this allowed for the expansion and sophistication of the human brain, in particular the cerebral cortex and grey matter, which resulted in the growth of human intelligence. Homo Sapiens are known to have disproportionately large brain to body size.

Our human ancestors have been on this earth for over six million years. Our early ancestors ate what we would today consider a mostly raw vegan diet with some fresh fish and occasional meat when the hunt was successful. It was when we started to increase our fatty fish (DHA) consumption (due to the ease of fishing compared to hunting) that the brain gradually became larger in size and more complex. It should come as no surprise then that the brain needs an abundance of plant-based foods AND a good supply of healthy fats in order to survive. A pescatarian diet is probably the most brain-boosting and brain-supporting diet on the planet due to its abundance of pre-formed omega 3s.

It is widely accepted that our recent collective decline in brain health (and mental health) is to do with the fact that our DNA hasn't adapted to the sudden deterioration of fats and other nutrients in our modern diets. The quality and quantity of brain-healthy foods has slowly depleted and diminished. The combination of refined grains, inflammatory dairy, processed meats, trans fats and high levels of sugar has been disastrous for neuronal longevity. Add to this the problems we have with industrial pollutants and toxins like mercury and aluminium and it's easy to see why dementia is crippling the fragile modern brain.

DHA is one of the most well documented brain protectors and makes up more than 90% of the omega 3 fats in the brain. DHA is a major building block of the brain and is critical for optimal brain health and development at all ages and stages of life. Numerous studies and systematic reviews have now shown that higher intakes of omega 3 reduce the incidence of common brain disorders such as Alzheimer's, vascular dementia and memory loss.[115] Furthermore, deficiencies in DHA have been linked to depression, suicidal tendency, addictive behaviour, reduced memory and reduced attention and learning.

The brain depends on a daily supply of healthy dietary fats. Omega 3 and omega 6 are essential fats: that means the body cannot make them and they need to be taken daily in the diet. Brain lipids (fats) are constantly being renewed and any drop in dietary intake can drastically alter them, which can affect the brain's functionality and long-term health by predisposing it to a multitude of brain disorders.

The importance of healthy fats in our diet was highlighted by a landmark study of 6,000 participants aged 65+ that showed that those who consumed low amounts of omega 3 had a 70% higher risk of developing Alzheimer's than those who consumed more. The study showed that people who consumed less than 1g of omega 3 per day had the highest risk of dementia and those who ate more than 2g per day were unlikely to develop dementia at all. The same conclusions were mirrored when researchers looked at brain MRIs of those with high omega 3 consumption. Brain scans of individuals who didn't consume much omega 3 showed accelerated ageing and brain shrinkage. MRIs especially identified the vulnerable memory centre (the hippocampus) as prone to neuronal loss with poor dietary fat intake. To reduce this risk, ensure that you eat healthy fats every day.

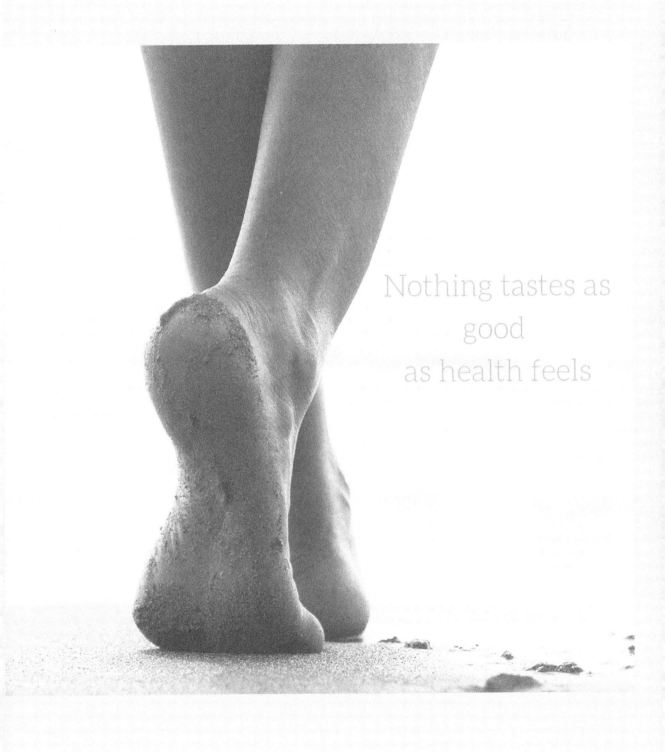

Nothing tastes as
good
as health feels

Foods that are rich in the kinds of fat that the brain thrives on include wild fatty fish like mackerel, salmon, sardines, anchovies and caviar (if you can afford it!). These all provide pre-formed form of omega 3 called DHA that the body and brain can use straight away. Vegetarian sources are tapioca, walnuts, oats, sunflower seeds, flaxseed, chia seed and hempseed - however, these don't provide pre-formed DHA and rely on the body converting them from Alpha Linolenic Acids (ALA) to DHA. Most people convert ALA to DHA weakly so strict vegetarians and vegans should supplement their diet with omega 3 from algal oil. Algae is what the fish eat in the first place to become so omega 3-rich. It makes sense then to eat them direct from the source.

Other nutrients that are highly important to the brain are proteins. Proteins are the body's building blocks and are made up of smaller units called amino acids. Amino acids are essential for just about every function in the brain and body. Their importance cannot be underestimated. Amino acids form the brain's chemical messengers or neurotransmitters. Neurotransmitters are in charge of how we think, feel, act and behave.

The human brain relies on a carefully orchestrated co-operation of over a hundred different chemical neurotransmitters that work with military precision. Some of the most important neurotransmitters are serotonin, dopamine, gamma-aminobutyric acid (GABA) and glutamate. They all have huge power over how we feel, think, behave and function. The brain's neurotransmitters are created from - you guessed it - the food we eat. So you can see it's absolutely vital that you eat well to nourish your brain.

Tryptophan is the sole precursor of the neurotransmitter serotonin. The body cannot make it so it must be consumed in your diet. Depression, anxiety and poor memory are all associated with serotonin deficiency states. The brain requires good levels of serotonin to preserve its status quo. Happiness depends upon good serotonin levels and the best thing is that non-pharmacological routes to increasing serotonin are plentiful because we can consume tryptophan-rich foods. Chia seeds are a wonderful source of tryptophan, a powerhouse food source for the brain. Edamame, prunes, spirulina and natural yoghurt are also rich tryptophan sources. You can also take tryptophan as a supplement in the form of 5-HTP, which I do sometimes myself.

Vitamin B6 is a co-factor in the tryptophan conversion process so make sure you are taking sufficient vitamin B6 too - they work in synergy. If you are feeling a bit low in mood, then check your diet includes enough sources of tryptophan and B6 and supplement if needed. (Try the delicious chia seed pudding at the end of the book for a simple brain-boosting, tryptophan-rich breakfast.)

Dopamine is manufactured in the brain by breaking down the amino acid tyrosine, which is produced from phenylalanine. Dopamine has been dubbed the 'motivation molecule' because without it we don't feel motivated and we don't experience pleasure and reward. Deficiency of dopamine is associated with depression, memory impairment, Parkinson's disease, Attention Deficit Hyperactivity Disorder (ADHD) and schizophrenia. Plant foods like soybeans, chia seeds, pumpkin seeds, peanuts, almonds and spinach are rich sources of phenylalanine, as are foods like salmon and sea bass.

Glutamate is the brain's main excitatory neurotransmitter - it causes us to get up and go, to act, to initiate and to do things. It gives us momentum and movement in life. And it also gives us learning and memory. 90% of the brain's neuronal synapses are glutamatergic, i.e. primed and programmed to release glutamate; that's how fundamental and vital it is. Virtually every food that contains protein contains some glutamate, but rich sources of glutamate include tomatoes, kidney beans, mushrooms, walnuts, soy and eggs. The brain needs good quality foods to make good quality glutamate.

Gamma-Aminobutyric Acid (GABA) is an important inhibitory neurotransmitter that is also made from glutamate. Our gut microbes help convert glutamine to glutamic acid into GABA. Given that most of us have gut imbalances secondary to modern western living, it's no wonder we have so many problems with sleep, mood and health in our society. A poorly functioning gut is a major cause of low GABA - and GABA helps us relax, helps us manage stress, helps to reduce blood pressure and helps shift the brain into a lower, calmer gear. It also facilitates sleep. GABA is vital in today's stressed out, fast paced, super stimulated world. Make sure you get your glutamate from quality sources and ensure that you eat good quality pre- and probiotic foods (or supplement if necessary) to support its production in the gut.

Vitamins are also vital players in brain preservation and function. The B vitamins deserve special mention. Without enough thiamine (B1) there is loss of functioning of the nervous system; without enough niacin (B3) there is pellagra, a condition that includes dementia, dermatitis and diarrhea; without enough pyridoxine (B6) there is the risk of both dementia and depression (serotonin, dopamine and GABA all require B6); and without choline the brain cannot manufacture acetylcholine, which further increases the risk of dementia. Diets that are poor and deficient in vitamins can have a huge impact on mental health and wellbeing. Given the importance of all of these nutrients for the brain it's difficult to believe that some people are still not convinced about the incredible healing and protective power of our diet. Without a doubt, food is medicine. When there are so many great reasons to eat good foods it's amazing that we eat so much junk.

Numerous studies have looked at supplementation of B vitamins and have shown how they can help to prevent dementia, maintain memory performance and reduce brain shrinkage in the elderly, as measured by MRI.[116] In one two-year study, for example, supplementation of folic acid, B12 and B6 helped reduce brain shrinkage by 53%. The study also found that when B vitamins were supplemented alongside good omega 3 intake, brains responded even better.

Minerals are also incredibly valuable to the brain. We primarily absorb them from the fruit and vegetables that we consume (or animal products that we consume) and they get them from the soil in which they graze or grow. There has been a lot of concern recently about soil overuse and depletion of the mineral content. Fast cropping and changing agricultural techniques are slowly depleting the mineral content of our foods. Minerals help the brain perform everything from nerve conduction to fluid regulation, hydration and metabolism. We need to be careful that nutrients don't vanish from the soil. We need to urgently employ sustainable farming practices to protect our precious soils - otherwise our bodies and brains will suffer. We also need to steer our agriculture away from toxic herbicides and pesticides otherwise our children will face a double whammy - they will be born with a chemical burden unknown to previous generations and eat nutrient-depleted food that makes them further vulnerable.

Metals such as mercury, arsenic, lead and cadmium are part of the Earth's natural crust but can be highly toxic to the body and brain. Heavy metals are everywhere and can accumulate in the body when there is nutritional imbalance. They can cause widespread inflammation and toxic stress. Many of these metals are found in the foods we eat - mercury in contaminated fish and arsenic in rice, for example. And they are found in industrial products, in our water supply, in cosmetics, in medicines, in cooking containers (e.g. aluminium cookware), toothpaste, dental fillings (mercury) - the list goes on and on. Heavy metals have become serious pollutants because their use is poorly regulated. There has long been a general disregard and indifference towards heavy metals and industrial pollutants by governments and the supposed regulating agencies. Some experts believe that heavy metal toxicity is one of the biggest threats to our future brain health. They can also mess with your thyroid and adrenal function, ruin your mitochondrial function and suppress your immune system. Foods absorb heavy metals from the water, air and soil in which they grow. In order to avoid issues with heavy metals it is important to eat mainly from the bottom of the food chain (metals and toxins bioaccumulate in animals), eat mainly organic foods, limit your consumption of farmed fish (to avoid mercury) and filter your water (to remove lead). A regular sauna session can help to sweat out heavy metals and chlorella and glutathione can be helpful as supplements to help with metal detoxification.

Plant-derived antioxidants also play a huge role in brain health. No organ is more sensitive to oxidative damage and stress than the brain and it takes a continual flood of antioxidants to combat the daily oxidative stress that the brain endures. Vitamin C and vitamin E are the brain's major antioxidant super players and need to be consumed in abundance. These two play an important role in keeping our brains youthful, vibrant and damage free. Once again, 'eating the rainbow' (i.e. eating colourful vegetables) will help you maintain good levels. The richer the colour of your food the more antioxidants they contain. Studies have found that antioxidants work best for the brain when taken through whole foods rather than supplementation, although supplementation is better than allowing deficiency.[117]

Fresh foods such as oranges, strawberries, blueberries, lemon, broccoli, spinach, flaxseed and almonds are all great sources of these two crucial vitamins. Keep a stock of them at home and make sure you sprinkle berries, flaxseeds, strawberries and lemons on foods when you can! And I mustn't forget to re-mention chia seeds - nature's incredible ancient Mayan seed that is literally a brain superfood.

Interestingly, it's important to eat well but not to overeat. Being overweight is just as bad for the brain as it is the body. Studies have shown that excess body fat increases not only insulin resistance but inflammatory chemicals that can directly damage the brain. A 2005 study looking at structural changes of the brain showed that increasing waist to hip ratio was associated with a direct decline in size of the hippocampus - the brain's memory centre.[118] And the hippocampus' function and performance is directly related to its size.

No chapter on the brain crisis would be complete without a mention of depression. Many years ago, the mainstream explanation of depression was that our brains were chemically imbalanced and that the way to treat it was with pharmaceutics that helped increase serotonin. This is too simplistic and reductionist. As time has passed, we have reviewed our views about depression and have realised that depression is more than just a chemical imbalance and likely reflects everything from our food choices, stress levels and lifestyles to our psyche and feelings of disconnect.

Some people are genetically more prone to depression if they have certain genes but often these are only 'turned on' with traumatic exposures and stressors in our lives. If you have this genetic picture and bad things don't happen to you, it seems you are no more likely than anyone else to become depressed. I guess what I am saying is that nobody is condemned to a life of depression and anxiety and genes don't totally determine your destiny. The biggest factors switching on depression are life events, long-term stress and disconnection. So, while biological causes exist, they certainly don't override the very issue of depression being a reaction to our stressful, modern lives.

Given that depression isn't an absolute chemical imbalance it seems insane that we primarily treat depression with potent and addictive pharmaceutics. A better focus would be to look at the context of a person's feelings and to reduce the stressors that cause it in the first place. Looking at the state of a person's diet and nutrition would also help in the treatment of depression. In the modern world many people have become socially isolated, disconnected and disheartened. Where vibrant communities once held people together there is now significant isolation and disconnect.

There are many flaws in the way we live today in the west. We could all do with consciously slowing down. We could all do with less hustle and hassle. Less pointless material stuff. Less stress. Less admin. Less social media. We need to stop pursuing happiness just for ourselves and switch the way we think about life. A less selfish approach to life could well be the route to improved happiness and purpose. In many other parts of the world people pursue happiness as a social and collective thing, not just as an individual thing. They don't just seek to achieve and thrive alone like we so often do in the west. Happiness is more a collective, familial or communal experience, because community is what life is about in many places. Sadly, we have lost this sense of community in the west and in the process somewhere it seems we may have lost ourselves. Thinking that a chemical pill can resolve all of this is reductionist and simplistic.

"Depression and anxiety might, in one way, be the sanest reaction you have. It's a signal saying you shouldn't have to live this way and if you aren't helped to find a better path you will be missing out on so much that is best about being human."

Johann Hari, author, Lost Connections

Regular socialising, meditation, yoga, exercise and intimacy are all great therapies for depression. Counselling and talking therapy are particularly effective in helping support people who are bereaved or depressed. Rather than immediately prescribe pharmaceutical and chemical therapy I am much more inclined to prescribe social and emotional therapy, meditation, yoga, exercise, regular time in nature or talking therapy - something that actually helps individuals find their purpose or *'joie de vivre'* again.

CHAPTER 6: The Food Crisis

"Let food be thy medicine."

Hippocrates

Over 2000 years ago Hippocrates recognised the importance of food with his famous words. Since these times we have departed significantly from the healthful, nourishing foods that used to connect us to the earth. The ultra-processed foods that intelligent man created to outsmart Mother Nature are now the foods that are causing us harm. We eat more foods from a packet than we do from the soil and we are suffering the consequences of this with our collective health decline.

We have to be accountable for the fact that many modern diseases are the unfortunate consequence of our poor food choices. As consumers, we have to take some blame. We want foods with long shelf lives, we want seasonal foods all year around and we want quick access to foods from all over the globe. What we have done is change the way we eat so profoundly that this has had a direct impact on our health. When we increase a food's shelf life it requires significant processing and results in nutrient depletion. In order to withstand the effects of time on a shelf, food needs to be low in nutrients. Otherwise bugs and bacteria alike tend to collect and feed on them. So that's exactly what food manufacturers do - take the nutrients out. The milling of wheat, refining of sugar and polishing of rice are all examples of how we have stripped our food of its vitamin, mineral and fibre content. Modern farming and mass agriculture have added fertiliser, pesticides and herbicides to our foods resulting in a fast and furious farming mentality that puts quantity over quality. The resultant pest-resistant pseudo-produce does not deliver the same quality of vitamins and minerals as it used to, plus risks a toxic, carcinogenic mix of herbicides and pesticides. How we have allowed this to happen is beyond belief.

Foods that are highly dense and nutritious don't have a shelf life or a label. They are straight from the earth (or sea) and come with an abundance of natural super substances.

PROCESSED FOODS

More than 50% of the foods consumed in UK homes are processed.[119] Put simply, this means that over half of what we eat is made in a factory or lab. My general rule is that anything with more than five listed ingredients falls into the 'processed' category. Gulp. That's most supermarket foods! Indeed, it is. Supermarket aisles are full of fake food with little nutrient value. The reality is that the modern western diet is desperately micronutrient-depleted and instead full of undesirables such as sugar, chemicals, preservatives, additives, trans fats, omega 6 and hidden salt. Eating these kinds of foods over a long period of time will absolutely and irrevocably affect your health. In my world it's called Collateral Damage.

Because our foods have become so adulterated and processed, rates of obesity in Europe are rapidly approaching those of the USA (currently one in three). In fact, in the USA, there are now more obese adults than there are overweight adults.[120]

When obesity rates go up a public health disaster always follows. Because humans were not designed to carry excess fat. This has been the sequence of events wherever traditional diets have been replaced with modern, western diets. First comes changes in the diet, with increasing levels of sugar, salt, refined carbohydrates and animal products. Then obesity, diabetes, cardiovascular disease and cancer. The UN recently announced that problems stemming from 'overnutrition' have, for the first time, exceeded problems stemming from undernutrition in the world. Isn't this a sad state of affairs? Gluttony is definitely getting the better of us here...

In remote parts of the world obesity, diabetes, cancer and heart disease are almost unheard of. Dennis Burkitt, who worked with many native populations in his lifetime, proposed that we call these diseases 'western' diseases because when native populations came to the west and adopted our diet and our way of life, these diseases soon followed. And he was right.

Simply by moving to places like America migrants quickly begin to 'acquire' chronic diseases. In the space of a generation we saw the Japanese, Africans, Pacific Islanders and many others lose their immunity to western diseases and acquire the same risks of diabetes and cancer as the rest of us. Either there is something present in the western diet causing this, or something absent from it. In fact, it turns out it's a combination of both. Heavy sugar and processed foods push vegetables, nuts, seeds and whole foods off the plate!

It's not just the food we are eating but the quantity of the food we are eating and the way we are eating. We currently spend half our food dollars on meals outside the home. We frequently eat at drive throughs, on our laps, in front of the TV, on the road and, increasingly, alone. Throughout history humans have enjoyed preparing and eating food in groups, sharing and socialising. Increasingly, we are being disconnected from the thousands of years of culture and civilisation that traditionally surrounded our foods as we eat processed, lab-made foods, alone, hurriedly and in large portions.

The other worrying thing is that as well as processed foods altering the way we eat and the amount we eat, they've also changed the way our bodies deal with the food we eat. Studies have shown that junk foods hijack the brain's neurochemical pathways and cause overeating. A 2015 study at the University of Michigan showed that people overeat junk foods in accordance with how processed they are - in other words, the more processed a food is the more likely we are to overeat it.[121] Highly processed junk foods like pizza and pastries overwhelm our biological and molecular signals and override our willpower on a biochemical level. Vegetables and fruit don't cause this kind of binge eating because they don't hijack the dopamine reward centre in our brain. People can become genuinely 'addicted' to junk foods.

There are five 'Blue Zones' across the world: these are longevity hotspots with the highest number of centenarians.[122] In these places it is common for people to live well into their nineties and hundreds in good health, with mental agility and a good quality of life. These longevity hotspots are Sardinia (Italy), Okinawa (Japan), Loma Linda (California), Nicoya Peninsula (Costa Rica), and Icaria (a Greek Island).

In these places people enjoy a diet that is healthful, they move daily, they enjoy community and personal support, they live meaningful lives and they manage stress efficiently. It is frequently noted that there is very little discontent in Blue Zones. And it is not technology and pharmaceuticals that keeps people alive here, but simple, healthy and active lives.

What epidemiologists have noted when they study the longest-living populations in the world is that they all eat diets that are high in a variety of plant-based foods. People in Blue Zones all eat different diets but what they have in common is that they eat plentiful fruits, vegetables, seeds and nuts (the 'good' stuff) and low amounts of dairy, animal protein and processed foods (the 'bad' stuff). They incorporate exercise into their daily routines and are much more physical than the average westerner. They don't need treadmills and gym memberships to achieve this level of fitness; they use their bodies physically in their daily lives, by tending the fields or walking the earth, and move far more than the sedentary office worker does. Their bodies are resilient and able to cope with stress. They have very few chemical toxins to fight off. They live in small communities with a strong tradition of religion or meaning and this affords them a feeling of happiness that seems to add to their sense of wellbeing.

We can learn a lot from these Blue Zones. I highly recommend Dan Buettner's book *The Blue Zones: 9 Lessons for Living Longer from the People Who've Lived the Longest,* and I love to follow @BlueZones on Instagram for the most wonderful stories celebrating longevity and long, happy lives around the world.

SUGAR

Sugar is a metabolic catastrophe for your health. Sugar has no nutritional value and adds nothing to our diet. It contains no vitamins, minerals, micronutrients or anything beneficial whatsoever. It is one of the few food substances that humans consume without any nutritional benefit. Alcohol is another.

Sugar is highly addictive and damaging to the body and is a major cause of disease through the problem of insulin resistance. Manufacturers of food have known for a long time that sugar is bad for us, but they have hidden the incriminating evidence and have continued to add it to our food because they also know something else - sugar is highly addictive. And if they can create a genuine addiction, they have a consumer for life. BINGO.

Manufacturers need to stop dodging the data that shows sugar is very bad for human health - they have an ethical duty to stop hiding it in our foods. Did you know there are conveniently 56 different names for sugar? It comes in many disguises and can be hidden in many different ways on food labels. Processed, ready-made supermarket foods are the biggest culprits of high and hidden sugar. Cooking sauces, bread, salad dressings, fizzy drinks, pastries, cereals, ketchup all contain significant amounts of sugar. Many foods masquerade as 'health foods' (think snack bars and the new trendy 'protein' bars) but are laden with sugar. We also need to understand that simple carbohydrates, such as white bread and pasta, are converted rapidly into sugar. Sadly, sugar is everywhere and it is a relentless effort to avoid it - for those of us who want to! Every kind of processed food has sugar in it, whether concealed or listed. The moral of the story is to boycott processed foods and eat foods in their natural state. This is the only way you can shun sugar and see your health dramatically improve.

A study published in *JAMA Internal Medicine* in 2014 examined sugar consumption in the USA (Americans are incidentally the world's highest consumers of sugar) and found that individuals who consumed more than one quarter of their daily calories through sugar were three times more likely to die of cardiovascular disease than people who consumed less than 10% of their daily calories in sugar. This is through the damaging effects of insulin resistance and pancreatic damage.

Food manufacturers have an ethical responsibility to reduce their use of sugar in processed foods to save us from the obesity and diabetes crisis (as well as all the other diseases). With 75% of supermarket foods containing hidden sugar, this will take a long time to ripple down. The best thing you can do is start to make simple changes in your daily diet that will help reduce your sugar dependence. I say dependence because sugar is one of the most addictive anti-nutrients in the modern western diet. The historian Sidney Mintz described sugar as the 'opiate of the masses' and studies have found it to be more addictive than heroin.

Sugar taxes on soft drinks, which came into play in 2018, are a positive step. Given that a can of cola contains the equivalent of nine sugar cubes - your entire day's sugar limit - this is an extremely important and sensible tax which will have huge implications for our nation's health.

Studies have also shown that 500ml of Pret a Manger orange juice has the same amount of sugar as 13 Hobnob biscuits! So Pepsi and Coca Cola are no longer the only bad guys. Commercial juices and smoothies are just as bad and are - in essence - liquid sugar. Some experts blame these kinds of drinks, often marketed as the healthier option, for our expanding waistlines.

If you are sitting here reading this and feeling shocked and guilty about eating too much sugar (or, worse, feeding too much sugar to your children) you are not alone. Many people aren't aware of how pervasive sugar is in our society. Cleaning up your diet and swapping sugary, processed foods for more whole foods will help you rapidly reverse any sugar-related damage. The human body has an incredible capacity to heal even after years of nutritional trauma. Diabetes, obesity, heart disease - they can all be reversed with powerful and positive food choices.

People often ask me about sugar alternatives. Stevia and xylitol are naturally-derived sweeteners whereas aspartame and saccharine are chemically derived and have been linked to cancer in animals. Many experts believe aspartame to be highly neurotoxic. The FDA originally refused to approve it due to concerns about its toxicity. I would seriously suggest that you avoid it.

Sugar Sugar

· · · · · · · · · · · · · · · · · · ·

In 2015 the US FDA examined 1,074 ready made infant and toddler foods. It found that 35% of their calories came from sugar.

National levels of tooth decay in the USA stands at a whopping 92% compared to 2% in Nigeria.

The WHO recommends that we get only 5% of our daily calories from sugar.

The average Brits consumes twice the recommended amount of sugar- equivalent to 14 sugar cubes a day.

Most Brits eat an excess of 200-300 calories per day due to sugar.

One Innocent Smoothie contains 30% more sugar than a can of coke. Not so innocent afterall.

One Pret A Manger Orange Juice has the sugar equivalent of 13 Hobnob biscuits.

Studies on artificial sweeteners and their links to cancer have been contradictory but several have suggested toxic effects on the brain. There are many other reasons to avoid chemical sweeteners. Whilst they do help cut down on the extra calories from sugar, sweeteners continue the sweet reward system in the brain. Numerous studies have now found that sweetness might actually desensitise the brain's reward system, confuse our neurobiology and result in increased food consumption, weight gain, glucose intolerance and diabetes.[123] [124] Honey, maple, agave and rice syrup are not sugar substitutes but are high in sugar and also hijack and activate the brain's dopamine reward system just as readily. It's much better to retrain your palate and adjust to very low sugar consumption. It only takes a few weeks to rewire the brain and to learn to enjoy foods and drinks without sugar. Soon you will wonder why you ever felt the need to add sugar in the first place.

SUGAR ADDICTIONS

Sugar affects the brain's reward system, the mesolimbic dopamine system. The neurotransmitter dopamine, a powerful chemical transmitter, is released in response to a rewarding event such as sugar consumption. Nicotine, drugs and sex also hijack this system so it's not surprising that dopamine is blamed for most of our sinful and addictive behaviours. Activating this system sets up a pathway that makes you want to get the reward again and again, contributing to the repeated behaviours seen so commonly in addiction.

Studies on rats have shown how sugar dependent they can become.[125] This anti-nutrient that we have introduced into the food chain is causing massive health problems across the globe and hijacking our brains and making it HARD to let it go... Clever.

There is no short cut or easy way around it. You just have to go cold turkey and cut out sugar. The health benefits will be magnificent in the long term if you can resist the temptations and sustain it. Sugar ages all tissues and organs through a process called glycation, so everything from your skin to your brain will benefit from dietary reductions. Your teeth will thank you, your waistline will be trimmer, your arteries will be less inflamed, your cholesterol will be lower, you will have fewer wrinkles and your chance of diabetes, cancer, Alzheimer's and cardiovascular disease will be significantly reduced. What better reasons to cut down on sugar could you possibly need?

CARBOHYDRATES

We have become a nation of 'carboholics'. We eat far too many refined carbs and adulterated carbohydrates and our collective health has suffered as a consequence. One of the main problems with the modern western diet is easy access to carbohydrate-based foods. If you are running around busy all day and put no thought into your food choices then carbohydrates are likely to feature prominently in your diet because of their super-abundance in our lives. A normal day for most people is cereal or toast for breakfast (carbs and sugar), a sandwich for lunch (carbs and sugar), and pasta and sauce for dinner (carbs and sugar). Snacks might include a snack bar (carbs and sugar) and a piece of fruit (fructose sugar). Sugars and refined, cheap carbohydrates have got us into this mess and avoidance of them will get us out of it. In the eloquent words of Dr Sarah Myhill, the problem is easy to diagnose: "Simply look in the supermarket trolley - if it's composed of bread, cereals, biscuits, pasta, fruit, crisps, chocolate and alcohol then its owner and his/her family will have (insulin resistance or) metabolic disease."[126]

For too long we have been telling the public to eat low fat foods, but when we take fats out of food they are generally replaced with carbohydrates or sugar. It is the removal of fat from our food that has caused skyrocketing rates of disease. Ironically the low-fat campaign coincided with a dramatic increase in the global incidence of obesity and diabetes. Many people cite the adoption of low-fat diets as the turning point when Americans (and, not long after, the rest of us) got really fat.

Excess sugar and refined carbohydrates make us overweight and fat. I always tell my patients to consider refined carbohydrates as 'pre-sugar sugar' because that is exactly how your body treats them. Your body turns white bread and white pasta into sugar.

Simple and refined carbohydrates are unhealthy. By simple and refined, I mean foods like white bread, white rice, pastries, cakes, cereals and biscuits. They have little nutritional value and rapidly turn into sugar in the body. In fact, white bread was one of the first 'fast foods'. Human health took a turn for the worse when we learnt how to refine our grains and make bread 'white' because we took out the fibre and the nutrients. As Michael Pollan says in his book *In Defence of Food:* 'White bread was the first fast food... [it] was the start of our love affair with simple carbohydrates. Not long after we refined rice and made it white too. And before we knew it fibreless food and simple carbohydrates were a staple in our diet.'[127]

Humans evolved over millions of years eating a diet that was low in sugar and had no refined carbohydrates. We were hunter-gatherers and existed on plants, nuts, seeds, fish and occasional meat. When primitive man did eat fruit it would have been seasonal and plucked straight off the tree - it would have been more of a bitter crab apple than the sweet Pink Lady of today. Primitive man didn't feed himself every few hours either. He would have had periods of fasting when food was scarce. Nowadays, because all kinds of foods are highly available, we enjoy an almost constant consumption of foods, especially sugar and carbs. And by now you should know where that leads...

Primitive man moved a lot more each day than we do, which would have helped to correct and mop up any excess sugar in the blood. The problem nowadays is that we eat an abundance of sugar and refined carbohydrates and we don't move enough to cope with the excess. Do this for long enough and the body won't be able to cope. Initially you will get insulin resistance and then insulin failure and then full-blown diabetes when the pancreas gets overwhelmed.

It's important to understand that there are different kinds of carbohydrates and that it's the refined (pre-sugar) ones that should be absolutely avoided. My general mantra for carbs is 'Brown is Beautiful' - so seek out whole grain carbs and colourful vegetables (these are good carbs) and that should generally keep you on the straight and narrow.

FATS

Over the years there has been much confusion about the fat in our diets. Does fat make us fat? Is saturated fat linked to heart disease? In short, there has been a lot of confusion and noise and we have been fed some bad and conflicting science. As a consequence we have demonised fats and were told to remove them from our diet. In the 1970s, we were advised to eat low fat foods and the food industry consequently removed a lot of fats from our foods. The problem is that when you remove fat it is generally replaced by something else - like sugar. So we all started eating low fat yoghurts, low fat cereals, low fat everything ... and sugar seeped into our food chain in higher and higher amounts, packaged as 'low fat' health food but actually far from healthy.

Another problem with reducing fat in our diets is that fat satiates and curbs hunger whilst sugar doesn't. When fats were reduced in our foods, we felt hungrier and, ironically, ate more. The simplistic reduction and demonisation of dietary fat in our foods has caused an epidemic of obesity and diabetes because sugar is the culprit for our obesity crisis - not fat.

Just as with carbohydrates, fat can be broken down into healthy and unhealthy fats - both can add to our waistline if eaten in significant quantities. Some fats are essential for health while others fuel inflammation and oxidative stress. It's important you know the difference between the two so you don't vindicate the wrong fats.

Trans fats

Trans fats are damaged fats and by far the worst type of fat to consume. These are the fats that raise your LDL cholesterol and cause inflammatory damage. Trans fats are cheap and have a long shelf life. They lurk in all kinds of packaged and processed foods and will often be labelled as 'partially hydrogenated oil'. Trans fats are found in many margarines, pastries, sauces, cookies, crisps and french fries. They are also used in most takeaway deep fryers. Avoid this fat if you care about your long-term health. The FDA in 2015 actually banned inflammatory trans fats which should mean that we see them disappear from our foods soon. This is a small victory for all of us and will protect our future generations.

Monounsaturated fats (MUFAs)

Monounsaturated fats are in liquid form at room temperature and can help reverse inflammation. Olive oil, avocados and many nuts (almonds and cashews) fit into this category. These are healthy fats and, in appropriate quantities, should form part of a healthy diet.

Polyunsaturated fats (PUFAs)

Polyunsaturated fats are the cause of much confusion. Some are healthy, such as the fats found in oily fish like sardines, anchovies and salmon, which give us brain- and heart-boosting omega 3. These fats are unprocessed and therefore retain their healthful qualities. Other PUFAs, like vegetable oils and margarines, are damaged during processing; they are unhealthy, high in omega 6 and can create inflammatory pathways. These should be avoided in order for us to correct our skewed omega 3 to omega 6 ratios to improve insulin resistance and cardiovascular disease (I will explain this fully later).

Saturated fats

We have almost a hundred years of research on saturated fats and we are more confused than ever! The debate has long raged around saturated fat. Saturated fats are linked to inflammation and high cholesterol, which can drive heart disease. Saturated fats are high in meat, dairy and cheese products. If you do eat these products you should choose lean cuts of meat and remove all fat from the meat.

I personally focus on natural fats derived from nuts, seeds, avocado and olives. If you do this, you manage to avoid any processed and manipulated trans fats and avoid turning your healthy fats toxic by heating and hydrogenation.

Fat is a macronutrient needed by the body. To remain healthy, we need to consume good fats. This is of critical importance to maintaining a steady state in the body and in the expulsion of toxins from the cells. Every single cell membrane in the body is made of fat (known as lipids) so fat regulates what gets in and what gets out of cells. Our bodies need fat for rebuilding cells and for hormone production. So healthy fats are good for us.

During the 1960s and 70s the food industry started using more vegetable oils. Agricultural surplus could be made into very cheap oil and the anti-saturated fat campaign of the time told everyone that because vegetable oils were derived from plants, they were the more healthful option. In fact, the rise of vegetable oil in the US and global food chain has been a public health disaster. Most vegetable oils are unhealthy (think sunflower, rapeseed and cottonseed oil) because they are commercially processed and oxidise easily. They also contain high amounts of omega 6 fats, which are pro-inflammatory and bad for human health.

We have gone from zero consumption of vegetable oils in the early 1900s to consuming it as 7-8% of our calories - making it one of the single biggest increases in any kind of food nutrient over the course of the 20th century. More than a hundred dangerous oxidation products have been found in a single piece of chicken fried in vegetable oil. Safer alternatives to vegetable oil include:

- Avocado oil - high smoke point of 270 degrees Celsius so ideal for cooking

- Coconut oil - doesn't oxidise when cooking (use expeller pressed versions to avoid the distinct coconut flavour)

- Palm oil – doesn't oxidise when cooking (seek out sustainable options)

- Cold pressed extra virgin olive oil (great for cold, non-heated dishes)

- Fats from nuts

- Fats from avocados

Let's look at omega 3 and 6 briefly.

We need to include essential fatty acids like omega 3 and omega 6 in the diet every day. They are both classed as 'essential' fatty acids because the body cannot make them. We need them in an ideal ratio of 1:1 omega 6 to omega 3. Anthropological research shows that our ancestors had omega ratios of roughly 1:1 but today most westerners have skewed ratios of up to 25:1.[128] This is staggeringly unhealthy and pro-inflammatory.

We get long-chain omega 3 fatty acids (EPA and DHA) exclusively from seafood and marine algae. The body can also synthesise EPA and DHA from the short-chain omega 3 alpha linolenic acid (ALA). ALA is found in plant foods such as flaxseeds, hempseeds, pumpkin seeds and walnuts. However, it is far easier for the body to use preformed DHA and EPA (from seafood or algae) than it is to convert it from ALA.

DHA is a major building block of the brain and is critical for optimal brain health and development at all ages and stages of life. Numerous studies and systematic reviews have shown that higher intakes of omega 3 reduce the incidence of common brain disorders such as Alzheimer's, vascular dementia and memory loss.[129] Furthermore, deficiencies in DHA have been linked to depression, suicidal tendency, addictive behaviour, reduced memory and reduced attention and learning.

Any drop in dietary intake can drastically alter brain lipids, which can affect the brain's functionality and predispose it to a number of brain disorders. Because the brain comprises a high percentage of fat, it is imperative that we nourish our brains with daily essential fatty acids. We need to do this throughout infancy and adolescence, adulthood and old age - otherwise we could face mental retardation (infancy) or brain atrophy and deterioration (maturity).

Death by Vegetable Oil

Vegetable oils include soybean, corn, safflower, sunflower, cottonseed, rapeseed oil and margarines.

Vegetable oils are chemically processed and adulterated oils that are often made with GMO's and pesticides.

Vegetables oils are found in most processed foods (salad dressings, cheeses, sauces, crackers & ready meals).

Vegetable oils contain high amounts of Omega 6.

Vegetable oils are highly unstable and inflammatory.

Vegetable fats oxidise easily.

Modern western diets are abnormally high in omega 6 fats and low in omega 3 because of our unhealthy reliance on vegetable oils. There is an abundance of omega 6 in commercially processed foods. Omega 3 and omega 6 compete for the same metabolic pathway so taking too much omega 6 means your omega 3 intake is reduced.

Omega 3 has a powerful systemic anti-inflammatory action in our bodies and is an excellent source of support for the brain, heart and skin. The only way we can correct the omega imbalance is to increase our consumption of omega 3 and reduce our consumption of omega 6. Almost everyone would benefit from this. To do this we need to avoid many of the cheap, processed foods sold in supermarkets that use vegetable oil and increase our consumption of omega 3 fats such as in oily fish.

In India, for example - a country with a high level of heart disease in urban areas - the ratio of omega 6: omega 3 fats is highly deranged at about 40:1. This, combined with a high level of smoking, accounts for India's very high rate of premature death (under age 65) from cardiovascular disease. In rural India, ratios are much healthier. This reflects the changes that occur to essential fatty acid ratios when a population starts eating processed and convenience foods instead of simple, unprocessed traditional foods.

Some studies suggest that some individuals get almost 20% of their daily calories from soybean oil alone and have a whopping intake of omega 6 that is 25 times in excess of evolutionary norms.[130] Since we now know that inflammation is pathogenic in almost all diseases, it is likely that pro-inflammatory omega 6 has contributed to the very significant rise of virtually every modern disease. It is hard to overstate the negative effects on health of too much omega 6.

Experts recommend we aim to increase our omega 3 consumption four-fold to profit from the health benefits it confers. By increasing your daily omega 3 consumption you will correct the skewed ratio and steer your body into a preferential omega 3 pathway.

One study showed that replacing corn oil and canola oil with olive oil helped participants reach a more healthful omega 6:3 ratio of 4:1 and led to a 70% decrease in total mortality.[131] Countless other studies have shown that DHA levels have now reached subclinical deficiency in many people, which is linked to increasing incidence of heart disease, inflammatory disease, mental health decline and suboptimal neurodevelopment.

DHA is likely to be the primary reason that populations where fish consumption is high are consistently healthier than populations where it is low. But nowadays fish are so contaminated with pollutants from the ocean, such as mercury, dioxins and polychlorinated biphenyls (PCBs), that they no longer offer the absolute health benefits they once did. It is important that we learn to nourish ourselves with foods that help us attain healthy fatty acid levels without adding to our disease risk burden through heavy metal contamination and pollutants. Eating wild-caught rather than farmed fish will help reduce your potential mercury and toxin exposure.

For vegans and vegetarians, it can be hard to achieve a good intake of omega 3 heathy fats because of weak conversion. Some studies suggest as little as 8% of ALA is converted to DHA.[132] This conversion is weakened even more if you are nutrient depleted or if your omega 6 consumption is high as it inhibits the conversion of ALA to DHA.

Fatty acid deficiency is often overlooked because it shares many symptoms with other conditions but as a nutrient deficiency it can have significant long-term sequalae, including brain atrophy and cognitive decline. I often recommend omega 3 supplements, especially if access to clean, non-contaminated fish is problematic. The body's need for healthy fats is so fundamental and their benefits so widespread that I tell all my patients to carefully analyse their fatty acid intake and supplement if there is any suspicion of deficiency. Studies looking at levels of contamination of fish oil supplements fortunately have shown very low levels of contaminants, certainly much lower than an equivalent serving of fish. Most tested supplements had contaminants ranging from one to six parts per billion per serving, which is far below the upper safety limit of 100 parts per billion set by the GOED[133] and significantly lower than fresh fish.

PROTEIN (ANIMAL)

Let's look at a high animal protein diet. The first thing to note is that a heavily meat-based diet often pushes plants and vegetables off the plate. By this I mean that meat eaters generally view vegetables as the 'side dish' and the meat as the 'main event'. So eating 100-200g of meat per meal soon becomes the norm, with a side serving of fries (think damaged trans fats) and a small amount of greens.

This ratio of meat to greens is unhealthy and is part of the bigger problem of portion control. Secondly, high consumption of meat poses some health risks including increased colorectal cancer. A systematic review of 21 studies and meta-analyses of 18 studies showed that consumption of processed and red meats is a risk factor for obesity, higher BMI and higher waist circumference.[134] These in turn are risk factors for higher rates of diabetes, heart disease and cancer.

High meat diets are associated with higher rates of colorectal and rectal cancer (18% increased risk) and pre-menopausal breast cancer (22%)[135]. Red meat has also been shown to raise Insulin-like Growth Factor 1 (IGF-1), an inflammatory protein linked to higher rates of most cancers. When we cook it in unhealthy ways it can also contains carcinogenic compounds such as heterocyclic amines (HCA) and polycyclic aromatic hydrocarbons (PAH) - both carcinogens. Processed meats contain toxic nitrites and all animal products contain saturated fats.

Commercially processed meat can also contain growth hormones, growth factors and copious antibiotics - none of which are healthful to humans but are used for capitalistic purposes to gain more profit from each kilogram of meat. Disturbingly, about 70-80% of the western world's antibiotics supply is used in the food chain (in animals) rather than used for treating human disease. Many factory farms that raise animals for human consumption use antibiotics to help their animals survive the inhumane and filthy living conditions which would otherwise kill them and are now the breeding grounds for superbugs.

Antibiotics are frequently used in intensive farming because the conditions are so cramped and squalid that infection spreads easily. They frequently live in their own and other animals' faeces with other animals dying and decomposing around them. The conditions for intensively farmed animals are truly appalling - and are kept away from prying eyes. Some animals have only a space the size of their body to move around in and, unsurprisingly, become distressed and depressed. The habitual squalor increases the likelihood of infections through the food chain.[136]

The antibiotics given to farmed animals are the same ones we give to humans to save lives and treat infection - penicillins, macrolides and tetracyclines. The more we use them in our food chain, the more chance we have of getting into problems with antibiotic resistance when our life might one day depend on them.

Antibiotics are used for several reasons in the food chain:

To treat infection - high output dairy cows often get mastitis
(infection of the milk ducts).

To control disease outbreak - if one animal gets ill the rest of the group will
often be given preventative antibiotics.

To prevent diseases - low level antibiotics are often given daily
in animal feed to prevent disease.

As growth promoters - this practice has been used since the 1950s. Agribusiness realised that antibiotics helped animals grow better and faster with less feed, making it a win-win situation for profit-intent farmers. Antibiotic use as growth promoters is now banned in 51 countries including the UK, although is still allowed in over half the countries of the world including the USA and Canada. Despite vast improvements in EU legislation, an EU 2012 study comparing antibiotic levels in animals and humans showed that animal anti-microbial use was higher than human.

Over-exposure to antibiotics can have terrifying consequences and the issue of antibacterial resistance is a very real threat, not only to individuals but to our entire civilisation. If antibiotics continue to be overused, both in medicine and livestock, then we face a bleak future of resistance and death from simple infections. This would mean death in childbirth, death from tuberculosis, amputations from simple things like cellulitis, death from commonplace infections like tonsillitis. Life as we know it would change. It would be an absolute disaster for human civilisation, so we really need to rein in our overuse of antibiotics.

If we act now and reduce our meat consumption, we will also be helping to stop our overdependence on antibiotics through our diets. Collectively, we should also purchase only quality, humane and pasture raised meats and vote with our forks. This would force livestock and animal farmers to stop using growth hormones, stop using antibiotics and stop feeding animals with GMO- and pesticide-laden crops that in the end only serve to poison us.

Unless meat is organic in origin it is likely to have been artificially stimulated in some form to deliver more flesh weight for commercial profit. Dead chickens are often injected with salt water to yield more weight at the checkout - sometimes up to 20%. A recent John Hopkins study showed everything from antibiotics, caffeine, acetaminophen, diphenhydramine and fluoxetine (an antidepressant) in chicken samples in the USA. Yikes...

There are other health issues with meat, aside from the increased cancer risk, increased saturated fats and increased antibiotic resistance. Fifty percent of all food-borne infections in the UK can be traced back to meat and about four out of five campylobacter infections come from contaminated UK poultry. Having been hospitalised for ten days in Australia once for campylobacteria food poisoning, I can tell you it's not fun.

In the USA the Centre for Disease Control estimates that almost 50 million food-related illnesses occur each year with 127,839 hospitalisations and over 3,000 deaths. They manage to isolate about 10 million cases to known pathogens; the other 40 million are from unknown pathogens in foods. Worrying, isn't it? Eating animal flesh and meat carries a high risk of contamination and illness and the burden from unknown pathogens is high. This is why you must be sure to cook meats well, adhere to best by dates and wash down cooking utensils appropriately.

It's worth noting also that meat-eaters are three times more likely to be obese than vegetarians, and nine times more likely than vegans. If the above reasons haven't resonated with you then it's wise to cut down your meat intake for the sake of the planet.

SEAFOOD

Seafood offers us health benefits in the form of healthy fats and omega 3. Since we can't all eat algae at the moment (algae is what the fish eat to become omega 3-rich) then it falls to fish or algal supplements to gift us our healthful omega 3. However, the problem is that most of our fish are now contaminated with toxins and our seas have been overfished.

Seafood is associated with significant contamination with heavy metals including mercury, dioxins and PCB (polychlorinated biphenyls). 90% of our total persistent organic pollutants (POPs) appear to come from eating foods of animal origin.[137] For example, dioxin is one of the nastiest pollutants in the human food chain and is thought to be responsible for 12% of cancers in the developed world. The Environmental Protection Agency estimates that up to 95% of our dioxin exposure comes from red meat, fish and dairy products.[138] Medium to larger fish at the end of the food chain can bioaccumulate toxins in their fat because they eat the smaller, more contaminated fish. And then we eat them and acquire all their bioaccumulated toxins. That is why eating from the bottom of the food chain (i.e. plant based) is safer!

The bottom line is that eating animal protein has a huge impact on our environment and carries significant blame for our current climate crisis. Eating animal protein is no longer a necessity for human survival. We can generally get all the protein that animal flesh delivers from plant sources. So, then it becomes an intellectual choice and a sustainability choice. And if you saw the brutal suffering that cattle and poultry endure before they get to your plate, I suspect most of you wouldn't actually eat meat once it was dished up. Watch the documentary *Earthlings* if you are ready to see what the animal industry is about.

The truth is that the meat, cattle and poultry industries are brutal. Animals live inhumane and cruel lives in dreadful conditions. And we all let this happen and are complicit in that brutality. The meat industry accounts for much of the damage that we are doing to this planet - experts agree that if we all reduced our meat intake we would have a chance of saving the planet. Very few people realise that making plant-based, whole food choices is one of the most impactful things we can do to save ourselves from ecological ruin.

Adopting a plant-focused diet and reducing meat consumption is a way of voting with your dollar and taking responsibility for our animal welfare and our delicate ecosystem.

DAIRY

Milk is species-specific and we are the only species that insists on drinking the milk of another species into our adulthood. Cow's milk is the perfect food for a nursing baby calf because it supports rapid growth but it is far from ideal for humans. Cow's milk contains growth factors and hormones that help turn a 40-kilo calf into a 200-kilo cow in the space of 12 months but these growth factors can be unhealthy for us.

Cow's milk was not designed for human consumption and when we insist on consuming cow's milk (even adult cows don't consume it!) we run into problems. The dairy industry has cleverly convinced us through their persistent marketing campaigns that we need milk for growth and strong bones but it is far from a natural elixir. This is 'the calcium conspiracy'. We do not need cow's milk for calcium; there is plentiful calcium in plant-based foods and in green leafy vegetables like broccoli, cabbage and okra. We don't have to rely on cow's milk for strong bones because studies on osteoporosis (a bone-thinning age-related disease) repeatedly show that countries with high milk consumption still have high rates of osteoporosis.[139]

We do not need cow's milk any more than we need dog's milk or cat's milk. And because of the growth factors and hormones in cow's milk we should probably keep our exposure to a minimum. Over 80% of us are missing the enzyme lactase that breaks down the sugar in milk (lactose). This is an evolutionary hint that our bodies are not designed to drink the milk of another species.

Furthermore, cow's milk and dairy products can be inflammatory. Dairy is one of the most inflammatory food groups that we consume - it is also one of the most common causes of food allergy. Inflammation from dairy allergens and lactose intolerance affects millions of people worldwide, causing everything from bloating, excessive wind, constipation and abdominal pain to acne, joint pain and eczema.[140] My five-year-old son (alongside many other children worldwide) is highly allergic to cow's milk. If he drinks it, within a few hours he will be engulfed by a nasty eczematous rash and have a bout of severe diarrhoea. When we remove all dairy from his diet he rapidly recovers. If you think you or your child has cow's milk allergy, go to your GP and request RAST testing for food allergens.

Casein, one of the main proteins found in dairy, is the major inflammatory culprit. In particular, the A1 beta-casein subtype (found in regular commercial milk) is particularly inflammatory. What we see in people who consume a lot of cow's milk and dairy is an increase in IGF-1 levels.[141] IGF-1 is a growth factor and a marker of systemic inflammation. Given that inflammation is pathogenic to most of the diseases that kill us it's probably a good idea to avoid it.

We know from studies that high IGF-1 from animal protein consumption can shorten the human lifespan.[142] Vegans have consistently been shown to have lower levels of IGF-1. Early exposure to cow's milk has also been implicated in juvenile or Type 1 diabetes and cow's milk cannot be digested easily by young infants. This is why your healthcare professional will always advise that infants are not fed cow's milk under the age of one.

Other issues with modern dairy are the use of antibiotics and synthetic hormones. Many industrial cows live in cramped and filthy conditions on industrial dairy farms. They are kept in a forced state of lactation to produce milk, with sore nipples and frequent bouts of mastitis (inflammation of the mammary tissue due to blocked milk ducts or infected milking machinery). Because of their close contact with other cows, low dose antibiotics are used daily in their feed to stave off the risk of mass infection. Many cows are fed corn instead of grass (their native feed) because corn is cheap and accessible and feeding corn reduces the amount of land taken up by grazing cows. Most corn nowadays is genetically modified and has been treated with pesticides.

The dairy industry is an environmental polluter and contributes significantly to greenhouse gases. Dairy operations contribute to water and soil degradation and cow manure adds toxic nitrous oxide to the environment - not to mention the huge amount of methane gas that cows produce, which is roughly 23 times more potent than carbon dioxide as a heat-trapping gas. Avoiding cow's milk is easy now that there are so many great plant-based milks.

ALCOHOL

Alcohol is listed as a known human carcinogen by the National Toxicology Program and by Cancer Research and as a definitive human breast carcinogen by the WHO.[143] The more alcohol you consume the more likely you are to develop certain types of cancer including oesophageal cancer, liver cancer, breast cancer, stomach cancer, cancers of the head and neck and colorectal cancer.[144][145]

The latest research shows that even regular light to moderate drinking can trigger cell change and increase your cancer risk. A large study that involved France, Canada and the USA showed that people who drank less than 1.5 alcoholic beverages a day accounted for less than one third of the alcohol-related cancer deaths, while those who drank more than 3 beverages a day counted for the majority of deaths.[146] Another study conducted in 2013 estimated that nearly 5,000 breast cancer deaths a year were attributable to light drinking.[147] The best thing to do is to remove the risk altogether.

Alcohol is essentially a sugar that causes inflammation, has toxic by-products and burdens the liver. We know that cancer and most other modern western diseases are caused by chronic, low grade inflammation. The best thing to do if you are concerned about your health is to cut out alcohol. The metabolites of alcohol (called acetaldehyde) are highly toxic known carcinogens. In addition to the extra cancer risk, alcohol consumption risks toxic damage to the liver and pancreas. Most wines these days are heavily contaminated with pesticides so if you do drink alcohol then choose organic, sulphite free wines and spirits.

THE BOTTOM LINE

The Global Burden of Disease Study (funded by the Bill and Melinda Gates Foundation) systematically analysed the causes of human death in our modern era. The findings were deemed of such great public health importance that they were published in the *Lancet* medical journal. The study looked at everything from processed meat consumption to fruit, vegetable, nut and seed consumption. The findings showed that eating more plant-based whole foods would save millions of lives from premature death. In particular, the study found that eating more vegetables would save 1.8 million lives, eating more fruit would save 4.9 million lives and eating more nuts and seeds would save 2.5 million lives. That's over 8 million lives per year saved by improving the number of plants in the diet.[148] Don't you want to be one of them?

The last hundred years have seen an abrupt and radical change in our relationship with food - changes that we haven't adapted to or evolved to cope with. Unless we rapidly develop some kind of superhuman system to cope with these changes, we will continue to damage our health with the foods we eat.

We need to change the way we eat and change our relationship with food. We need to start nourishing ourselves and our families with organic, whole foods that are nutritious, delicious and life-sustaining. The more of us that change our ways of eating the more demand there is for superfoods and the more available they will become. We have seen this recently with the vegan movement - vegan foods are much more widely available today than they were ten years ago. We have also seen it with the organic movement. You see - it works. We have the power to exert change. Our choices matter. Embracing a diet that is rich and diverse in vegetables, nuts, seeds and beans and low in sugar and processed foods is by far the best way to reverse the very modern problems of obesity, diabetes, heart disease and cancer.

These dietary changes are the key to our future health and are also the very foods that will help create sustainability for our beautiful planet. There is great joy to be had in aligning your personal food choices with those that will save our world.

CHAPTER 7: The Inflammatory Crisis

Even the most casual observer can see that in the space of a few decades and generations drastic increases have occurred in the numbers of food intolerances, food allergies, general allergies, inflammatory conditions and autoimmune disorders. Because it's happened so fast it's unlikely to be due to our genetics. Rather, it's highly likely that something in our diet, lifestyle and environment has made us vulnerable.

Inflammation is the natural process by which the body tries to heal itself after physical, metabolic, microbial or autoimmune insult. It can be caused by physical trauma (bites, cuts, wounds etc.), by pathogens (viruses, bacteria, fungus etc.), by chemicals (cigarette smoke, toxins etc.) or by the body getting confused and attacking itself (autoimmune). Inflammation is a vital part of the body's immune system and is necessary for our survival.

The inflammatory response starts a complex chemical pathway through which the body attempts to heal. Uncontrolled inflammation sustained over a long period of time can be harmful to the body and plays a role in almost every major disease of our time. Inside our arteries, inflammation contributes to atherosclerosis. Inflammation can trigger mitochondrial damage and DNA mutations that trigger cancer. It can cause localised joint destruction as in arthritis. And in Alzheimer's, inflammation of vulnerable brain tissue is pivotal to the pathology. So chronic inflammation matters. Metaphorically speaking, we are going up in flames.

The human immune system is incredibly complex. The inflammatory system has adaptive capacity but once you stress it out repeatedly (as we do in our modern lives) it can become faulty and go into overdrive or become suppressed, causing vulnerability to infections and cancer. Neither a revved up immune system or a flaccid, underactive immune system are good for your health.

So why are we experiencing such profound issues with allergy, inflammation and immune problems? Well, we don't yet know *entirely* but experts think the problems stem from changes in the way we eat and live. What we do know so far is that it's not just one thing causing the problem but a complex interplay of many factors.

The hygiene hypothesis suggests that our sanitary modern lives, where we are no longer in close contact with the earth and nature, means we are 'too clean' and our immune systems haven't sufficiently developed. Our declining gut health is also thought to be responsible for our modern immune problems because the microbes in our gut drive and steer our immunity. Another theory is that as we pollute our bodies with our dreadful diet the toxic load cannot be managed. Another factor could be our over-reliance on delivery methods like Caesarean sections, where infants miss out on important bacterial inoculation from their mother's birth canal. We have also introduced a lot of grains into our diet in recent history. Many people are sensitive to these grains, such as gluten, and suffer an immune response if they eat them. In reality, it's likely a combination of all these things that tips us over the edge.

The number of people suffering from diseases caused by allergies or an imbalanced immune system is increasing[149] and is at an all-time global high. The transformation of previously rare allergies and immune conditions into common health problems suggests we have a serious problem on our hands. Food allergies, for example, have skyrocketed in the last 50 years. Peanut allergies have doubled in the western world and food allergies now affect up to 10% of children and up to 5% of the adult population.[150] Food allergies can be very serious and can kill. One in fifteen children currently have an intolerance to one type of food or more. Since 1990, admissions into hospital in the UK for food allergies have increased by 500%, admissions for anaphylaxis have increased by 700% and angio-oedema admissions have increased by 40%. In addition, prescriptions written by doctors for allergy medicines (e.g. anti-histamines and steroids) have significantly increased.[151]

Asthma was relatively rare of at the beginning of the 20th century but nowadays is considered 'common' because it affects over 150 million people worldwide. One in thirty children wouldn't be able to breathe without the help of asthma drugs. Figures from the World Allergy Organisation reveal the global prevalence of asthma has increased by an astounding 50% every decade for the past 40 years.[152] Allergic rhinitis (hay fever) and eczema have trebled in the last three decades, with GP consultations increasing by 260% and 150% respectively.[153]

Autism wasn't even a disorder at the turn of the last century and was only given a name in 1943 when it was described for the first time. Official medical records for autism only really start in the millennium and even back then it was half as common as it is now. Nowadays 1 in every 68 children have a diagnosis of autism or autistic spectrum disorder. Coeliac disease (an auto-immune response to wheat) has doubled in some parts of the world compared to rates reported in the 1950s. And Multiple Sclerosis (MS) affects more people than ever - favouring the western, caucasian populations - and is growing by 2.5% per year.

These conditions are considered so normal and standard nowadays that many people don't even realise they are 'new'. Clearly something is causing our bodies to misinterpret its external and internal threat level, interfering with its basic immune and defence tasks causing system dysfunction. It's not rocket science - something serious is going on. What we need to know is what is causing our body's immune systems to overreact and misfire? It may well be there is a common thread connecting all of these 'new' problems. Could chronic inflammation, driven by poor microbial health and poor nutritional intake, be driving us into new and catastrophic realms of illness? Could obesity, Crohn's, autism, Type 1 diabetes, MS, anxiety, IBS, asthma and eczema all have a common gut and food related cause? Autistic patients struggle with loose stools, Irritable Bowel Syndrome and depression are linked and obesity has its origins in the food that passes through the gut. Although the gut and the immune system have always seemed unrelated and somehow separate, modern science has now connected the two in very powerful ways.

Most people think of their immune system as lymph nodes and white blood cells but 80% of the body's immune cells actually reside in the gut. And our gut wall is one of the most important immune barriers defending us from outside invaders. Although it's on the inside of the body, the gut wall is a meeting place where the outside and inside worlds cross over and meet. Only a couple of cell layers separate the outside of the gut wall from the blood and circulatory system inside. So the defence and quarantine of invaders in the gut wall needs to be extremely robust.

The gut wall is an incredibly important barrier to outside pathogens, chemicals and toxins. The modern gut wall has to contend with a constant barrage of pathogens, toxins, chemicals, pesticides, heavy metals, processed foods, alcohol and much much more. Our gut steers our immunity and it may well be that these 'new' diseases have their origins in our habits that overwhelm the gut. We are 10% human and 90% bacterial. Our gut harbours over 100 trillion microbes who aren't just hitching a ride but have co-evolved with us over millions of years and have helped form and shape us. Without them we cannot exist. All of a sudden it doesn't seem so far-fetched to think that some of this immune excitation might be to do with our food, our guts and their constant interaction with the immune system.

"We know Roundup, the commercial name of glyphosate-based herbicide, contains many other chemicals, which, when mixed together, are a thousand times more toxic than glyphosate on its own." Dr Robin Mesnage, Kings College London

Professor Aaron Lerner from Carmel Medical Centre in Israel has led some important studies[154] that suggest that loss or impairment of tight junctions in the epithelial part of the gut lining may be a cause of the increasing auto-immunity we are seeing. Tight junctions are like check points in the gut wall that protect the entry of foreign macromolecules and invaders. Think of them like Border Control. Tight junctions are critical for the maintenance of equilibrium and balance of the immune response. Damage to them means the gut wall is leaky and permeable to bacteria, toxins, allergens and carcinogens. Tight junction dysfunction is at the heart of new research into autoimmunity and processed, industrialised foods seem to weaken the tight junctions. Researchers have found that common food additives such as 'glucose, salt, emulsifiers (fat solvents), gluten, microbial enzyme transglutaminase and organic solvents' all weaken the tight junctions in the gut.[155] The food industry, especially the additive market, is poorly regulated so avoidance of processed foods is strongly advised if you suffer from auto-immune or allergic disease. Whilst more studies need to be undertaken, we see once again a bigger (and scarier) price tag than previously thought to time-saving and convenience foods. The solution is to eat organic, whole foods and to heal the gut.

"

If you don't recognise
an ingredient your
body won't either

"

An unhealthy diet destroys us from the inside out and stresses the body in numerous ways. When we eat a diet high in chemicals, toxins, damaged fats, salt, sugar and animal proteins (as in the typical western diet), we are directly feeding the body's inflammatory overdrive. The immune system becomes activated when it detects something foreign. Think of the immune system as the body's internal army - ready to take action to prevent threat from foreign bacteria, chemicals, toxins and pathogens. This immune reaction is necessary and protects us on a daily basis from the hazards of our environment. But sometimes the immune system stays switched on even though the threat has been dealt with - this causes harmful internal inflammation.

Many modern diseases such as arthritis, cancer, heart disease, auto-immune disease and Alzheimer's have been linked to a chronic internal inflammatory process.

The gut, brain and body cannot function normally with continual exposure to toxins, chemicals, metabolic waste and free radicals. If our exposure to toxins outstrips our ability to detoxify then we end up storing harmful toxins in our bodies, which can result in profound and permanent damage to our DNA. These small, systematic, daily cellular insults are resulting in an inflammatory crisis of unknown proportions.

Many health educators now feel that the best way to calm excessive inflammation and help the body out of this faulty over-firing is to eat an abundance of anti-inflammatory and gut-supporting foods that allow the body to heal and detoxify.

Inflammatory Insults

Elevated blood sugars → inflammation in the blood stream

Elevated blood sugars → glycation (sugar damages molecules)

Processed and synthetic foods → reduction in beneficial bacteria

Altered gut microbiome → tight junction dysfunction

Altered gut microbe → altered nutrient absorption and deficiencies

Altered gut microbiome → leaky gut - toxins seep into the blood stream

Altered gut microbiome → disrupted metabolic homeostasis

Altered gut microbiome → impaired blood-brain barrier ('leaky brain')

Poor gut bacteria → reduced levels of neurotransmitter e.g. serotonin, GABA, BDNF

Excess inflammatory foods e.g. detrimental omega 6 fats → stirs up further inflammation

Exposure to environmental toxins → heightened immune response

Reduced dietary fibre → prolonged transit time → toxin accumulation

Chemical and toxin exposure → toxic metabolites → mitochondrial damage, DNA damage, chronic inflammation

Excess body weight → stimulates inflammatory pathways

We make over 2,000 immune cells every second. If this process becomes dysfunctional it can have huge ramifications for your overall health. The good news is that the foods that help support the immune system are the same foods that keep us healthy in all the other ways - fermented foods, berries, vegetables, nuts, seeds and beans. Mother Nature is superbly clever and manages to give us foods that are disease and inflammation fighting - they are nature's way of protecting us. The gradual loss of these foods from the modern diet and their replacement with industrialised, processed foods is one of the underlying reasons we have become so chronically ill. The foods that help protect us against heart disease, diabetes and cancer are the same foods that help us avoid excessive inflammation and immune response. The reason for this is that the common denominator tying all these diseases together is inflammation.

By now you should know that inflammation always causes collateral damage, the extent of which might not be obvious until you succumb to some serious pathology. Inflammation, oxidative stress and the accumulation of toxic metabolites including free radicals becomes the cellular norm in people frequently consuming processed foods.[156] The more fast foods and convenience foods you eat, the more your toxic load increases and the more you impair your body's ability to function optimally and inhibit inflammation. It's also worth noting that obesity causes its own inflammation - so it's a lose-lose situation to be overweight.

It is thought that we have created and added in excess of 14,000 chemicals into the human food chain in recent years. Many are not listed on food labels, are not regulated and have never been human-approved or tested. We likely eat about 3kg of untested chemicals directly from our foods each year - more if you eat a lot of processed foods. And that doesn't include the environmental toxins that leak into the food chain from plastics, pesticides, herbicides and chemical contaminants. Add to this our over-reliance on potent medications that have significant toxic potential and it's easy to see why most of us are losing the chemical battle. The solution is to eat real foods and minimise our toxin and chemical exposure as much as possible.

Inflammatory Toxins in Food

• • • • • • • • • • • • • • • • • • •

Cow's Milk - antibiotics, bovine growth hormone, A1 beta casein.

High fructose corn syrup - high blood sugars, accelerated heart disease, raised cholesterol & triglycerides, increased blood clotting, an accelerator of cellular ageing.

Hydrogenated fats - diabetes, cardio-metabolic syndrome, heart disease and cancer.

Emulsifiers - used to give texture and body in foods. Emulsifiers are known to effect gut health by reducing beneficial bacteria.

Heterocylic amines - formed when cooking meat and fish at high temperatures and linked to inflammation and colon cancers.

Polycyclic aromatic hydrocarbons - meat cooked at high temperatures, linked to colon cancer.

Lipid peroxides - meat cooked at high temperatures e.g. frying, grilling and barbecuing.

Nitrates & nitrites - used as preservers in processed meats, known to be carcinogenic and linked to colon & pancreatic cancers.

Theobromine - found in chocolate, soft drinks, baked goods - in animal studies it has been liked to problems with endocrine and reproductive development.

Mercury - found in food colour additives like Yellow 5, Yellow 6 and also in high fructose corn syrup, farmed fish & many types of shellfish. Can harm unborn babies and retard neuro-development.

Cadmium - often found in rice (absorbed from the environment) and linked to cancer, heart disease, diabetes and kidney disease.

Lead - found in unfiltered water supplies. Can cause lead poisoning.

Aluminium - eg. sodium aluminium phosphate (E541) and sodium aluminium sulphate are used as food stabilisers. Aluminium can also seep out of cookware. Aluminium has been linked to toxicity and Alzheimers.

Dioxins - bioaccumulate in the fat of animal protein, many seafoods are highly contaminated. Linked to cancer, can interfere with hormones and damage the immune system.

Sodium benzoate - often added to milk & meats, can inhibit digestive enzymes & can cause headaches, stomach upset, asthma & hyperactivity.

Sodium phosphate or phosphoric acid - Is added to most fast foods and deli meats, baked goods, canned foods, microwave meals etc to thicken and stabilise food. Should be avoided by people with kidney disease and cardiovascular disease.

Food colourings - Red 40 and Red No 3 are both derived from petroleum and are linked to hyperactivity in children and cancer in animals.

Artificial sweeteners eg aspartame - chemicals linked to obesity, migraine, tachycardia, joint pain, depression, memory loss, seizures & brain damage.

Herbicides (eg. glyphosate) - Roundup is the commonest herbicide used in agrochemical farming worldwide. It is linked to human cancers but has not been banned. Sadly the EU just renewed its 5 year license. Monsanto (USA biggest producer of Roundup which is glyphosate) was successfully sued in 2018 for $289m for causing non Hodgkins lymphoma. This toxic weed killer is found in most foods in the USA according to FDA testing.

CHAPTER 8: The Gut Crisis

"All disease begins in the gut."

Hippocrates

GUT HEALTH AND THE MICROBIOME

The human digestive tract is teeming with trillions of bacteria, fungi and other micro-organisms. In fact, bacterial cells far outnumber human cells in the body by about ten to one and it is thought that for every human gene there are in the region of 360 microbial ones.[157] These incredibly diverse micro-organisms, with all their collective genetic material, make up what we call 'the microbiome'. The microbiome is responsible for human health because it helps us digest our food, prevents unfriendly bacteria from taking up residence in the gut, and works to keep the gut balanced, healthy and free from toxic build-up.[158] Micro-organisms also play another pivotal role - the by-products of their metabolism help to control inflammation as well as the body's immune response. The profound (and relatively recent) connection between the gut, our immune and inflammatory systems is causing huge ripples in the health sector because finally we are starting to understand the missing pieces of the puzzle that underpins human health.

We have more than 100 trillion microbes inside us - that's more bugs in one body than humans have ever inhabited this Earth. These essential microbes help guide, steer, mingle, feed and even 'hijack' our own genetic material. Whilst our genome has remained relatively stable in the last hundred or so years our microbiome has changed radically.[159] With depletions in the diversity of our gut microbiome comes depleted health. And I will tell you why…

In the last 15 years we have learnt significant amounts about the importance of the microbiome and how its dysfunction can lead to a huge array of human illnesses. From the knowledge we have gained we know that the good, protective bacteria in our gut need to outnumber (or at least balance) the bad and harmful bacteria otherwise disorder, dysfunction and disease ensue. Abundant and diverse gut micro-organisms are pivotal to every conceivable aspect of our health and longevity.

"

10%Human
90%Microbe

"

Micro-organisms have inhabited this planet for millions of years and over those millions of years we have developed a symbiotic and beneficial relationship with them, such that our life now depends on them as well as vice versa. Bugs are part of our natural flora and are everywhere from our skin to our ears, nose, mouth, anus and genitalia. As we move from the mouth, to the stomach, to the small and then large intestines, the number of bugs grows exponentially. Each environment has its own separate and unique micro-organism population which can be altered by our diet, lifestyle and environment. No bugs are more important than the ones that inhabit our digestive tract and gut. It is these organisms that are most closely connected to our health - or the loss of it.

The very first exposure we get to micro-organisms is when we leave the protected, sterile environment of the womb during the process of childbirth. Passage through the mother's birth canal is one of the first (and most important) exposures that an infant gets to micro-organisms. Natural vaginal childbirth allows the mother to pass on trillions of beneficial bacteria to her baby - one of the most important events that determines the later state of microbial diversity, and incidentally the later state of health. Some experts suggest that the 'set point for inflammation may be an individual's method of birth'[160] because a number of important studies have now shown that those individuals who do not pass through their mother's birth canal and are instead born by Caesarean section miss out on this vital inoculation.

With UK Caesarean section rates nearing 25% (and up to 50% in places like Brazil and China), this poses a potential public health threat.[161] Altering the way women give birth may essentially change humanity at an evolutionary level through its impact on the microbiome. A huge proportion of our children are now missing out on the important gut bacteria that are needed for the provision of health and immune resilience for the rest of their lives. Studies have shown that babies born vaginally have many more disease-preventing beneficial microbes, such as Lactobacillus and Bifidobacterium, than their Caesarean-born counterparts.[162] This puts them at a significant advantage.

Studies also link a huge variety of modern diseases and disorders to Caesarean delivery, including increased allergy, autoimmunity, cancer, autism, coeliac, obesity and Type 1 diabetes.[163] Do not despair if this is you or if this is the way your child was born. There are many ways to reinoculate and repopulate the gut with beneficial bacteria.

Simple adjustments to what you eat and the way you live can repopulate the gut to such an extent that a C-section delivery becomes less relevant. By the end of this chapter you will be familiar with measures you can take to superboost your gut health and in the recipe section at the end of this book there are lots of wonderful gut-boosting recipes for you to enjoy.

I myself was born by Caesarean section, as were my three children. I don't let it worry me but I am glad that I understand the significance of this and know how to nurture a healthy biome. I also had nine months of quadruple antibiotic therapy when I had a shock diagnosis of advanced Pulmonary Tuberculosis aged 25 whilst in medical school. The extensive TB antibiotic regime undoubtedly saved my life but it also totally annihilated my beneficial gut bacteria, which took years to restore. Studies have shown that virtually everyone born after 1950 will have a deranged microbiome. It's just the nature of modern life. Modern western living creates an extremely hostile environment for our good bugs. For those who missed out on gaining our mother's beneficial bacteria during birth or for those who have had extensive antibiotics (like me) we just have to be extra diligent.

C-sections, formula feeding and antibiotic use in infants have all significantly increased in recent years and are linked to poor adult gut health and immunity. Diabetes has increased 700%,[164] autism twenty-fold [165] and obesity has doubled since the 1980s. The evidence seems to be mounting to show that the method of your birth affects your early microbiome, which in turns affects later microbiome diversity, which drives almost every aspect of your health. Epigenetics is one of the most exciting and dynamic areas of medical research. It looks at how our environment influences our gene expression. From the day we are born until the day we die our environment, our diets and our lifestyles are influencing our genes. The foods we choose and the lives we live play a huge role in determining our disease risk and ultimately dictate how long <u>and</u> how well we live.

So to some extent the foundation of your microbiome is laid down in the first few days of life. The first few years of infancy are particularly important because as you grow you acquire more bacteria from the environment - both good and bad. The idea is that the beneficial ones like Lactobacillus and Bifidobacterium cancel out the effects of the bad ones like Staphylococcus and Streptococcus.

Our membranes provide them with food and vital nutrients whilst they help us to digest our food, manufacture vitamins (vitamins B1, B7, B9, B12, vitamin K), fight pathogens and support neuro-chemical production. If things tip in the wrong direction and the bad bacteria overgrow (dysbiosis) then your health can become compromised through a complex pathway of inflammation and immune deficiency.

Interesting studies are now appearing regarding obesity and the microbiome. Obese people have been found to have less diverse gut bacteria than people of normal weight, likely due to the ingestion of bug-depleting processed foods, fats, excess sugars, carbs and even alcohol. Identical twin studies have shown that when bugs are transplanted from an overweight identical twin into lean mice the mice get 17% fatter than the mice who are inoculated with bacteria from a lean twin.[166] Studies like this are starting to help us understand the complex pathway to weight gain and obesity. It may well be that obesity is a combination of chronic overeating, metabolic disruption, genetic tendency AND microbiome imbalance. The simple calories in and calories out model may soon be obsolete and future weight loss programmes may need to include probiotics as well as exercise and dietary changes.

We have also learnt in recent years that some micro-organisms are able to draw more calories from the foods we eat than others, which is clearly unfavourable in the current climate of recreational overeating. In 2006, a US research group showed that obese people have nearly 20% more Firmicutes bacteria (*Lactobacillus, Clostridium, Enterococcus*) than normal weight people. Firmicutes are known to hijack our metabolism and try to help us retain and extract more calories from our foods. Whilst this may have been beneficial and advantageous for our primitive ancestors, who went through regular periods of food shortage, it is not helpful for us now because we live in a world of food glut. The same study found that obese people have 90% less of the Bacteroidetes strains - these beneficial bacteria specialise in breaking down plant fibres and starches. Bacteroidetes and Firmicutes make up 90% of our gut bacterial population[167] and the ratio of the two (F:B) are seen as obesity biomarkers. The studies suggest that if you have more Firmicutes then you are more likely to be or become overweight and if you have more Bacteroidetes (like populations in Africa and rural Asia) then you are more likely to maintain a healthy weight and be slim. Clearly it would be advantageous to increase the Bacteroidetes population if you are overweight.

Of course, this then begs the question: has antibiotic overuse partly exacerbated the problem of obesity in modern society through depletion of beneficial weight-maintaining bacteria? We know that when lab mice receive low dose antibiotics, they suffer 15% more increased body fat than mice that aren't fed antibiotics. Given that about 80% of the world's antibiotics end up feeding livestock[168] (useful because they promote growth and weight), if you are looking to lose weight it's an idea to reduce animal-based foods like meat, poultry and dairy because those very antibiotics return to haunt you through the foods you eat. So, remember this - if antibiotics are used to fatten livestock, they are likely to also fatten you![169] Yet another reason to cut down meat or at the very least seek out organic meats to avoid microbial damage.

Don't fret if any of the above information applies to you. You can easily tweak and boost your microbiome to correct bacterial deficiencies. We can do this effectively and simply by adjusting our diets and lifestyles. Just increasing your intake of dietary fibre and eating more probiotic foods can drastically improve your Firmicutes to Bacteroidetes ratio[170] which will in turn improve your chances of weight loss, reduced blood sugar, improved mood and reduced inflammation. Worth trying, don't you think?

Fibre is found in lots of plant-based whole foods like fruits, vegetables and beans. Fibre is only partially digested so once it gets all the way down to your colon or large intestine it feeds your good bugs, which, in turn, feed you back. The body is unbelievably clever - this symbiotic relationship is incredibly important. It's very much a case of feed them well and they will feed you well.

If you want to really boost your gut health, then add both fibre and 'super-fibre' to your diet. Super-fibrous foods contain Fructo-oligosaccharides (FOS) and Inulin. These are found in raw asparagus, dandelions, Jerusalem artichokes, garlic, leeks and onions. Another type of super-fibre is Galacto-oligosaccharides (GOS), found in the superfoods broccoli, Brussels sprouts, kale, cabbage and collard greens. Yet another reason why greens are the healthiest food on the planet! In the wise words of Jeff Leach, founder of the Human Food Project: 'Increasing the diversity and quantity of whole plants [in your diet] will be a big help. Fibre from veggies is enough - it's all we've had through human evolution. Your colon is a bioreactor and the bacteria are the workers.'

KNOW YOUR ENEMY

Exposure to certain chemicals, pesticides, medicines and foods can adversely affect your intestinal microbes. Medicines like antibiotics, the pill, NSAIDs (e.g. ibuprofen, neurofen) and acid blockers like omeprazole all deplete your good bacteria. Antibiotics kill both good and bad bacteria so they decimate the general bacterial population and it can take months to years to recover and regain a healthy balance. Antibiotic overuse has significant implications for our collective gut health (and waistline!), so we need to exercise prudence in their use. Chlorine in water, alcohol, chronic stress and exposure to pesticides can also harm our beneficial bacteria. Filter your water, reduce your alcohol intake and eat organic to improve your gut's functionality. Pesticides are designed to kill bugs so it's no wonder they destroy our gut bacteria. They are also extremely toxic to your mitochondria, the powerhouses of your cells and the place where most cancers start.

Lack of gut-boosting micronutrients like fibre alters the microbiome diversity because bacteria require foods like fibre for their fuel. That is why fibre is called a 'prebiotic'. Prebiotic is a term used to describe foods that feed the good bacteria in our gut. They in turn control what nutrients we absorb from our diet and what nutrients we manufacture. Remember from Chapter Two that Brits eat woeful amounts of fibre, averaging only 18g a day rather than the recommended 30g. It's no wonder our microbiome is struggling. It certainly pays dividends to keep your microbes happy. Eating more fibre will not only boost your biome but also reduce your risk of digestive cancers.

Stress negatively affects the microbiome and impacts the ability of the biome to maintain its harmony. Stress stimulates elevations in the hormone cortisol (the stress hormone) which directly depletes protective bacteria. Cortisol also increases permeability of the gut wall, meaning toxins from our food and drink can unintentionally seep through the intestinal wall and get into the blood stream causing low grade inflammation. This movement of toxins through the weakened gut wall is called Leaky Gut. Stress and leaky gut are a toxic combination.

*"When you take antibiotics, you are doing to your body
what the farmer does when he sprays his fields with pesticides."
Geoffrey Cannon author, Superbug*

I like to think of the gut as a garden where you don't want your weeds to overgrow. Getting the balance right between the good and bad bacteria can be challenging in a modern world but the importance of doing this cannot be underestimated. Studies show that if you were born post 1950s then it's likely your gut balance is disturbed. This is because we live in an age of excess antibiotics, stress, alcohol, chemicals, medicines, sugar, artificial hormones and processed foods. All of these have negatively affected our collective gut bacteria and had an adverse outcome for our health. Modern western living starves our microbial self.

Signs of a disturbed microbiome are bloating, wind, abdominal discomfort, constipation, sluggishness and general malaise. In terms of how gut dysfunction affects the rest of the body, these kinds of symptoms may be the warning signs that other more serious problems might be brewing.

The reason you don't want to overlook the state of your gut health is because it drives everything: your immunity, detoxification, nutrient absorption, mood, libido, metabolism and brain health.

Gut dysfunction (or dysbiosis) is now thought to be related to all the following conditions:

Food allergies & sensitivities	Insomnia and sleep disorders	Small bowel overgrowth	Irritable bowel syndrome (IBS)
Joint pain and arthritis	Headaches/ migraine	Constipation/ diarrhoea	Halitosis (bad breath)
Leaky gut	Alzheimer's	Coeliac disease	Gum disease
Candidiasis	ADHD	Obesity	Dental problems
Chronic fatigue	Autism	Diabetes	Mood disorders e.g. depression and anxiety
Rosacea	Eczema	Acne	

Leaky Gut

When I was in medical school over 20 years ago, we learnt very little about nutrition, nothing about the microbiome and the term 'leaky gut' didn't even exist. Most doctors out there practise with little knowledge or understanding of these two latter issues. However, it's almost impossible now to ignore their importance.

Leaky gut is where the intestinal lining's tight junctions, which hold together the cells of the wall, become weakened and more permeable.[171] What this means is there is a failure of the normal intestinal barriers that stop foods, toxins, pesticides, hormones and unwanted pathogens[172] from seeping into the body through the gut wall and into the blood stream.[173] It's a bit like a security guard falling asleep at your front door and robbers sneaking in.

Normally a healthy gut wall will stop unwanted diffusion of foods and toxins into the blood and lymphatic system but in many people cumulative changes in the microbial ecosystems and accumulation of chemical toxins can severely compromise the intestinal wall. Once they seep through, these materials act as toxins and send signals that excite the immune system to mount a response.

If we bombard our body with more toxins than we can eliminate then we will store toxins, which damages cells and stimulates a widespread immune response that can penetrate even the blood brain barrier.[174] For this reason, it's important that we adopt a diet that won't threaten or harm our gut wall. Eating gut-healing foods will help prevent leaky gut. Gut boosting measures include avoiding gluten if you are sensitive to it (it's a relatively new addition to our diet), avoiding processed foods, eating organic, increasing fibre intake, reducing alcohol, reducing antibiotics, avoiding unnecessary medications and reducing stress.

If you are worried about leaky gut then speak to your doctor. A test (known as the Lactulose and Mannitol Test) can be performed to investigate your intestinal permeability by checking the levels of two sugars in your urine. You can also check the health status of your microbial population with stool tests from your doctor.

Immunity

80% of the body's immune tissue is found in the digestive tract. The gut is a huge hub of immune cell activity and the place of interaction between our symbiotic microorganisms and our complex immune system. I will save you the heavy science but the 'crosstalk' between these two systems may well hold the answers to many of our modern diseases. Gut microbiota help to regulate immune homeostasis - providing a fine balance between eliminating invading pathogens and toxins and maintaining health.

A huge number of studies are currently being conducted in this area to try to pinpoint and better understand the role of gut health in human immunity. These studies often involve using germ free (sterile) animals and manipulating their microbiota with either antibiotics or reconstitution (inoculation) of the normal microbiome.

Depression and mood

Diagnoses of depression and anxiety are soaring. The WHO estimates that depression now affects more than 350 million people globally and is the leading cause of disability worldwide. WHO predicts that by 2020, depression will become the costliest disease to treat. Prescriptions for antidepressants have skyrocketed in the western world - 64.7 million items of antidepressants were prescribed in the UK in 2017, up from 31 million in 2006 (NHS Digital).

The gut is often referred to as our second brain. Depression and anxiety are strongly linked to disruption in gut microbiota, and gut and brain health are intimately connected. The communication between the gut and the brain is called the gut-brain axis and occurs through both physical and biochemical pathways. The gut contains over 500 million neurons that are connected to the brain through the nervous system, the biggest connection of all being the vagus nerve, which sends signals in both directions.

As well as the physical connections to our brain through nerves, the gut is connected to the brain through chemicals called neurotransmitters. Interestingly, a very large number of chemical neurotransmitters are made in the gut rather than the brain, which is why gut health is so vitally connected to brain health. For example, 80% of serotonin (the brain's 'happy' hormone) is made in the gut,[175] not the brain, and a significant proportion of the anxiety-controlling neurotransmitter GABA (gamma-aminobutyric acid) is produced in the gut too. Gut microbes also produce short chain fatty acids such as butyrate, propionate and acetate by digesting dietary fibre. Butyrate is important for maintaining the blood brain barrier which protects seepage of toxins into the brain known as 'Leaky Brain'. When the gut biome is disturbed and disordered it can cause too much production of LPS (Lipopolysaccharide), an inflammatory neurotoxin. LPS is implicated in depression, dementia and schizophrenia.[176] So you can see how connected these two organs are.

What this means is that what we eat has a remarkable impact on the brain's functionality and mood. At the end of the day, humans cannot survive without these colonies of bugs. Although miniscule in size, invisible to the naked eye and comprised of only one cell, their power is enormous. Micro-organisms have predated us by millions of years and will most probably survive the end of the human era too.

The good news is that there is a lot we can do to boost and support the microbiome and it all starts with - you guessed it - diet and lifestyle. Through a few simple changes we can go about repopulating our guts with beneficial bacteria. The Americans call this 're-florestation' - a term I simply love!

If, like me, you were born by C-section, or were formula-fed as an infant, or have had lots of antibiotic exposure (also me), then it's especially important that you repopulate your gut bacteria. How long you have on this earth most likely depends on it - the effort you make now will buy you time later. The great thing is that the superfoods you need to empower and enhance your gut are absolutely delicious and widely available. At times when your access to fresh foods is severely restricted (e.g. if you are travelling) then get in the habit of taking a good probiotic supplement.

PREBIOTIC FOODS THAT FEED YOUR BENEFICIAL BACTERIA	PROBIOTIC FOODS THAT REPOPULATE THE BENEFICIAL BACTERIAL
Raw Jerusalem artichoke Raw asparagus Dandelion Jerusalem artichoke Raw garlic Raw leek Raw and cooked onion Broccoli Brussels sprouts Cabbage Collard greens Kale	Kimchi (one of the best probiotic foods) Live cultured yoghurt (or coconut yoghurt for vegans). Pasteurisation kills off the good bacteria, so it needs to be live or unpasteurised. Miso Kefir (or coconut kefir for vegans) Sauerkraut (fermented cabbage) Apple cider vinegar Pickled vegetables (look for unpasteurised pickled foods in brine, not vinegar) Kombucha (fermented black tea) Tempeh (fermented soya beans - a complete protein)

GUT HEALTH GUIDELINES

Lower your calorie intake. Lower intake of calories prolongs life and reduces ageing through reduced oxidative stress, improved blood sugar control and improved beneficial gut organisms.[177]

Avoid sugar. Sugar fuels unwanted bacteria and increases the risk of leaky gut, mitochondrial damage, insulin resistance and immune compromise.

Avoid alcohol. It kills the good bacteria and is full of empty calories, sugar and toxic metabolites with little nutritional value.

Eat high fibre prebiotic foods e.g. nuts, seeds, whole grains, melon, pears, asparagus, onions, leeks, Brussels sprouts, sweetcorn, carrots, broccoli and leafy green vegetables. They feed the good bacteria and modulate stress hormones positively.[178]

Consume more fermented foods. Humans have eaten fermented foods for thousands of years and studies have shown that fermented foods positively modulate brain activity through improvements in the microbiome.[179] Fermented foods have been virtually lost in the modern western diet. Their benefits are enormous so let's change that. Eat more kimchi, miso, natto, tempeh, kefir and live yoghurt.

Consume polyphenols e.g. green tea, cocoa, coffee, olive oil. They improve beneficial bacteria, improve cognitive capacity[180] and reduce oxidative stress. Polyphenols slow down the cellular ageing process. Black and green tea have been shown to increase Bifidobacterial numbers and green tea has the added benefit of crowding out harmful Clostridial bacterial species.[181]

Consume tryptophan-rich foods. Tryptophan is an amino acid that is converted into the mood-boosting neurotransmitter serotonin. Tryptophan-rich foods include chia seeds, oats, tofu, dried dates, chickpeas, lentils, beans, spirulina, sunflower seeds and peanuts. For non-vegetarians, eggs, fish and poultry also contain tryptophan.

Swap unhealthy fats to healthy fats in the form of nuts, seeds, avocados, olives and coconut oil.

Increase omega 3 intake and reduce omega 6. Studies have shown that omega 3 can increase good bacteria in the gut. Eat wild oily fish or take algal supplements.[182] [183]

Prioritise sleep. Sleep is a super nutrient and is needed for the body and brain to heal and repair. Good quality sleep supports a healthy gut.

Filter your water. Filtering tap water removes pesticides, pharmaceutical residue and chlorine. Chlorine kills the good bacteria in your gut. Pesticides like Roundup are widespread in our foods and environment. They are known to negatively impact microbial diversity.

Avoid unnecessary medications. Aspirin, ibuprofen, the pill, omeprazole, antibiotics and many other medicines harm gut bacteria. Avoid taking them where possible. If you take a course of antibiotics increase your intake of gut healthy foods and take a probiotic supplement simultaneously and for a month afterwards.

Consider a daily probiotic supplement - look for lots of different strains and a high CFU count, ideally 10-20 billion.

Reduce and manage your stress. Stress reduces gut health and has a whole host of other negative health effects. Most notably it causes chronic, low grade systemic inflammation that is central to the pathology of most western diseases.

Exercise 4-5 times per week. Bugs need exercise too. They thrive when we exercise regularly.

L-glutamine is an amino acid that is particularly helpful at healing the gut wall. In cases of 'leaky gut' driven inflammation glutamine is of phenomenal benefit. It is best taken at night, when the gut rests, and in cold water, as heat can potentially destroy it. It nourishes, rebuilds and repairs the small intestine and helps reduce gut permeability and leakage of food and toxins into the blood. Digestive enzymes and probiotics can also help calm intestinally-driven inflammation. The French routinely give probiotics with antibiotics, as do other populations around the world. If your doctor ever gives you antibiotics then take it upon yourself to increase your intake of the gut-friendly superfoods like fibre, sauerkraut, miso and kimchi AND take a high calibre probiotic supplement for the duration of your antibiotic course and for at least four weeks afterwards.

For a great quick reference chart on a huge variety of probiotic benefits based on evidence from clinical trials, see www.usprobioticguide.com.[270]

Here is a quick summary that you may find helpful for specific strains of bugs. It can help guide your choice of probiotic supplement.

Lactobacillus acidophilus helps boost the immune system, curbs candida, helps maintain cholesterol levels and manufactures lactase and vitamin K. Lactobacillus acidophilus is also evidenced for eczema/allergy in children and for treating C Difficile infections.

Lactobacillus brevis boosts cellular immunity and BDNF, the vital brain growth hormone. It also crowds out bad gut pathogens and enhances killer T-cell medicated immunity.

Bifidobacterium longum is one of the first bugs to colonise us at birth and C-section babies like me may miss out on its protective benefits. It is readily available in supplements. Bifidobacterium longum helps improve lactose tolerance and reduces the incidence of food allergies, IBS and diarrhoeal illness. Bifidobacterium longum can also reduce anxiety through its impact on intestinal neurotransmitter production and is evidenced to reduce the damaging effects of oxidation. Other studies have suggested it may play a role in the suppression of cancerous tumours, but more studies need to be completed to confirm this.

Lactobacillus rhamnosus has been shown to reduce diarrhoea in children and supplementation of this probiotic has been shown to reduce the incidence of eczema and allergies in Finnish babies and infants.[271] Lactobacillus rhamnosus is evidenced for improving symptoms of bacterial vaginosis and candidiasis in women.

Combinations of **Streptococcus thermophilus, Bifidobacterium breve, Bifidobacterium infantis** and **Bifidobacteria longum** have been shown in trials to kill common food-borne pathogens such as Listeria and Clostridium.[272]

L reuteri is evidenced for improving atopy, constipation, reduction of tonsillitis and antibiotic-related diarrhoea in children. Combinations of L reuteri, B bifidium, L planetarium and Lactobacillus rhamnosus are evidenced for antibiotic-related diarrhoea illness.

A Note on Supplements

Probiotics are not all created equal. Their effectiveness is determined by their diversity of organisms, the number of organisms and their delivery method. Generally speaking, the more bacterial strains a probiotic has the better and the higher the number of CFUs (Colony Forming Units), the better chance it has of delivering a significant number of good bacteria to the gut. The delivery method is also important. Many advanced formulas now come with special micro-encapsulation that allows the bacteria to survive the harsh acidic stomach and gastric juices that would otherwise destroy the bacteria.

Look for a brand that tests its probiotics for survivability and comes with laboratory certification. Many cheap probiotics will be broken down by the gastric juices of the stomach and will never actually introduce any new bacteria into the intestines.

I give all my patients probiotics and consider it a universal supplement (alongside vitamin D3 and omega 3). In my clinical practice it has become clear that there is no one who wouldn't benefit from boosting their beneficial bacteria. From acne and rosacea to leaky gut and depression, probiotics are the new 'must have'.

THE FUTURE

The future is exciting when it comes to the research and understanding of the microbiome. Everything from immunity, skin health, brain health and even autism can be linked to gut dysbiosis so the vastness of optimisation of the microbiome as potential therapy is truly profound. What we are learning is that the gut may actually be the epicentre of many modern and 'new' diseases and repairing our gut health may be a new frontier for treatment. I predict that faecal transplants will become the norm in the future, where diseased gut will be repopulated with healthy bacteria from a faecal donor. Watch this space.

CHAPTER 9: Big Pharma and the Medical Crisis

"By staying healthy you deny the pharmaceutical industry
the profit it expects to harvest from your disease."
Mike Adams, The Health Ranger

One of our greatest oversights is to think that we can medicate our way out of our poor diets and lifestyles. Treating bad food and lifestyle choices with drugs and chemicals is always going to be flawed and will never be the most effective solution. If doctors continue to dish out drugs instead of inspiring changes in our diet and lifestyle, we become complicit in the flawed thinking that drugs are better than lifestyle changes - which is simply not the case. It's like colluding with your patient if you allow them to ignore the power of positive dietary and lifestyle choices. Drugs often mask the symptoms of disease and allow us to ignore the signs that tell us that something is wrong.

If we had no drugs or pharmaceutic agents, we would have no choice but to adjust and change our collective behaviours. The problem is that drugs are everywhere; they are even advertised on the TV if you live in the US, which is something I totally abhor. Medicines don't stop pathology. They don't correct cause. They simply hide or mask our symptoms so we can ignore them a little longer. This is not good medicine or good practice. Your body can heal itself if you give it time, cut out the toxins and give it the nutrients it needs. We seem to grow up with the crazy and conditioned belief that chemicals heal but foods don't. Something has gone very wrong indeed.

Symptoms are your body's way of telling you that something is going wrong. And once you have 'symptoms' it means that the pathological (damaging) process is well underway. Many of the interventions I am advocating are easy to make, cheap and come with no side effects. Reducing excess sugar, reducing salt, reducing toxic fats, reducing dairy and reducing fast foods will definitely help, plus getting up off the couch and doing some exercise will add further benefits. None of these come with a prohibitive price tag and they can all afford you incredible health benefits.

Every year we all pay hundreds of pounds for our cars to be MOT'd. A mechanic looks at the car, does a thorough inspection and advises interventions and replacements we can make to optimise our car's performance and longevity and to keep us safe. Isn't it funny that we don't even give our own bodies the same level of care and respect? Or that we find a few hundred pounds spent on better quality food unsustainable? It's time to wake up and start prioritising our health because if we don't pay now, we will pay later.

Why have pharmaceutics become the option of choice? Well, remember this. GPs in the UK are paid for the interventions they make, not the lifestyle advice they give. Many GP surgeries are run as small businesses and the more pills, interventions and procedures they do the more they can earn. It's the same in the States. No one profits from lifestyle medicine except you and most western medical systems are not set up to promote preventive interventions. So, it follows that a system that is not set up to reward lifestyle measures will not validate lifestyle measures either. Add to this the fact that GPs often have less than 10 minutes face to face with a patient and you soon realise that it's almost impossible to cover everything. It becomes more a case of troubleshooting until the next crisis rather than being able to offer a complete and holistic approach to health. And that is not the fault of hard-working and generally conscientious doctors but is a fault with the system.

As a GP myself, I know the constant tug of war that I face between tending to the acute problem and trying to educate about the long-term. If you are always time-poor, all you get time to do is treat the current crisis - but it never solves causality or the root cause of the problem. Add to this the fact that it takes time to educate people about diet and lifestyle and it's easy to see why quick-fire pharmaceutics have become the treatment of choice. Until we all value lifestyle and nutritional medicine and make time and space for it in our consultations, it is unlikely that things will change.

Many doctors fail to stress the importance of lifestyle and dietary changes in their dialogue with patients. They know the current practice of pharmaceutic dependence is far from ideal but assume that the alternative - changing lifestyle and diet - is probably too hard for patients to action. Failing to mention and educate them on the enormously positive power of nutrition and lifestyle does our patients a huge disservice.

Meditation is the new medication

Patients rely on us doctors to give them the latest science and to guide them to make sensible, healthful, evidence-based decisions. The evidence points heavily towards the positive benefits of changing our diets and lifestyles. All patients have the right to know how they can help fix and reverse their conditions without the side effects of pharmaceutics. If a patient chooses not to follow their doctor's advice, that decision should rest with them. The doctor should not withhold important health information based on the assumption that the patient will find it too hard to do. Having access to the information is vital. Breakfast, lunch and dinner is where it needs to start. And what doctors learn at medical school needs to be dramatically updated and overhauled to include optimum nutrition.

One of the biggest problems we face in the west is how to reprogramme and restructure our medical system to include preventative, functional and lifestyle medicine. This really needs to start in the institutions that train healthcare workers, such as medical schools and nursing colleges. If the next generation are taught the value of nutrition and lifestyle medicine, then we will have a better equipped workforce that can help to positively guide and steer the public. We need to bridge the gap between pharmaceutical and preventative medicine and ensure the public understands the potential benefits of changing their diet and lifestyle to stave off disease. Once we do this, we will realise that food really is one of the most powerful drugs on the planet! What you eat and how you live each day has a huge impact on your general state of health and we need to return this power back to the individual.

For far too long now we have prioritised pharmaceutical and chemical medicine over preventative medicine. We have invested in technology to repair heart disease, cancer and stroke but have forgotten that the better (and cheaper) thing to do is to prevent it in the first place. Yes, the surgeon can cut things out and chemotherapy can kill cancer cells, but neither address the root cause of the problem. Looking at WHY we develop illness and disease is the sensible way to move forward; marrying the practice of lifestyle and preventative medicine with modern technology and pharmaceutics is surely the most comprehensive way to treat disease. If we are ready to end our dependence on prescription medicines then a nutrient-dense, whole food, low sugar diet is what we need.

"As a nation we have lost touch with the role we should play in our own health and wellbeing, expecting the NHS to pick up the pieces."
Dr John Giles, Medical Director, Benenden Health

DRUG MONEY

The pharmaceutical industry is a trillion-dollar business and patients are the industry's ATM. Thousands of studies on nutritional and lifestyle science are published every year but we choose to ignore them because we are conditioned to think that pharmaceutics are the answer. That conditioning comes from the pharmaceutical companies themselves but let's remember that they have a huge vested interest in keeping our beliefs this way. Our illness is driving their business and increasing their share price and they stand to lose a lot if we all start to get healthy and fit. They can't sell us dietary changes, but they can sell us costly medicines.

It's important that we understand the relationship between pharmaceutical companies and doctors. Pharmaceutical companies invest millions into developing new drugs in the hope that they will one day make them billions. Just to get a medicine from creation to FDA approval in the USA costs an average of $1.3 billion[184] and doctors are therefore very important middle men - the drug dealers, so to speak. Up until recently pharmaceutical companies could wine and dine doctors and take them away on all-expenses-paid trips whilst telling them about their marvellous new medicines.

Doctors are generally time-poor so they often take the information given to them by pharmaceutical companies and act on it in good faith. Very few will take the time to riffle through the mountain of evidence and look for publication bias in the trials. It worked nicely for a long time. Only recently, the wining and dining of doctors has been banned and deemed inappropriate, like a form of collusion. So, for many years doctors have been unintentionally complicit with Big Pharma in supporting the dark side of the pharmaceutical industry.

What doctors often don't know is that the information they receive regarding drugs and their efficacy is heavily biased by the drug and pharmaceuticals companies themselves. Often papers that show very little efficacy or impact for a drug are conveniently buried underneath alternative studies that show beneficial impact and clinically significant outcomes. Negative trials often aren't published; the positive ones are. This practice of cherry picking the data is dangerous because it means that doctors are practising without full access to the facts.

The other thing that happens is the benefits of a drug are often greatly exaggerated and the side effects semi-concealed. This is definitely what happened in the case of statins. We are starting to realise as doctors that the side effects of statins were much more common than we were led to believe and the positive benefits much less clearly defined. Incidentally, statins are one of the most prescribed drugs in the west, accounting for $35 billion annually.[185]

Here is the craziest thing - the FDA doesn't actually conduct independent trials on the drugs submitted for approval but relies on research done (more often than not) by the pharmaceutical companies themselves. If ever there was a way to influence study outcomes with commercial bias, this is it. It's a win-win for Big Pharma. They conduct the drug trials, get doctors to ghost write marketing materials or lend their name to them, submit only the positive trials to the FDA for consideration and then make billions from the consequent drug sales. It's time this kind of practice ended.

We need neutral, unbiased, evidence-based medicine that is not caught up in politics and corporate greed so that physicians can make sensible decisions to best improve their patients' health. Unfortunately, the current environment is one which is severely distorted by Big Pharma's cheque book.

This is the dark side of medicine. Big Pharma companies make millions out of us being sick. They are benefiting enormously from the current global epidemics in heart disease, diabetes, cancer, arthritis, auto-immunity, dementia and obesity. Given that all these diseases have sky rocketed over the last 50 years, we have to ask ourselves if we are getting value for money from drugs. Personally, I don't think so. Big Pharma has a vested financial interest in keeping us diseased and sick and is driven by the pursuit of profit. Their primary goal is not our health. We have to remember this.

Whilst most doctors serve their people honourably and with the best of intentions, some doctors have been complicit in the money making and have abandoned their humanitarian and altruistic service in pursuit of a fast buck. Private medicine is particularly open to abuse by greedy individuals. Numerous doctors have been found guilty of over-prescribing medicines, investigations and treatments in a bid to gain extra revenue. Once again, no one makes money out of diet and lifestyle improvements - which is why few doctors are plugging them. What is really interesting is when we get access to unpublished reports. An interesting meta-analysis of published and unpublished trials showed that placebo (dummy) anti-depressants worked just as well as the drug 82% of the time and 52% of anti-depressant drug trials failed to show any benefit.[186]

Professor Peter Gotzsche is a huge critic of our current pharmaceutic approach and claims that modern anti-depressants cause up to half a million deaths per year in the western world.[187] In his book *Deadly Medicines and Organised Crime,* Peter blames drug companies for corrupting healthcare with publication bias, overstatement of drug benefits and downplaying of side effects. If you are interested in looking into these ideas further, then I can highly recommend Ben Goldacre's *Bad Pharma,* and Peter Gotzsche's book *Deadly Medicines and Organised Crime* makes for an interesting read.

So are we becoming 'Prescription Thugs' and should we pull back on the medicines we are taking? This is a very complex and multi-factoral question and I ask that you read this chapter cautiously and that any decisions you make are made in conjunction with your doctor or healthcare provider.

There are many different drugs available on the market these days. Some are undoubtedly beneficial and positively life-saving. I am not advocating that we don't use drugs - what I advocate is that we try lifestyle and dietary measures FIRST and in conjunction with medicines to help to actually reduce causation.

Just remember that doctors are often overwhelmed by heavy workloads, pharmaceutical choice and ever-increasing data to interpret. As a patient, what you need to ask your doctor is how safe are the proposed medicines? What are the potential side effects? What are the potential interactions? What are the alternatives? What happens if you don't take the drug? Before you commit to any new medicine you need to satisfy these questions for yourself. The NHS is increasingly time and resource poor so it falls upon patients to take responsibility for their own health and be active participants in their own medical and healthcare decisions. Becoming your own healthcare advocate is empowering. Taking the time to educate yourself about your options is truly invaluable.

Death by Drugs

UK doctors issue 2.7 million prescriptions per day and over 1 billion per year.

Prescription drugs and medical interventions are the third leading cause of death after heart disease and cancer in the western world.[277]

Approximately 66 million medication errors occur in the UK per year.[278]

In the UK, 1,700 deaths per year are caused by avoidable drug reactions.[279]

In the USA, over 127,000 people per year die from taking a prescription drug at exactly the right dose the doctor prescribed.[280]

The United States - which makes up 5% of the world's population - now accounts for 42% of the money spent on prescription drugs.[281]

Since 2010, there have been more overdoses resulting in death in the United States from prescription opioid pharmaceuticals than heroin and other street narcotics.[282]

More than 80 million prescriptions for psychiatric drugs are written in the UK each year.

Over 60 million antidepressant prescriptions are written in the UK each year.

More than 1 in 10 UK women takes an anti-depressant.

Prescriptions for Ritalin (for ADHD) have more than doubled in the last decade, with 922,200 prescriptions written in 2014.[283]

"Virtually everything we know about drugs is what the companies have chosen to tell us and our doctors... The reason patients trust their medicine is that they extrapolate the trust they have in their doctors into the medicines they prescribe. The patients don't realise that although their doctors may know a lot about diseases... they know very, very little about drugs that hasn't been carefully concocted and dressed up by the drug industry."

Peter Goetzsche, Deadly Medicine and Organised Crime

PART TWO
How to save your life by changing what you eat

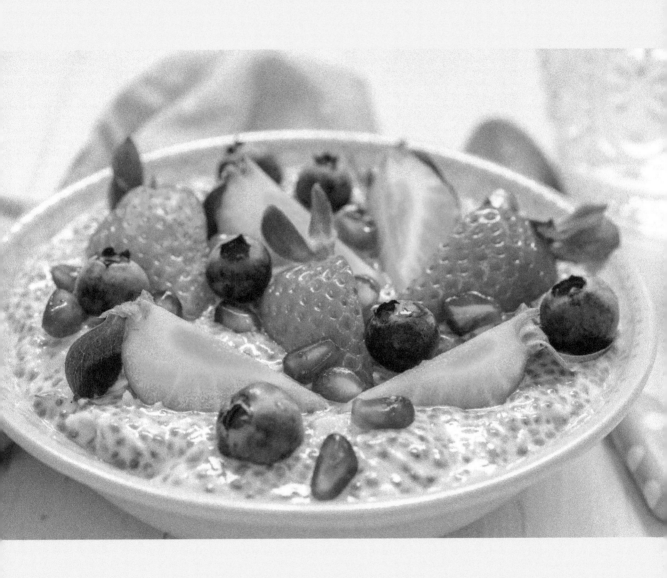

CHAPTER 10:
How to Save Your Life by Changing What You Eat

The first part of this book should have convinced you by now how unhealthy the standard western diet and lifestyle is. The health and financial implications of our current diet and our current way of living are hard to exaggerate or overstate. The western diet which is slowly taking over the whole world, is killing and bankrupting us simultaneously.

A low GI, whole food, plant focused diet is the one universal diet that will reduce your risk of not just some but all of the modern inflammatory diseases because it's the diet we were designed to eat. A low GI whole food diet is supported by a mountain of clinical evidence that tells us it's the best diet for preventing the diseases most dreaded in our society - cancer, heart disease, diabetes, stroke, autoimmunity and dementia. It is the healthiest diet because it reduces the common thread that connects all modern disease - insulin resistance and inflammation. As a consequence of eating better you will trim down and lose weight, improve your gut health, improve your heart stats and achieve a better sense of mental clarity and focus.

The food you eat is the most important factor that influences your future health and longevity. It trumps genetics. Everything you put into your mouth and onto your plate is either fighting disease or feeding it. The body can only perform its complex cellular duties of protection, maintenance, detoxification, renewal and repair if you feed it the right nutrients. Everything you consume is what you eventually become.

Dietary choices determine your cellular fuel and predict your future health. So, if you want to be on superfuel, you need to be on superfood. It's that simple. Eating delicious, dense, nutrient-packed superfoods is the only way to achieve true health. Over time, it becomes your way of life - and it feels great. It delivers far more than you think. Eating well can be pricey but eating badly will cost you even more. And only when you have lost your health will you ever truly appreciate it. Hospitals are full of people gasping for breath or yelling in pain, full of regret that they didn't take better care of themselves. Don't let this be you.

"If I had known I would live this long
I would have taken better care of myself."

Good health requires a lifelong commitment to great and nourishing food choices. It's like an ultra-marathon not a sprint. The ceiling of human existence is no longer clearly defined. We don't even know how long we could all live if we took better care of ourselves!

Diets often focus on short-term shifts in your macronutrient or calorie balance but studies show that only 2% of dieters ever keep off the weight they lose; the other 98% put it all back on.[188] What diets do is favour short-term weight loss at the expense of long-term, sustainable, healthful living. They are also a catastrophe for your metabolism and affect your body programming such that the next diet is even less likely to succeed. The problem with counting calories is that we have been taught that that's the thing that matters most. Well, actually it isn't. Food is very much a case of quality over quantity. A day's worth of calories derived from fast foods, refined carbohydrates and junk is not the same as a day's worth of calories derived from superfoods. Calories DO matter. But they need to be nourishing calories. The wrong foods eaten continuously, day after day, cause the majority of western disease and disability through the process of chronic inflammation. The typical western diet drastically shortens your lifespan and reduces the quality of your life in later years. Nutritional excellence is the best way for you to guarantee a long, healthful and happy life. And to be honest, there is no excuse. Nowadays we have almost instant access to the most beautiful, nutrient-dense superfoods imaginable. We don't have to hunt and gather for three days to find good food. It's there at the farmers' market, in the health food store or at the click of a button.

This is not a diet book. This is about changing the way you eat and live forever. Diets often fail. And they make us feel miserable because we then feel that we 'failed'. They reinforce our deepest insecurities and this feeds negative thoughts. The $175 billion diet industry is making a profit out of messing with our relationship with food and is messing up our metabolism and self-esteem in the process.[189] That's not what we want. The answer is not a fad diet. The answer is changing what we eat in the long term and learning to enjoy foods that have a low impact on the environment too. I call this Intelligent Eating.

WHAT IS A PLANT-BASED, WHOLE FOOD DIET?

A plant-based, whole food diet is a low GI diet based on foods derived from plants and includes fruits, vegetables, nuts, seeds, beans, legumes and whole grains. As long as it's low GI (low sugar) and centred around minimally processed, whole foods featuring diverse plants then I am happy that it is healthful and beneficial. Whole foods are foods that are still in their natural state and that are minimally processed. When you eat whole foods, you are eating foods in their most nutritious form. All plants are superfoods because they have an abundance of different vitamins, minerals, antioxidants, phytonutrients and fibre that literally flood your cells with nourishment.

A whole food diet based on plants will deliver an abundance of nutrients that will provide your body with the daily fuel to thrive and not just survive. We need to embrace healthy, nourishing, disease-preventing diets that are sustainable in the long term. Ways of eating that can follow us through our lives and enrich our experiences. Food has long been connected to the human experience and a healthful relationship with food is key to happiness, vitality and maintaining long-term health. So, while weight loss is important because being overweight increases the risk of many diseases and causes inflammation in itself, weight loss is not the overriding goal. If you strive for great health instead of weight loss the weight will more than likely fall off and stay off. The most effective healthcare is self-care and the healthiest foods for your body are also the healthiest foods for your weight.

There is no such thing as eating everything in moderation. Forget that. Forget eating little and often too unless your doctor has specifically directed you to do this. The moderation myth has been propagated for too long by too many and moderation is not the key to healthful, nutrient-dense living. We should not be eating sugar in moderation or refined carbohydrates in moderation, nor should we be eating trans fats in moderation. Even moderate amounts of these foods can be harmful and can bring about premature disability and death.

THE **PROBLEM** WITH OUR FOOD SYSTEM

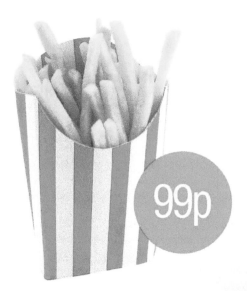

99p

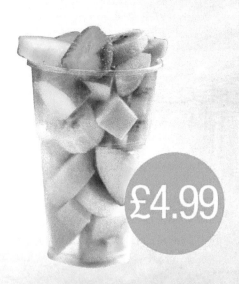

£4.99

Our entire society is set up to allow us to quickly and conveniently indulge in unhealthy foods. It's easier nowadays to find a Big Mac than it is to find an apple or pear. Supermarkets, high streets, airports and canteens are full of high-calorie, energy-dense, nutrient-deficient foodstuffs that only further perpetuate our unhealthy relationship with them. The more of us that vote with our forks and pressure and lobby for easy access to healthful foods, the more likely it will happen. Where there is a possibility for profit there is possibility for change.

Food diversity is incredibly important for our health and for food sustainability. Our recovery from these toxic foods starts in the home, in our cupboards and in our fridges. Take an honest look inside your fridge and see if it really looks healthful. As a junior doctor, I was appalled to work in a busy hospital that had a Burger King in its lobby with queues always halfway out of the door. It's this kind of infiltration of junk food into the very fabric of our society that has caused such huge health problems. Junk food doesn't belong in places of healing like hospitals.

A hundred years ago people were lean and slim. But now overweight and obese is the new 'norm'. Fast food sales globally in 2016 reached $540 billion[190] - a whopping growth of more than $533 billion since its advent in the early 1970s. It's time to fight back and stop letting these foods drive us into early graves.

If you have children, make sure you lead by example. If you don't want them to eat junk foods, don't bring junk foods into the house. Children will always take the path of least resistance and cannot rationalise the way an adult can about the dangers of junk foods. It is up to us to care for them and teach them to enjoy the taste of natural foods. Healthy choices and health habits start in our youth. As parents we play an incredibly important role in shaping our children relationship with food. Get it right early and their life will be far healthier and happier as a result of your input. Start a superfood chart for your children where you get them to eat in colours - red, yellow, green, purple and blue - and get them to tick off the colours they manage to eat every day. It becomes fun! Let the winner each week pick a treat or a game to play and you will soon see them enjoying their fruit and veg. Take them to cookery class or better still teach them in the home how to make healthy recipes. Show them through your food choices that you are choosing health and longevity and explain to them that mummy and daddy choose to eat well so they can be around for longer. That's what I tell my kids and they love that I am doing something that will help keep me in their lives longer.

With repetition and positive reinforcement your children will eventually understand that these are life-affirming choices to be made each day. Much like children nowadays understand that smoking is bad for you and kills you, so too they will learn that junk foods and sedentary behaviours are also killers. Be proactive at the school. Make sure the school menu is healthful. I have had to have many conversations with my children's school over the years about the quality of foods on offer, but the teachers realise it is only me wanting the best for my children.

My kids used to get a snack box at their after-school club that consisted of a sandwich (white bread), a KitKat, a packet of crisps, a carton of orange juice and a piece of fruit. I was aghast when I learned of this. Needless to say, my children tried to hide it from me because kids will always want what everyone else has. No one wants to be different or left out.

So I spoke to the school and pointed out how a snack box like this contributes to a future of insulin resistance, heart disease, cancer and stroke. Very quickly, the school adapted the box contents and now the kids happily munch on healthier foods and they don't feel any less happy because of it.

Jamie Olivier has done a lot in the UK for raising awareness about the health of children's meals in schools and we all need to thank him for trailblazing because it's always hard to be the first to speak out against the crowd.

'Every time we chose to buy an organic product,
we're voting for a better food system'
Jamie Oliver

YOU'VE GOT TO NOURISH TO FLOURISH

Transforming your diet will allow you to earn back your health and can add up to 20 years onto your life. Who doesn't want that? In real terms, that could mean the difference between dying in your late 50s when your children are young, missing out on future weddings, future grandchildren, future friends, future travel, future retirement plans and all the wonderful things that could have been.

Or living a longer, healthier life to see your *grandchildren* into adulthood and your children safely into their middle age or beyond. Travelling the world and enjoying your retirement, enjoying your mature years with health and vitality on your side. I know which one I choose, and I know which one your future self would want you to choose.

How to get started

In order to rewire your brain into healthy mode you have to accept that it is going to be hard initially. You will need to make an active commitment to healthful living. You have to recalibrate and reset. And you need to throw away all the ultra-processed junk foods in your fridge and cupboards and make a strong commitment to reducing your sugar, sodium, damaged fats, dairy, processed meats, gluten and refined carbohydrates. You need to become your own health and wellness advocate and invest in yourself as a priority.

I promise you nothing tastes as good as healthy feels and it's never too late to recapture your health and reset your biological clock. Where the mind goes, the body will follow. Make the commitment today - we always think we will do things tomorrow but the reality is that another birthday, date night or party will delay your most important move: the move to better health and the chance to earn a better life.

*** If you have any medical problems consult your doctor first and ask them to help support and guide you to a better way of eating ***

Your dietary focus needs to be on maximising your micronutrient intake. Too many of us miss the connection between food and nutrients. Food is our cellular FUEL. It is our means of life. Sustenance. Health. Cellular function. Without it, we die.

Habits are hard to break. We are all to some extent creatures of habit and find auto-pilot easier than carving a new path. The problem comes when the habit is causing disease so needs to be broken. Habit is incredibly powerful; it is the reason many of us go to the fridge over and over again despite not being hungry. Habit is the reason why we buy the same groceries each week, the same brands, eat the same ten meals and indulge in the same ice creams or donuts over and over again.

Junk food is an addiction. We are hardwired via the brain's dopamine pathway to return time and time again to foods that are bad for us but that taste pleasurable. It's no different chemically to an alcohol or drug addiction. It's just more acceptable to eat junk foods than it is to shoot up drugs.

Ever wondered why Pringles are SO hard to stop eating? Or why you can't just eat one French fry? The food industry is complicit in creating deep and enduring food addictions that we all find incredibly hard to break. In fact, it is actively engaged in designing foods in a lab that utilise our inherent dopamine weakness, making us want more and more. For food scientists the key is to catch us early in our childhood and get us addicted for years. In 2006 $10 billion was spent on advertising food and beverages to America's youth and 44 major food and beverage marketers spent over $1.6 billion promoting their products to children in the United States.[191] McDonalds spent more than any food and beverage company on advertising in 2016 at £85 million.[192]

So yes, the transformation is going to be hard and yes, the odds are stacked against you. Many people have made deep-rooted connections with addictive foods as a means of coping with the highs and lows of life. In these instances, the joy of good, proper, nutritious food has been replaced with something far more complex.

But the victory is sweet - and the quality and quantity of your life depends on it! When it gets tough, hold onto the thought of the 20 years of life that you may gain from doing this. Surely your life is worth that? Enlist the help of your doctor, a nutritionist or a counsellor if your addictions are really ingrained. We know from studies with tobacco and drugs that beating addictions is more likely when you have professional support.

I promise you once you are a few weeks into a whole food, plant-based diet you will no longer crave your old pseudo-foods and you will learn to anticipate the foods that nourish your body and respond best to its biological needs. Making heathy food choices will cease to be hard and will become one of the most intensely pleasurable and satisfying way of 'creating and gifting yourself future health'. In the eloquent words of Dr Joel Fuhrman, 'Earning it back - meal by meal'.

"If you want to know what health is worth then the best person to tell you will be someone who has lost it."
Dr Joel Furnham

On your journey you will meet with sceptics. People will try and tell you all kinds of things. But hold tight and remind yourself that low GI whole foods and plant foods are like the water that quells the inflammatory fire. Ignorance is bliss - up to a point. But when your health, your life and the future of this planet depends on it - it suddenly has more meaning.

"We can't tell people to stop eating all meat and all dairy products... Well, we could tell people to become vegetarians... if we were truly basing this only on science we would, but it's a bit extreme."
Director of Harvard's Cardiovascular Epidemiology Program

The problem with so much of society is that the food industry often colludes with the government and vice versa creating deep conflicts of interest. The truth is that the meat, dairy and food industries are so influential that everyone is worried about the fallout if they speak out against them. Afterall, the Texan Cattle Industry once tried to sue Oprah Winfrey and 'muzzle her voice' because she said live on her TV show that she never wanted to eat a hamburger again after learning about cannibalistic feeding techniques and CJD risks! All of us doctors who have ever dared to suggest that cow's milk is inflammatory and shouldn't be a dietary staple have been accused of 'scaremongering'. I am trolled frequently by people who have a vested interest in the dairy industry but that doesn't deter me. Someone has to speak up. Just because the dairy industry wants us to believe that milk is good for us doesn't mean it is. It reminds me of Mahatma Gandhi's wise words: 'First they ignore you, then they laugh at you, then they fight you, then you win'. As anyone who has come along with new ideas that challenge the status quo knows - it's not easy.

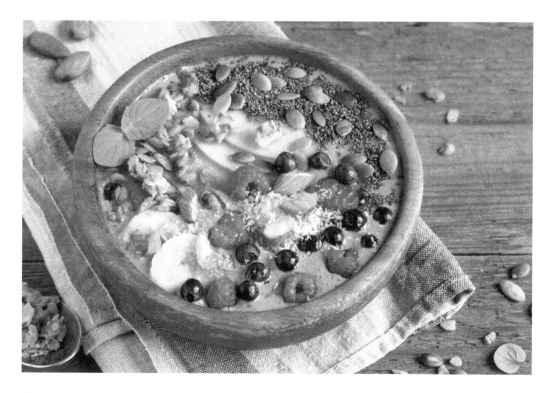

My own journey back to health took a while. I spent my teenage years as a vegetarian but by the time I was 20 I gave up because it was too hard to sustain at university. I am not proud to say that my undergraduate days consisted of consuming far too many microwave meals and far too much Diet Coke. Now in my forties, I eat for health and nutrition so the foods I eat are ones that align me with health. I don't categorise myself with any food activist group nor do I food shame those who make different choices. I just make choices based on the science that I know. I take supplements where I am deficient to bridge the gap and to optimise my immune and mitochondrial function, but I am not rattling around taking hundreds a day. Real foods will always trump isolated synthetic nutrients.

I am not obsessive or fanatical about food, but I enjoy feeding my body nutritious superfoods and I enjoy eating clean, green foods. Sometimes I fall off the wagon. When I do, I just try to get back into heathy eating with the very next meal rather than the next day or the next week. My tuberculosis diagnosis in my early 20s and the resultant problems it caused to my immunity have meant that eating healthily has always been a focus for me.

So, although I haven't always been a total angel, I've never strayed too far off a healthy path either. The hardest thing I find in my day to day life is finding time for daily exercise. I have had to make a HUGE effort to get daily exercise into my busy life and even sometimes that's been a real push. With three young children and a busy work life, finding the time to do some form of daily exercise is always a challenge! But I know it's vital for my health so I now prioritise it.

The most important thing to know is that no one can sustain perfection all the time. No one. As long as you eat really well most of the time and exercise as much as you can you will be winning. What you do every day is far more important than what you do every once in a while, so don't beat yourself up if you indulge every now and again or you skip the gym from time to time.

This is a guideline and something to aim for. It's not intended to make you feel bad, inadequate or like a failure. The diet industry has done that enough for us all! Think of this book more as an inspiration to get your life in order but remember to commit to the change too. Try all of my recommendations for at least 3-6 months - it takes that long for your tastes, your habits and your body to adjust. Tell your family and friends you are committing to a new food regime and exercise regime and try to stick with it no matter what. Take before and after photos of yourself and watch the weight drop off. Remember that slim people can be unhealthy too so don't think this is solely about weight loss. It's for health gain. Some people are slim despite eating anything and everything (including lots of sugar) and doing little or no exercise. That's not really healthy, is it? Imagine their inflammation levels! Make a food and exercise diary, track your progress and tick off the colours of the rainbow. Tell everyone you know about what you are doing and ask them to join or support you.

Most importantly, don't give up if you are met with cynicism from others. Conditioned behaviours, recreational eating and following what everyone else did got you in this mess in the first place. Don't be disheartened if people don't understand why you want to do this. It may very well be that they only come to understand your choices years later.

Most people lapse when they are travelling or on holiday and away from normal routine. If you lapse occasionally, don't get fanatical about it; just try to get back on high-nutrient foods as soon as you can. To prevent this, you can anticipate your food requirements and prepare things in advance that you can take on the road or on your travels.

ACT NOW

Stop buying unhealthy foods.

Buy new superfoods to replace your old foods.

Choose and plan recipes for your coming week (see the recipe section for inspiration).

Forward plan each meal (until it becomes easier).

Cook in bulk and freeze the leftovers to reduce your workload.

Eat three nutrient-dense meals a day and try to limit snacking or grazing.

Eat your evening meal no later than 6pm and try to delay breakfast until you are truly hungry. Preferably after 10am.

Brush your teeth after eating so you aren't tempted to graze.

Drink water plentifully.

Limit juices, milky drinks and alcohol.

Exercise at least 5 times per week - mix up sessions of cardio training, weight training and toning/core exercises like yoga or pilates.

Write yourself some motivational post-it notes and scatter them around the house.

Tell yourself you now eat for nourishment and health.

Try to get your family and friends to support you or - even better - to join you.

Connect with others in your community or on social media for inspiration and support. Connection makes a huge difference. Humans were made to connect.

Make a superfoods chart, put it on your wall and tick it off each time you eat veg, nuts, seeds, beans etc. It becomes fun and whole families can do this!

There are many different versions of healthful diets, but I can tell you that the modern western diet isn't one of them.

I am not advocating that you all become vegetarian or vegan. There are some very unhealthy vegetarians and vegans out there, trust me. It's not so much about categorising yourself and your diet. I don't even do that myself. This is about more than that. It's about embracing a diet where disease prevention is prioritised. It's about eating a diet centred around minimally processed, low GI foods because the best available science today tells us that this is the way to best optimise health. What this is really about is increasing your intake of superfoods for the benefit of your lifespan and healthspan and reducing your consumption of foods that don't serve you positively. In terms of the planet and sustainability, every small reduction you make to your factory meat and dairy consumption helps reduce the impact of these industries on our planet. It all counts, and it all adds up. With over seven billion people in the world all our small actions, good and bad, compound and mount. Never assume that your actions don't have impact. THEY DO.

"Your body wants to regain its health if you let it. But if you keep re-injuring yourself three times a day you interrupt the healing process."
Dr Michael Gregor

Personally, I found that, after reading all the science and understanding the impact that my food choices had on my health and the health of our planet, these changes came very naturally. Nowadays I love to feed my body nutrient-dense plant based whole foods.

CHAPTER 11: The Evidence for Plant-Based Diets

Diet is the single biggest factor that predicts how long we live.

Globally, 17.7 million people die each year from heart disease, 6 million people die from strokes and 8.2 million from cancer - and we still don't care? To make improvements in our lifespan we don't need scalpels or drugs - we need knives and forks. What is on your fork each day is what matters the most in the end. Making the change today will be one of the best things you ever do. We only have to look at developing countries to see how cancer and chronic diseases thrive in urban food environments. Countries that used to have some of the lowest rates of cancer (breast cancer in China and India; colon cancer in Japan) now have rising rates. These cancers are concentrated in the newly urbanised centres of India, China and Japan where people are most exposed to fast and processed foods.[193]

Other studies have showed the rapid negative impact that occurs when people start consuming the Standard American Diet (SAD). In 2015, a study took 20 African Americans and 20 South African tribespeople and made them switch diets for two weeks. When the South Africans ate Western foods, they quickly had changes in their microbiome and intestines that promoted inflammation, whilst the African Americans experienced positive improvements in their gut health and inflammatory markers.[194] This study shows you how quickly both positive and negative changes can take hold and impact your body. Another study, this time involving a huge number of people (800,000) showed that eating a diet consisting of inflammatory foods caused increased risk of colorectal cancer — a 51% increased risk for men and a 25% increased risk for women.[195]

Numerous studies now highlight that animal-based diets cause more heart disease and death than plant-based diets. Indeed, a large study of over 43,000 Swedish women showed that the more women ate animal protein the more their risk of cardiovascular disease went up. The reason for this is that high consumption of animal protein equals high IGF-1, which increases vascular risk, but it also means less intake of plant-based food that have enormous protective properties.

Remember from Chapter One that the endothelium of our vessels need protecting. Well, a constant supply of nitric oxide can help to protect them and prevent inflammation. Nitric oxide rich foods are generally plant based. These findings were consistently reproduced in other studies that showed that heart disease risk goes up when animal product intake goes up.

Colin Campbell, in his famous book *The China Study*, examined thousands of inhabitants of rural China and compared them to Americans eating a Standard American Diet. He noted repeatedly that the rural Chinese in his study ate very little animal protein (less than 10%) and had very low rates of heart disease. We see a pattern over and over again in that whenever a society leaves its traditional diet and embraces a modern western diet, its rate of heart disease and stroke increases.

Another well-known study looked at the Mediterranean diet (PREDIMED study) and showed that longevity and health can be improved when eating is plant-based. In this study each serving of plants consumed extended lifespan and each serving of animal-based protein reduced it. In fact, the study showed that reducing consumption of animal products by two thirds reduced deaths by more than 40%.[196] The Iowa Women's Health Study also showed this.[197] It studied 33,000 women for a whopping 18 years and concluded that if you ate more vegetable protein in your diet you had a 40% reduced risk of cardiovascular disease than those eating animal protein. What is more, they isolated these benefits specifically to plant-based foods like vegetables, seeds, nuts and beans and noted that potatoes, rice and bread did not afford the same benefits.

A study in *JAMA Internal Medicine* studied in excess of 70,000 people and noted that vegetarians live longer than meat eaters. Six to ten years longer, in fact. For six years from 2002 to 2007 the study followed a large group of Seventh Day Adventists in the USA, who are known to follow a vegetarian diet. The study observed that vegetarians were 12% less likely to have died in that period than their meat-eating peers. The vegetarian and vegan groups also had lower cardiovascular risk factors (thought to be due to lower saturated fat levels and higher fibre consumption), fewer deaths from diabetes, fewer deaths from renal (kidney) disease and fewer from metabolic syndrome.

According to the study (Adventists Health Study 2) vegetarian men live to an average of 83.3 years, compared with non-vegetarian men, who live to an average of 73.8 years. Vegetarian women live to an average of 85.7 years, which is 6.1 years longer than non-vegetarian women. We have to be careful with this study as Seventh Day Adventists are vegetarians who also avoid alcohol - so if you want to get these health benefits and these extra life years then cut out alcohol too!

In terms of cancer, we now have a mountain of evidence to show that a plant-based diet is both protective and beneficial. In 2014, a study looked at Americans aged 50-65 on a diet that included 20% animal protein derived calories. The study found that these individuals were four times more likely to die of diabetes or cancer than those eating a plant-based diet and were two times as likely to die of any cause in the next 18 years. These increased risks were primarily due to increases in IGF-1, which occur with animal protein consumption. The plant-based eaters didn't increase their risk at all.[198]

The rate of breast cancer in western women is approximately five times the rate of Asian women. Protective dietary factors have been identified that explain these differences. In 2009, Chinese researchers noted that Chinese women who had more than 15 portions of mushrooms in a month plus 15 cups of green tea had a 90% reduced rate of breast cancer compared to Chinese women who didn't include these protective plant-based foods.[199] It had long been postulated that green tea alongside other protective dietary factors was the reason for the low rates of breast cancer in Asian women.

Dr Dean Ornish has conducted some of the most famous studies on cancer and plant-based diets and has shown that we can reverse both heart disease and cancer with low GI plant-based diets. In 2005, he treated 44 patients with prostate cancer with a plant-based diet, prescriptive daily exercise and stress reduction techniques. It resulted in cessation of the progression of prostate cancer, as measured by the tumour marker PSA. He compared this to another 49 patients in a control group who didn't make any dietary or lifestyle changes and who saw an increase in their tumour activity.

When we consume high animal products the effect is twofold. Firstly, we increase IGF-1, which directly increases our risk of many diseases because it's an inflammation promoter; and secondly, increased animal intake pushes plants off our plate - this is a problem primarily because plants have the most enormous power to protect us. Plant based diets have protected humans for millenia.

Plants contain an incredible combination of vitamins, minerals, fibre, phytochemicals and antioxidants that work to protect humans in an exquisite biological feat of nature. Plant focused diets are not only healthful but are what we were designed to eat and any movement away from this diet, even if slight, has a huge impact on our longevity and disease risk. We could save an enormous amount in health care costs, let alone endless human suffering, if we all reduced our consumption of unhealthy foods and increased our consumption of plant-based foods. They need to be low GI of course though else they risk insulin resistance. The science is pointing more and more in the direction of plant-based foods because they quell inflammation, nourish us the most and afford us protection from most disease.

BLUE ZONES

What epidemiologists have noted when they study the longest living populations in the world is that they all share a diet that is high in a variety of plant-based foods. In the five Blue Zones people live well into their 90s and 100s in good health, with good mental agility and a good quality of life. These longevity hotspots include:

Sardinia (Italy)

Okinawa (Japan)

Loma Linda (California)

Nicoya Peninsula (Costa Rica)

Icaria (Greek Island)

In these places people enjoy a diet that is healthful, they move daily, they enjoy community and personal support and they live meaningful lives that manage stress efficiently. They use technology and pharmaceuticals minimally.

If we look at the Blue Zone of Okinawa in Japan the people are slim, active and engaged in their community well into their later years. The Okinawa Centenarian Study showed that they have low rates of heart disease and cancer, even stomach cancer which is typically high on the Japanese mainland. They eat virtually no processed foods and enjoy a deep sense of purpose through making lifelong communities of friends called *moais.* These are thought to play a pivotal role in their longevity, in addition to their healthy eating.[201]

When we look at Loma Linda, the sunny Californian hotspot of longevity, we can see that it is possible for Americans to enjoy long, healthy lives too! Loma Linda is inhabited by about 9,000 Seventh Day Adventists who don't drink, don't smoke and eat a largely vegetarian diet. They also enjoy a deep sense of community and purpose and live well into their 90s and 100s.

In Icaria in Greece, one out of three people live into their 90s and they have 20% less cancer, 50% less heart disease and virtually no dementia compared to standard westerners.[202] They epitomise optimal diet, daily movement and stress-free living.

What Blue Zones show us is that there isn't just one healthy diet but many. The problem is that the modern western diet isn't one of them. All Blue Zones show us that a diet incorporating plants and whole foods, combined with a simpler and more natural way of living, is the key to living a long, fulfilled and healthy life. So it's actually super easy to wipe out almost your entire risk of heart disease, cancer, dementia, diabetes and stroke with one diet and one set of changes.

WHAT YOU NEED TO DO

Cut out processed foods

Reduce meat and dairy intake (ideally < 5-10% calories)

Reduce salt intake (< 6g per day)

Reduce and minimise sugar intake

Reduce refined carbohydrate intake

Reduce alcohol intake (occasional use only - drink organic and sulphite free)

Increase plant intake, especially leafy greens and berries

Increase nuts, seed and legume intake (daily intake of all three)

Increase filtered water and green tea consumption

Exercise daily for 30 minutes (moderate level)

Reduce caffeine

Give up smoking

Sleep well

If you can do this most days, you are well on your way to experiencing optimum and renewed health and wellbeing. Rewiring your brain can take a while but you will learn to seek out nutrient-dense foods because they will make you feel full and satisfied. Your reward will be better mental clarity, better skin, better health, better energy, better libido and a better chance of living long and living well.

We all need to return to the diet that serves us best. It's not just for health nuts! The last hundred years have seen a huge change in our food environment with the market flooded with cheap, mass produced, nutrient-deficient foodstuffs. We have introduced thousands of new chemicals into our food chain and now experience a deep divide between the way we have eaten for thousands of years and the way we eat today. The only way you can claw back your health is to do it daily with better food and lifestyle choices. Meal by meal.

If switching to a whole foods diet is a dramatic change for you then that only serves as a powerful reminder of how far you have drifted away. Aim for it even if you don't achieve it each and every day. Not everyone wants to change everything at once; it's not all or nothing. Each incremental step in the right direction has a cumulative and compounding effect. You may not want to give up certain things totally but every negative food that you eat less frequently has an impact and when you understand the benefits of cutting back the results can be profound.

INTERESTING PLANT-BASED FACTS

Risk of colon cancer in daily meat eaters compared to those who eat meat less than once per month: 250%.[203]

Risk of colon cancer for people who eat poultry four times per week compared to those who don't: 200-300% greater.[204]

Risk of colon cancer in people who eat poultry once per week compared to those who don't: 55% greater.[205]

Risk of lung cancer (most common cause of cancer mortality globally) among people who consume a lot of fruit (especially apples, grapes and bananas): 40% reduction.[206]

Risk of lung cancer in people who consume a lot of colourful green, orange and yellow vegetables: 20-60% reduction.[207]

Vegan women have 34% lower rates of female-specific cancers, such as breast, cervical and ovarian cancer.[208]

Smokers who do not eat carrots have a three times greater risk of developing lung cancer than those who eat carrots three times per week.[209]

Risk of prostate cancer decreases by 5% for each serving of carrots consumed per week.[210]

Risk of prostate cancer in men who consume high amounts of dairy: 70% increase.[211]

Risk of prostate cancer in men who consume plentiful lycopene (found in tomatoes): 45% reduction.[212]

Risk of prostate cancer in men who eat high amounts of cruciferous vegetables (broccoli, kale, cauliflower): 41% reduction.[213]

Breast cancer incidence in Italian women consuming lots of animal-based products compared to Italian vegetarians: three times greater.[214]

Breast cancer rate for Japanese meat-eating women compared to Japanese vegetarian women: 8.5 times higher.[215]

Risk of colon cancer for men who eat beans and lentils twice per week compared to those who don't: 50% lower.

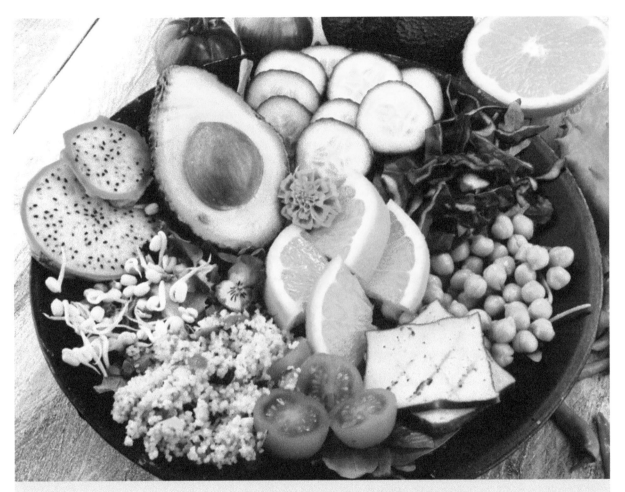

'If I'd known I was going to
live this long I'd have taken
better care of myself'
Eubie Blake

CHAPTER 12: How to Connect the Dots

Awareness is the first stage of healing and will help propel you into positive action. In life there are always events, stresses or reasons why we delay healthfulness. It's far easier to continue the way you are than it is to commit to and effect a dramatic change. That's why so many diets fail and so many people end up unwell. We are all time-poor, information-overloaded and overwhelmed with convenient temptations like fast foods that fall so easily and seductively into our laps. Once they are in reach it's almost impossible to say no so we just eat what's put in front of us. Once you recognise these patterns of behaviour, you can put into place a plan that will help you change these behaviours. I drive the long way home from my children's school every day just to avoid driving past a McDonalds, Subway, Costa and KFC. If I drive past them every day, I am much more likely to give in to my children's pleas than if we were to never see them in the first place. It's recognising things like this that help us remap and readjust our daily behaviours. And all the little things add up.

If you have decided to change the way you live and eat, then there is a double benefit ahead for you! The diet that is most healthful for you is also most healthful for our planet. Switching to a plant-based, whole foods diet will allow your body to be flooded by protective food substances and antioxidants daily and will cut out the disease-promoting substances like damaged fats, sugars, salt additives and toxins. In plant-based foods there are literally thousands of substances that have powerful anti-cancer, anti-ageing and anti-heart disease substances. These include antioxidants, phytochemicals, carotenoids, isoflavones, vitamins, minerals, retinols, bioflavonoids and polyphenols. With a few exceptions, these super substances are found wholly in vegetables, fruits, nuts, seeds, beans and legumes.

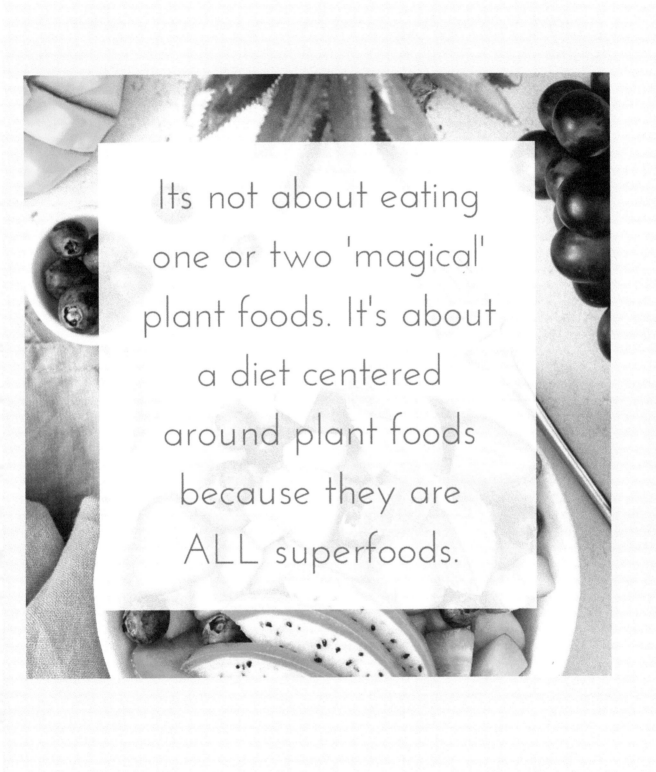

Its not about eating one or two 'magical' plant foods. It's about a diet centered around plant foods because they are ALL superfoods.

WHAT THE PROFESSIONALS SAY ABOUT PLANT-BASED WHOLE FOOD DIETS

"What is remarkable about the diet-cancer story is the consistency with which certain foods emerge as important in reducing risks across the range of cancers. Millions of cancer cases could be prevented each year if more individuals adopted diets low in meat and high in fruit and vegetables."

Cummings J, British Medical Journal

"All animal products ... are rich in substances associated with cancer and heart disease... Animal protein stimulates the rise of cancer-promoting hormones within the body, especially insulin-like growth factor 1(IGF-1)."

Dr Joel Furnham

"A low-fat plant-based diet would not only lower the heart attack rate by about 85% but would lower the cancer rate by 60%."

William Castelli from the Framingham Health Study, one of the largest and most reputed studies of long-term human health

"Eating processed meats or a diet high in red meat is a cause of cancer."

World Cancer Research Fund

"A vegan diet is probably the single biggest way to reduce your impact on Planet Earth, not just greenhouse gases, but global acidification, eutrophication, land use and water use."

Oxford University Study 2018

"If you step back and look at the data [on beef and cancer] the optimum amount of red meat you should eat should be zero."

Walter Willett MD, Harvard School of Public Health

"It was only a few years ago that vegetarians were relegated to the margins of society and had not yet been recognised as being on the leading edge of movements toward health, ecological sustainability and social justice."

John Robbins, author, *The Food Revolution*

"Eat fruit and vegetables as if your life depended on it - because it probably does."

Michael Greger MD, author of *How Not to Die*

CHAPTER 13: Superfuel with Superfoods

Whilst many plant-based foods deliver incredible health benefits there are a few foods that can be singled out for special recognition. These are Superfoods.

Superfoods are foods that have the special ability to nourish, fortify and drive us towards greater human health. They are highly nutritious, low GI and contain an abundance of different micronutrients that help support everything from detoxification to cellular renewal and repair. They provide vitamins, minerals, antioxidants, phytochemicals, fibre, lignans, polyphenols, catechins and much much more.

Eating a superfood diet will superfuel your health. Make sure every meal offers your body a diverse range of superfoods and you can't go wrong.

Superfoods are real, whole foods. They are best if they are organic and sourced locally - this reduces the risk of GMOs and pesticides. You will find them in your local farmers' market or in your local grocery store. Even the more unusual superfoods can be purchased online at the click of a button. Just make sure they are sustainably sourced.

Aim for at least 10 varieties of superfoods per day. A 2017 study concluded that ten servings of vegetables and fruit per day was better than the UK's suggestion of five a day. In the study, eating ten servings of fruit and vegetables a day (equivalent to 800g) was associated with a 33% reduced risk of stroke, 24% reduced risk of heart disease, 13% reduced risk of cancer and an overall 31% reduction in premature deaths.[216]

Due to space constraints I can't list every superfood in this book but have listed some of the most powerful and readily available ones that come with mountains of clinical evidence to support their superfood status. All the recipes featured at the end of this book contain a wonderful mixture of these powerful, life-affirming foods.

Greens

Greens are the healthiest foods on the planet and top the list of superfoods. Every single day you should aim to eat a number of different leafy greens or have a large green salad. Greens contain calcium, folate, iron, fibre and thousands of different phytonutrients and antioxidants, which flood your cells with protective antioxidants that reverse and neutralise oxidative stress. Every single day we need to consume abundant antioxidants because oxidative stress is how all tissues are damaged and how the body ages. Oxidative stress occurs when free radicals outnumber available antioxidants – kind of like a biochemical rusting. If you take an apple, cut it open and leave it out on the kitchen bench for 30 minutes it will turn brown. This is an example of oxidation. The exposure to oxygen damages the sensitive apple tissue. The same happens if you cut open an avocado, a banana or a pear. Well, the same also happens inside our bodies every day and it happens in an accelerated fashion if we don't eat enough antioxidant-rich foods. If you trickle lemon juice all over the apple slices this enzymatic browning doesn't happen, because lemon is rich in vitamin C, a powerful antioxidant. This is the power of antioxidants and greens are some of the best!

A study published in the *American Journal of Clinical Nutrition* showed that greens perform better when mixed with at least 3g of fat.[217] The beta-carotene, lutein, vitamin K and zeaxanthin in greens all require fat to liberate their health benefits and to allow for better nutrient absorption. So why not try a walnut and avocado salad dressing next time to improve that status of your greens?!

Kale is probably one of the most beneficial greens so try and get it into as many of your dishes as possible. It can taste a bit like grass(!) so I like to conceal it in smoothies and salads. Kale is an immune-boosting superfood with significant antioxidant power. In a study of 32 Japanese men, daily kale juice for only three months reduced their bad cholesterol and improved their good cholesterol as much as an hour of exercise daily would.[218] Now that's not bad for a food, is it?

NB: The only people who need to limit their intake of raw kale and raw cruciferous vegetables (alongside soybeans) are those who have problems with their thyroid because they can contain thyroid blocking compounds called goitrogens. Ask your doctor if this will affect you.

Broccoli is one of the healthiest greens you can eat. It belongs to the cruciferous family and contains an abundance of vitamins, minerals, phytonutrients and antioxidants, not to mention the incredible sulforaphane. This was found to be in the top 10 anti-cancer foods in a 2009 study published in the journal *Food Chemistry*. It is thought to be particularly effective at reducing the risk of breast and aggressive prostate cancer.[219] [220]

Sulforaphane is mainly found in cruciferous vegetables so you need to eat them every day to get the amazing health benefits. Sulforaphane supports liver detoxification and has been shown to reduce the size and number of breast cancer cells in mice, blocking tumour growth. It also helps fight infection by reducing levels of cytokines and NF-kB, which all drive inflammation.[221] [222]

Numerous studies (both animal and human) have shown that regular broccoli intake is associated with a decreased risk of heart disease and cancer.[223] Two large studies looking at a total of 134,796 Chinese adults found that fruit and vegetable intake is inversely related to mortality in men and women and that a dose response pattern is particularly evident in those eating lots of cruciferous vegetables. What this means is that the more fruit, vegetables and particularly cruciferous veg you eat (think broccoli, kale, sprouts, collards) the less likely you are to die from heart disease and cancer.

Sulforaphane is created by a chemical reaction that only happens when you chop or chew broccoli. So, if you plan to cook cruciferous vegetables make sure you chop them 30-40 minutes before you cook them to allow the reaction to take place. Broccoli sprouts are particularly rich in sulforaphane with approximately 20 times more than mature broccoli, so chose sprouts where possible. They can be eaten raw on green salads - just don't eat more than about 2-3 cups per day as it can make you feel sick.

Anyone with cancer or recovering from cancer should make sure that broccoli sprouts feature in their daily diet.

Spinach is a super all-rounder when it comes to nutrient delivery. It is packed with vitamins A, C and the much-forgotten vitamin K. It also has abundant manganese, magnesium, iron, calcium, folate and potassium. It's loaded with antioxidants and phytonutrients and is particularly effective at fighting free radicals in the colon.[224]

Several studies have found spinach to reduce arterial stiffness (and hence the risk of heart disease),[225] reduce the risk of cancer [226] and boost brain health.[227] Like broccoli, spinach contains sulforaphane and a multitude of antioxidants too. Sulforaphane helps the body to naturally expel pesticides and studies have shown that sulforaphane can block up to 60% of heterocyclic amines (from grilled meats) that cause cancer.[228]

As always, choose organic spinach to avoid toxic DDT that is still found in soils despite being banned in 1972. I like to either steam spinach or lightly heat it in a pan with a dash of olive oil for a few minutes and then squeeze lemon juice on it - this preserves the nutrients and iron and adds a little fun to the taste.

Bell peppers

Bell peppers are rich in quercetin, flavonoids, carotenoids, vitamin c and ferulic acid - all antioxidants and phytonutrients that work to combat renegade free radicals and reduce inflammation.[229] Bell peppers contain over 30 different phytonutrients so their nutrient capacity is simply phenomenal. They have been tested even after 6 months of freezing and the carotenoid benefits remained. A study from Poland showed that organic peppers have 10% more carotenoids and vitamin c than conventional peppers and about 30% more phenolic acid. Yellow peppers appear to have more carotenoids than red peppers whereas red peppers have more lutein and beta-carotene. So make sure you eat the full variety and colours of peppers in your foods. Aim for a minimum daily intake of 1 cup from the yellow/orange plant group. This would include carrots, sweet potato, squash and corn to help you reach your daily yellow-orange total.

Mushrooms

Mushrooms are another superfood, especially for vegans and vegetarians as they are abundant in the B vitamins and zinc which are of great nutritional value. Only a few types of mushrooms are edible, including field, portobello, truffle and shiitake varieties. They are low in calories and dense in micronutrients including B vitamins, zinc, selenium, copper, phenols and cancer-fighting antioxidants.[230] Mushrooms are considered a functional food which means that they play a role in human health beyond just nutrition.

Mushrooms are thought to be one of the most researched anti-cancer agents, hence the term 'medicinal mushrooms'. The shiitake mushroom has been singled out as being the most beneficial mushroom in human health and is thought to play a role in protecting against more than 200 conditions.

Shiitake mushrooms are rich in a unique alkaloid called eritadenine - a phytonutrient that inhibits the activity of an enzyme called angiotensin-converting enzyme. This enzyme is useful because it prevents unwanted constriction of blood vessels that causes high blood pressure and resultant vascular disease. You can understand why ancient civilisations called mushrooms the plant of immortality.

The anti-cancer benefits of shiitake mushrooms are thought to come from alpha and beta-glucans. These glucans are known to be 'host mediated' anti-cancer agents. What we mean by this is that they boost our immune function to help combat cancer. In particular they seem to boost natural killer cell and T cell function. Preliminary tests on animals have shown that beta-glucans can inhibit the spread of cancer. Some experts believe that if we fail to consume enough beta-glucans we become more susceptible to cancer. You can also get beta-glucans in whole grains (oats, barley) and nutritional yeast.

Eat mushrooms lightly cooked - raw mushrooms contain a toxin called agaritine that cooking destroys.[231]

In 2009, a study of Chinese women found that those who ate 15 mushrooms per month, along with 15 cups of green tea, had a whopping 90% reduction in breast cancer compared to women who didn't.[232] Clearly, it's an amazing superfood combination.

Garlic

Garlic use has been well documented by most major civilizations including the Egyptians, Greeks and Romans. There are even records of Hippocrates (the father of modern medicine) using garlic on his patients for healing. Garlic belongs to the allium family and is closely related to leeks, shallots and onions. Garlic is considered a superfood and features top of the list of anti-cancer foods listed in 2009 *Food Chemistry* journal.[233]

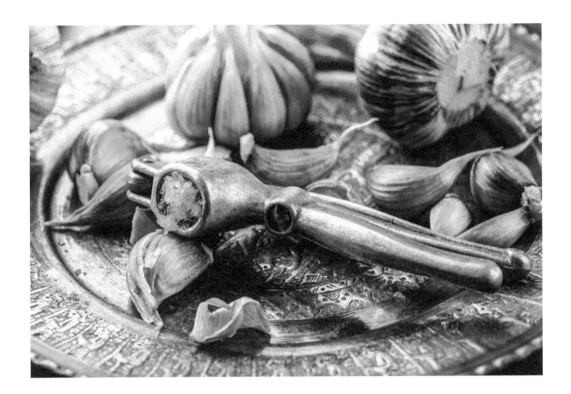

Garlic's health benefits are due to its sulfur compounds formed when it is chopped, crushed or chewed. Garlic is particularly helpful in reducing blood pressure, boosting immunity and reducing oxidation.

In one study, 600-1,500 mg of aged garlic extract was just as effective as the blood pressure drug Atenolol at reducing blood pressure over a 24-week period.[234] Studies using garlic supplements have also shown good effects against high blood pressure, high cholesterol and vascular-induced dementia.[235] It has even been shown to reduce heavy metal toxicity, with three doses of garlic a day outperforming the drug of choice D-penicillamine in reducing lead poisoning symptoms.[236] Believe me - food is medicine.

Legumes

Many people don't know what legumes are but they are a type of plant based food that come from the family Leguminosae. You would recognise them as kidney beans, soybeans, lentils, chickpeas and navy beans to name a few. The most famous legumes are baked beans! They are full of natural goodness including zinc, iron, folate, potassium and fibre and are low calorie sources of healthy fats, protein and fibre. One of the most comprehensive cancer studies published looked at over half a million studies and concluded that we should be eating either whole grains (unadulterated) or legumes (beans, chickpeas, split peas, lentils) at every meal to prevent cancer.[237] They have also been shown to reduce heart disease through reductions in total and LDL (bad) cholesterol.

Legumes have had a controversial history because they contain compounds called anti-nutrients such as phytic acid and lectins which can interfere with nutrient absorption. Proper preparation techniques can reduce the anti-nutrient load. Soaking them for 24 hours in water, straining them and then leaving them out to 'sprout' reduces anti-nutrient content significantly. Fermentation is another technique that reduces anti-nutrients.

If you need ideas then look at the recipe section at the end of this book. You can enjoy the avocado and beetroot hummus recipe for a serving of chickpeas at lunch time, or the cannellini bean wellington or the red lentil soup. All of these are delicious and will help you move towards increased consumption of beans.

Soya is a popular bean, but it is heavily processed and unfortunately most commercial soya is contaminated with GMOs nowadays. Try tempeh instead or edamame (young soya beans still in their pods). There are recipes for both at the end of the book. Lentils are a great choice because they are high in fibrous prebiotics and support your microbiome. Remember we are 10% human and 90% bugs! When sprouted, the antioxidant capacity of lentils doubles.[238] If you are running low on time then low salt tinned beans are considered a healthy option so always have them on hand in the cupboard. The benefit is that you don't need to pre-soak tinned beans and you still get the nutritional and cancer protection properties but in a convenient form.

How to soak beans, seeds and legumes

Inflammatory lectins and phytates need breaking up by soaking. Here's how to soak your nuts and seeds:

- — Pour water over the nuts, seeds or beans

- — Add 1 tablespoon Himalayan sea salt

- — Cover the bowl and let them soak for 6-8 hours

- — Rinse thoroughly to remove the salt

- — Spread them out to dehydrate

- — Dry them in a dehydrator or roast them in the oven at a low temperature

If you don't have the time then buy ready soaked nuts, seeds and beans.

Go Nuts

Countless studies show that people who regularly eat nuts have less incidence of cancer, heart disease and stroke.[239] They literally are nutritional powerhouses. Some studies have even shown that regular consumption of a handful of nuts can add up to two years to your life.[240] So you had better get eating some nuts! Nuts are great because they are a healthy source of fat and are packed with protein; they are the ideal snack for plant-based eaters who are in their ideal weight range. I wouldn't suggest anyone with weight issues eat too many nuts though as they are high in fat and energy dense. A number of large and reputable studies such as the PREDIMED study have shown that regular consumption of nuts can reduce the risk of stroke (by a massive 50%[241]) and heart disease.

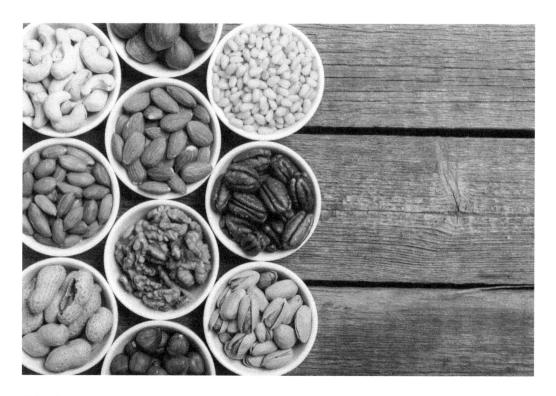

Of all nuts, walnuts seem to have the best health profile and cancer-preventing benefits. Your risk of cancer can be cut in half with only three servings of walnuts per week.[242] The antioxidants in walnuts are so remarkable that they have also been shown to reduce chemically-induced liver damage.[243] If you don't like the taste of walnuts, why not hide them in a salad dressing or sprinkle them on top of soups?

Macadamia nuts are also a great choice. They have roughly the same oleic acid levels as olives so they're a great snack for those who want to boost their heart and brain health.

Almonds are super rich in antioxidants, especially in their coat - a 200g portion contains as many polyphenols as a cup of green tea or a cup of steamed broccoli.[244] But almond production is incredibly water intense - it takes a gallon of water to grow each almond. You don't need me to tell you that this is totally unsustainable so try to eat almond alternatives. Over 82% of the world's almonds come from California, and the growing process uses so much water that it is putting the salmon in the Klamath River in jeopardy because of low water levels.

Almonds are the most consumed 'nut' in the world - we now consume ten times the amount of almonds that we did back in 1965 - and because of the trend for almond milk we now use 44% more land to farm almonds than we did ten years ago. Choose sustainable almonds or try and eat a diversity of different nuts, such as walnuts, pecans, pistachios and hazelnuts, to take the pressure off almonds for a while.

Just five Brazil nuts a day gives you your daily selenium, which can be hard to fulfil otherwise. Peanuts (technically a legume but often counted as a nut) are also superstars; they have high levels of folate that helps prevent the formation of beta-amyloid Alzheimer plaques in the brain and can prevent depression.

One word of caution, however: nuts are high in protein so don't overdo it. Most of us consume 2-3 times the amount of protein we need, which places an extra strain on our kidneys. In addition, commercial nuts are often bleached and chemically treated (e.g. pistachios) so buy organic nuts to avoid pesticides and chemical bleaches.

The very best way to eat nuts is to soak them. Soaking nuts reduces their phytic acid content that can block zinc, iron and calcium absorption. Most nuts should be soaked for 6-8 hours to reduce the phytic acid; the exception is macadamia nuts, as their levels are minimal.

Flaxseeds

Flaxseeds are powerful superfoods. The health benefits of flaxseeds are derived from three main factors - they are high in ALA omega 3, contain high levels of lignans and have high levels of soluble and insoluble fibre. A tablespoon of flaxseed contains roughly 1.8g of plant omega 3 and up to 800 times the lignans of other plant foods.[245]

Adding a few tablespoons of flaxseeds into your food each day can have profound health benefits. Flaxseeds are the richest vegetarian source of omega 3 but they also have a multitude of other health benefits including lowering blood pressure, reducing atherosclerosis, protecting against breast and prostate cancer,[246] reducing systemic inflammation, improving blood sugar (glycaemic) control[247] and improving triglyceride profile. That's a pretty magnificent superfood!

In a double-blind placebo-controlled randomised trial undertaken in 2013, flaxseeds were shown to work as well as the leading classes of blood pressure medications without any of the nasty side effects. The one-year trial gave participants either a placebo or 30g daily of flaxseed (concealed in foods). After six months the group that consumed 30g per day of flaxseeds saw their systolic blood pressure drop by an average of 10mmHg and their diastolic blood pressure drop by 8mmHg. The improvements were roughly equivalent to the results delivered by commercial blood pressure drugs and in real terms would result in 45% fewer strokes and 30% less heart disease.[248] This study confirms flaxseed's status as a superfood. In a Canadian study involving more than 6,000 people, those who ate flaxseeds regularly were 18% less likely to develop breast cancer.[249] And a large review of 27 studies involving more than 250,000 people published in the *American Journal of Clinical Nutrition* showed that those who ate higher amounts of dietary ALA experienced reduced risk of heart disease.[250]

Flaxseeds don't just have vascular benefits; they are high in phytoestrogens and have been linked to reduced breast cancer rates and reduced menopausal hot flushing.[251] A 2007 study looked at hot flushes in menopausal women and showed that two tablespoons of ground flaxseed added to food each day reduced their incidence by 57%. The women in the study reported the benefits started in the first week and peaked by two weeks. Other studies have been less conclusive but it's worth a shot if you suffer hot flushes and want to avoid HRT whilst also reducing your cancer risk!

Make sure you eat the whole flaxseed and not just the oil (which only contains part of the seed). The best way to get the benefits is to consume it as ground flaxseed or as 'flaxmeal', because if you eat the whole seeds, they can go through the body undigested. Ground flaxseeds can be sprinkled over salads, soups and placed (or concealed!) in virtually any meal to add texture, flavour and health benefits. Aim for 1-2 tablespoons of ground flaxseeds a day.[252]

Chia Seeds

Chia seeds are among the healthiest foods on the planet. 'Chia' is derived from the ancient Mayan word for 'strength'. Chia seeds have been consumed in abundance in parts of the world like Mexico and Central America for centuries. Recently they have experienced a boom in popularity in western countries because of their superfood and 'trendy' status.

Like flaxseeds, they are a superb source of vegetarian omega 3 and are loaded with nutrients, calorie for calorie. They are rich in fibre, magnesium, manganese, zinc, phosphorous and calcium. They contain abundant antioxidants and have a good balance of amino acids (the building blocks of tissue). Chia seeds are a great source of protein so for vegans and vegetarians, chia is a great option. Because of their high soluble fibre content (40% fibre), chia seeds can absorb 10-12 times their weight in water, filling your belly beautifully and leaving you with a deep and lasting sensation of fullness. In a double-blind randomised controlled trial of overweight type 2 diabetics, daily chia consumption was positively associated with significantly more weight loss compared with a placebo over a six-month period.[253]

As mentioned in the brain health chapter, chia seeds are a great source of tryptophan, an important and essential amino acid needed for serotonin production. Try the Mango Chia Seed Pudding in the Recipe Section for a fantastic antioxidant-rich breakfast or dessert option.

Grapes

Grapes contain anthocyanins, which are known to reduce inflammation. They also contain the much sought-after antioxidant resveratrol. Grapes are clinically evidenced to reduce the risk of several diseases, including heart disease, diabetes, Alzheimer's and eye disorders. It is thought that much of the positive health and cardiovascular benefits are derived from resveratrol.[254] The protective effects of resveratrol is thought to be why the French as a nation can smoke so much but still have low rates of cancer - because they drink lots of red wine! It is the red (not green) grape that contains the most resveratrol. In nature, as a general rule, the more colourful the plant the more micronutrient rich it is. So always choose colour when shopping.

Cherries

Cherries are rich in antioxidants such as anthocyanin and catechins, which fight inflammation and reduce free radical load. In one study when people ate 280g of cherries per day for a month their levels of inflammatory marker CRP reduced. Even more impressive is that their CRP levels stayed down for 28 days after they stopped eating cherries.[255]

Pomegranates

Pomegranates contain an abundance of beneficial and super-healthy micronutrients. They are rich in phytochemicals and are known to be potent antioxidants that are clinically evidenced to reverse some serious pathology, including atherosclerosis, cholesterol, inflammation, blood pressure and oxidative stress.[256] Pomegranates contain anthocyanins, catechins, quercetins and punicalagins - all of which act as powerful neutralisers of oxidative stress.

Studies have put pomegranates to the test with incredible outcomes. One study took patients with severe carotid artery blockages (a main artery that feeds the brain) and gave them 28g of pomegranate juice daily for one year. The participants experienced a 12% reduction in blood pressure and a 30% reduction in plaque. The participants who did not get the pomegranate juice daily experienced a negative 9% increase in carotid artery plaque. The carotid artery runs through the neck up into the brain to deliver vital oxygen and nutrients to the brain. Many strokes occur as a result of carotid artery blockage or narrowing due to plaque build-up so these impressive studies make pomegranate a wonderful and healthful addition to your daily diet.

Berries

Berries deserve special mention because they are one of the most powerful superfood groups out there. Eat them fresh when in season or straight from the freezer when out of season to benefit from their life extending nutrients. Berries do not lose their nutritional value when frozen so you can and indeed should eat them all year around.

Blueberries are powerful anti-ageing and anti-cancer allies. Try and eat one serving (a half cup) every day because they are rich in antioxidants, polyphenols and anthocyanins (these give blueberries their beautiful blue colour). The key health promoters in blueberries are phytochemicals, phenolic, anthocyanins, myricetins, quercetins and delphinidins. The great thing about blueberries is that they are native to Europe so we can eat them fresh and local and don't have to ship them halfway around the world, leaving a trail of diesel and carbon.

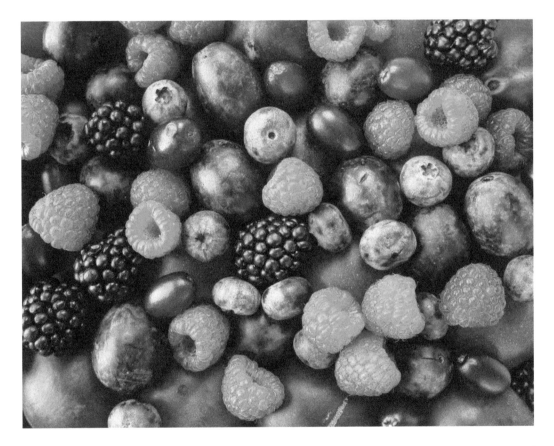

A 2008 study found that organic blueberries contain more phenols, anthocyanin and antioxidant capacity than conventional blueberries, so support your local organic farmers with your blueberry purchases. The darker the blueberry, the more antioxidants so choose dark, rich-coloured berries to enjoy.

Researchers at the Harvard School of Public Health reviewed the berry eating habits of 93,600 women between the ages of 25 and 42 over an 18-year period. The study (part of the Nurses' Health Study 2) showed that women who ate three or more servings of blueberries and strawberries each week reduced their risk of heart attacks by one third.[257] Women who ate other fruits and berries did not get the same cardiac benefits - so make sure you eat either blueberries or strawberries on a regular basis.

I love using blueberries in my daily smoothies. They cancel out some of the flavours of the greens like kale and spinach and give it a lovely creamy texture.

In a smaller trial, blueberries were found to lower blood pressure. The trial was a double-blind, placebo-controlled trial on 48 post-menopausal women with blood pressure problems (either pre-hypertension or hypertension). Every day, half the participants were given a cup of blueberries (freeze dried) and the other half received a placebo cup.

After just eight weeks on the trial the group who received the blueberries daily had significantly lowered their systolic (5.1%) and diastolic (6.3%) blood pressure. Those on the dummy or placebo dose experienced no change. In addition, the blueberries group experienced a 6.5% reduction in arterial stiffness and the placebo group experienced none. Arterial stiffness is relevant because it's a symptom of heart disease and a predictor of cardiovascular risk. The researchers in this small trial attributed the improvements in arterial wall thickness to a phenomenal 68.5% increase in nitric oxide, because nitric oxide helps to increase blood vessel flow and lower blood pressure. Those on the placebo dose had no change. Once again, we see the incredible benefits of super-nourishing foods on our health and wellness.

Another study published in the journal *Nutrition Research* found that daily blueberry consumption increases natural killer cells (NK cells) which are white blood cells that play a very important role in the body's immune defence against viruses and tumours.[258]

NK cells scan the body for abnormal cells and destroy them before they can develop into cancers. The study participants were divided into two groups. One received 250g of blueberries daily and the other a blueberry substitute. They all received their intervention in powder form so the placebo group weren't able to tell that they were not receiving blueberries. After only six weeks of daily blueberry consumption the blueberry group saw significant increases in their NK cell numbers and experienced reduced oxidative stress.[259] This has a huge knock-on effect on immunity. Without enough natural killer T-cells a minor infection can turn into something major and cancer can slip through the net. Hopefully I have convinced you to eat a daily portion of blueberries.

Strawberries are a superfood and a sustainable superfood at that. We grow them plentifully in the UK. Whenever we look at food we need to be thinking about sustainability and ensuring that our food choices are low impact for the planet. Strawberries have a very high anthocyanin content, which is anti-inflammatory and helps reduce oxidative stress, blood pressure and even improves our cholesterol profile. Eating just eight strawberries provides you with 120% of your daily vitamin C intake (higher than oranges) and an abundance of antioxidants and phytochemicals. Strawberries are a good source of potassium, which counters the effects of sodium in the body and helps to reduce blood pressure and related cardiovascular disease.

As well as anthocyanins, strawberries contain the flavonoids quercetin and kaempferol as well as ellagitannins, flavonols, fisetins, terpenoids, phenolic and ellagic acids that act as a defensive line against the development of cancers and tumours. For example, the flavonoid fisetin in strawberries can kill breast cancer cells without harming normal breast cells. Other studies show it can bring about programmed cell death in human colon and prostate cancer cells[260] and have significant activity against liver cancer cells.[261]

Per 100g, strawberries have minimal sugar and only 33 calories. For a guilt-free but indulgent snack try dipping strawberries into antioxidant-rich melted dark chocolate and cover with coconut flakes.

The UK strawberry industry is currently considered to be worth around £79m (2011) with around £45m of additional strawberries being imported from overseas each year. Strawberries are one of the most heavily sprayed foods and are featured regularly at the top of the Dirty Dozen. This is a list of heavily sprayed pesticide-laden fresh produce published by the Environmental Working Group. Strawberries frequently feature top of the list as the most contaminated fruit so only buy organic and local strawberries. Better still, go and pick your own strawberries and freeze them for the winter. Organic strawberry production currently only accounts for around 0.02% of the UK market so more needs to be done to make strawberries a sustainable, toxin-free option.

Acai berries are a Brazilian superfruit and an important part of the traditional diet of many indigenous tribes in the Amazon region. They grow on acai palm trees in the rainforests of Central and South America. Acai's most powerful health benefits come from its plant compounds, notably the anthocyanins that give it its deep purple colour. Besides being associated with cardiovascular health, acai berries have ten times the antioxidant capacity of grapes and three times that of blueberries. Per 100 grams of frozen pulp, acai has an antioxidant rating (ORAC) of 15,405 compared to blueberries at 4,669.[262] While no one food can act as a magic shield against cancer, some foods are known to stop cancer cells from forming and spreading. Acai is one of them. In test tube and mice studies it has been shown to have significant anti-cancer effects. It has been proven effective against colon cancer[263], bladder cancer[264] and breast cancer cells.[265] In addition, acai berries are profoundly neuro-protective and help boost memory and cognition. They also protect the brain against age-related degeneration.

In animal studies acai consumption has been shown to help a process called autophagy, where the brain cleans itself of toxins and debris. Acais are known to help support this vital brain function.[266] Acai also contains 19 different amino acids and fatty acids, making them great superfruit for your heart.[267]

Since fresh acai berries need to come all the way from the Amazon the best and most sustainable way to eat acai is as a puree or powder. Remember though that the more removed from the fresh fruit we get, the less the benefits. Look for a high-quality organic acai powder, harvested and produced in the right way.

Goji berries have the third most potent antioxidant effects of all the dried berries (pomegranates and barberries win!). Goji berries have had a long run in traditional medicinal therapies linked to longevity, strength, mood and sexual vigour. Studies show goji berries have beneficial activity for diabetics, are heart protective, can improve sexual function and benefit your brain.[268]

They are also a superfood for your vision because of an antioxidant called zeaxanthin which has been shown to protect against a common condition called macular degeneration.[269] Gojis have about fifty times the zeaxanthin of eggs so are a great option for vegans. Eat gojis in granola, sprinkled on salads or as a quick snack on their own. See our Goji Granola recipe for an easy, home-made, low-sugar option.

Avocado

Avocado is the fruit of the avocado tree, known as Persea Americana, and is often referred to as the 'alligator pear' because of its coarse outer shell. Avocados are highly nutritious fruits that are rich in healthy fats, fibre and contain over 20 different vitamins and minerals. Avocado contains more potassium than bananas and is loaded with heart-healthy monounsaturated fatty acids such as oleic acid, which reduces inflammation in the body. These are the same fats that are found in olive oil. In fact, 77% of the calories from one avocado comes from good fats making it one of the fattiest plant foods in existence. Oleic acid is clinically evidenced to reduce risk of heart disease, diabetes, metabolic syndrome and certain types of cancer. Several human studies have shown that avocados can help reduce total cholesterol[270], reduce blood triglycerides, lower LDL (bad) cholesterol and increase HDL (good) cholesterol[271].

In a 2013 study published in *Nutrition Journal,* avocado consumers were shown to have higher nutrient intakes, higher HDL (good) cholesterol, lower Body Mass Indexes (BMI) and less metabolic syndrome than non-avocado eaters[272]. Avocados also help you absorb fat soluble nutrients from other foods too, especially antioxidants like lycopene and carotenoids. A 2005 study from the *Journal of Nutrition* found that the addition of avocado enhanced lycopene and carotenoid absorption 4.4 and 2.6 times respectively[273]. So get eating avocados with your other favourite fruit and veg and know that their absorption will be vastly improved!

Avocados are amazing to cook with and give a recipe a luxurious, creamy and buttery texture. They are without doubt a fabulous and nutrient dense superfood and should feature regularly in your diet. They are also one of the 'cleanest' fruits, with fewer than 1% of conventional avocados testing positive for pesticides (EWG). A word of warning, however - from 2000 to 2015 global avocado consumption increased by over 400% to 4.25 billion avocados a year. This boom in avocado popularity has caused deforestation in Mexico, which is the biggest avocado producing country in the world. It takes 1000 litres of water to grow 1kg of avocados - by contrast, 1kg of broccoli uses only 45 litres of water. If you live in Europe it is much better to buy Spanish avocados that have travelled a lot smaller distance and are not contributing to the illegal pine forest deforestation in Mexico.

Avocados are also seasonal fruits so make sure you buy them when in season and eat walnuts, olive oil, anchovies and other healthy fats when the season ends. Buying Fairtrade avocados will also help by improving workers' conditions and remuneration.

Sweet potato

Sweet potatoes are an antioxidant and nutrient packed superfood grown all over the world. They are loaded with fibre, antioxidants, phytonutrients, vitamins and minerals which makes them great for combatting renegade free radicals that otherwise could damage your DNA. Studies have also found that the antioxidants found in sweet potatoes can promote the growth of healthy gut bacteria including Bifiobacterium and Lactobacillus species[274].

Vitamin A deficiency is a huge problem in many parts of the world causing many cases of premature blindness - including in children. Sweet potato consumption could help correct this because they are so rich in beta-carotene that readily converts to vitamin A. Beta-carotene is what gives sweet potato their characteristic bright orange colour. Just 200g of baked sweet potato provides more than seven times the amount of beta-carotene that an adult needs in a day.

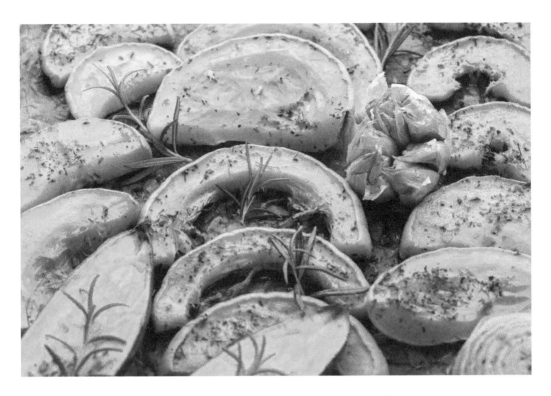

The anthocyanin (a group of antioxidants) found in abundance in sweet potatoes have been shown to slow the growth of certain cancer cells in test tube studies including bladder, colon, stomach and breast cancer cells. So sweet potatoes have an incredibly protective health effect. Their skin contains 16 times the antioxidants of the flesh so make sure you leave the skin on for your recipes to get the full nutritional benefits. Sprinkle sweet potatoes with turmeric and olive oil and bake them in the oven, serve with humous and you have a tasty and healthy instant super snack.

Kefir

Modern diets have virtually lost their probiotic content leaving our guts perilously low in healthy bacteria. Kefir is a yoghurt-like fermented drink and is a wonderful source of probiotics. It can be found in dairy-free forms such as coconut kefir for those who are vegan or intolerant of dairy. I love to add coconut kefir to my daily smoothie for an instant gut boost.

Depending on how it's made kefir may deliver up to 30 different yeasts and live bacterial strains including the major strain *Lactobacillus*. Studies are now emerging linking obesity and inability to lose weight to poor gut health so get eating some gut-healthy superfoods. Other great choices are sauerkraut, kimchi, tempeh, pickles, natto and miso. See our Superfood 'Superbug' Smoothie recipe or our Miso Roast Aubergine with Tempeh recipe for great gut-boosting food inspiration.

Herbs and Spices

Herbs and spices are powerful anti-cancer allies. It is really important that you learn to cook with herbs and spices (instead of salt!) because their health benefits are so profound. Herbs and spices deliver high levels of life-affirming antioxidants and help create incredibly rich food flavours. Once you master using herbs and spices in your foods nothing will taste bland.

Turmeric has potent anti-cancer and anti-inflammatory benefits and has been used for centuries in Ayurvedic medicine and cooking in Asia. It is made significantly more bioavailable with the addition of black pepper and healthy fats.[275] For example, studies have shown that a quarter of a teaspoon of black pepper increases its bioavailability by 2000%.[276] Turmeric has huge benefits for both body and brain and is a great example of Hippocrates' 'Let food be thy medicine'. The active medicinal compound in turmeric is curcumin. Most studies on the health benefits of turmeric use concentrated extracts of curcumin. Curcumin is a strong anti-inflammatory and competes with some of our best pharmaceuticals for reduction of inflammation but without the side effects of gastric irritation and bleeds.[277] Without getting too heavily into the science, curcumin blocks NF-kB, a molecule that travels into your cells and switches on genes related to inflammation. This is significant because NF-kB is believed to play a major role in all the chronic inflammatory diseases.

Curcumin is bioactive at the molecular level for oxidation. This means that it is a powerful antioxidant that delivers simultaneous blows to the oxidation cycle. Firstly, it blocks free radicals directly and secondly, it stimulates your body's own antioxidant defences, making it a powerhouse for tissue protection and anti-ageing.[278]

Curcumin is also a brain booster with the ability to support BDNF brain protein levels. This helps protect the brain against deficiencies that can cause depression and Alzheimer's.[279] By influencing BDNF, it may be effective at preventing and even reversing brain pathology and disease.

Another major benefit of curcumin is its anti-angiogenesis effect. Angiogenesis describes the way tumours and cancers ingeniously develop their own blood supply to survive. Multiple studies indicate that curcumin can reduce the growth of cancerous cells in the laboratory and inhibit the growth of tumours in test animals. Even more exciting is its potential anti-cancer action in humans - curcumin has been shown to help reduce pre-cancerous colon lesions by up to 40% with a 4g daily dose.[280]

Obviously more research needs to be done but curcumin holds incredible health potential. I generally take curcumin as a supplement because in turmeric, the curcumin content is only about 3%.[281] It would be very difficult to reach the concentrated levels used in clinical trials using just the turmeric spice in your foods, although I recommend you do this anyway.

A supplement helps tap into the benefits better with a more concentrated dose. Make sure it has black pepper in it to increase bioavailability. Another great way is to have it in turmeric matcha tea - one cup of this tea is equivalent to about fifteen green teas. Another powerful combination!

Oregano, which can be used in most dishes, is an antioxidant-rich herb with anti-inflammatory and anti-cancer benefits. It is a culinary and medicinal herb from the Lamiaceae (mint) family. In one study oregano was found to inhibit colon cancer cells[282] and in another study it inhibited colon cancer cell growth.[283] Oregano is also a great anti-inflammatory and is easy to add into your diet.

Other herbs and spices with powerful health benefits are **ginger, sage, parsley, chilli, cayenne pepper, cumin, rosemary, mint** and **cinnamon.** They all have anti-inflammatory and anti-oxidant benefit and have been used in the human diet for centuries. All our recipes at the end of this book feature lovely herbs and spices to try and help you get them into your foods regularly. They all deliver a huge number of diverse micronutrients and have dwindled considerably from our modern diet. Get back in the kitchen and start experimenting with their flavours and tastes. It really will be good for you!

Spirulina

Gram for gram, spirulina may well be the most nutritious superfood on the planet. It is simply amazing and is one of nature's most perfect foods. Spirulina is a highly nutritious biomass of cyanobacteria, a type of blue green algae eaten by native Africans and Americans and is packed with vitamins, minerals, high quality protein (with ALL the essential amino acids) and omega 3 yet is very low in calories. It became famous after is was used by NASA as a supplement for Astronauts. It is a freshwater plant that gets its colour from its main active, the phytopigment phycocyanin. Phycocyanin protects the brain, heart and immune system and is a wonderful antioxidant.

Several studies have shown that 1-2g of daily spirulina consumption is associated with up to 16% reduction in LDL cholesterol and 10% triglyceride reductions - both huge positives for lowering heart disease risk.[284] Research in animal models also shows that it can reduce tumour growth rate and tumour size.[285] [286] Spirulina's effect on cancers of the mouth have been particularly well studied and show an exciting potential for regression. A study in rural Southern India looking at precancerous oral lesions in pan tobacco chewers in Kerala showed that consumption of 1g of spirulina per day completely reversed 45% of the supplemented subject's lesions.[287] This is exciting stuff.

Spirulina has also been used to shield from and treat radiation excess and is highly effective for heavy metal detoxification. Phycocyanin is a nitrogen storage molecule and the nitrogen atoms can bind heavy metals (caesium-137, strontium-90, and potassium-40) and cleanse the body of radioactive metals. Because of its ability to help reduce radioactive substances, children who had unintentional radiation exposure after the Chernobyl disaster were treated with a 5g per day dose of spirulina. It accelerates the evacuation of radionuclides from the human body and is particularly effective at reducing radioactive caesium.[288] Now that to me is a truly remarkable superfood.

Spirulina is best taken as an organic powder or tablet. Choose organic because certain harvests are heavily contaminated due to the Japanese Fukushima event.

I add organic spirulina into my daily smoothie - you can find a great Vitality Smoothie recipe at the end of the book. If you want a great superfood powder with all of these things in then try Superfoods Blend available from www.zenii.co.uk. I know it's a high quality (and organic) supplement because I created it! It has a blend of 35 organic whole superfoods (greens, berries, veg, flaxseeds, turmeric, spirulina and broken cell wall chlorella) in a vegan powder formulation. A smoothie powder makes it easy to get every micronutrient box ticked daily, especially on days that you don't eat as well as you'd like.

Chlorella

Chlorella is another great marine superfood. It is sourced from freshwater algae and deserves special mention because it's loaded with antioxidants and vitamins but is also a uniquely powerful detoxification aid. It is especially active against heavy metals (such as mercury), chemicals and pesticides in the digestive tract which, if left in situ, can intoxicate the blood stream. Chlorella is a true multi-tasker and boosts the immune system,[289] improves blood sugar control,[290] promotes better metabolism,[291] improves brain function[292] and helps detoxify heavy metals.[293] [294] In mice studies, mice given chlorella along with methylmercury were found to excrete almost twice the amount of methylmercury in their urine and faeces as those not treated with chlorella.

The best way to take this powerful supergreen is as a powder or capsule - this way you can get an accurate dose and conceal the slightly bitter taste. About 3-6g a day is ideal for mercury detoxification but start slowly and work up to that. Your ideal dose depends on your age and weight. You can add it to virtually anything like mashed avocado, smoothies, porridge, coconut bursts and protein balls. Make sure you buy organic chlorella with a broken cell wall so it can be digested, otherwise you are throwing your money away.

Cacao and Cocoa

Despite the similarities in their spelling, cacao and cocoa are two very different ingredients. All chocolate products that we eat are derived from cacao seeds in some form or another, which are derived from the cacao plant. The cacao plant is an evergreen tree that grows in South America and parts of West Africa.

Cacao is a pure form of chocolate that comes very close to the raw and natural state, whereas cocoa is processed and roasted with high heat.

Cacao is a true superfood, containing more antioxidants than blueberries, but it has a strong aftertaste that is bitter, a bit like eating coffee beans. The higher the cacao in a dark chocolate, the more bitter the taste. The higher the cacao percentage the healthier it is because there's less space for additional ingredients like sugar. Dark chocolate containing more than 75% cacao delivers great antioxidant benefits. Just a few pieces will suffice though (!!) otherwise the benefits are outweighed by too much sugar. Cacao contains flavanols, a form of antioxidant. 100g of 75-85% contains 11g of fibre, 67% of your daily iron, 58% daily magnesium and 98% of your daily manganese. It also has the very important iron, zinc and selenium. One recent study showed that cacao and dark chocolate had more antioxidant activity, polyphenols and flavanols than fruits that were tested, including the super-potent blueberries and acais.[295] The flavanols in cacao can also stimulate the endothelium lining of vessels to produce nitric oxide (NO) which is extremely beneficial for vascular health. Nitric oxide sends signals for blood vessels to relax, reducing blood pressure and preventing arterial stiffness.[296]

Green Tea

Green tea is one of the healthiest drinks on the planet and should definitely feature in any longevity and anti-cancer diet. I try to drink at least three cups a day. I don't have a natural fondness for green tea but the more often you drink it, the better it tastes. It helps to remind yourself of its health benefits as you are drinking it, so any taste is counteracted by a positive mental surge. Green tea contains the anti-cancer phytonutrients catechins so it's about 15 times more powerful in antioxidant activity than blueberries are. It is evidenced to reduce heart disease, cancer, obesity and Alzheimer's disease.[297] [298]

Most of its benefits comes from its antioxidant and anti-inflammatory capacity, especially a substance called epigallocatechin-3-gallate (EGCG). EGCG inhibits inflammation by reducing cytokine production (pro-inflammatory)[299] and reduces damage to the protective fatty acids in the cells.[300] EGCG and other antioxidants found in green tea act in very specific ways to prevent cancer cells from growing. EGCG does this is by triggering the activity of so-called pro-death proteins, causing cancer cells to commit apoptosis or 'suicide'.

It also inhibits angiogenesis which is where cancer cells develop their own blood supply. If they cannot do this, they cannot spread and grow. Studies show that EGCG prevents the expression of a growth factor that is necessary for new blood vessels to form and grow.

Just remember, however, that green tea is high in caffeine so it might not be suitable for everyone. There are decaffeinated versions available but make sure these are organic. Clipper Organic Fairtrade Green Tea is my favourite high street brand.

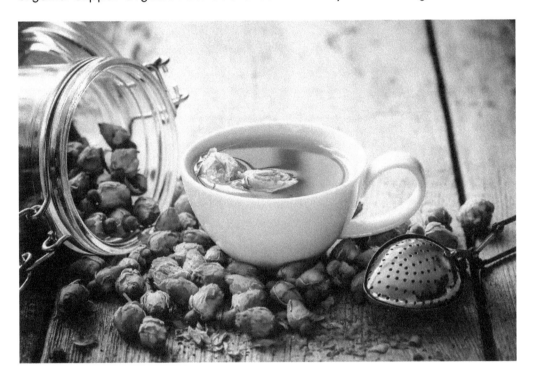

Other beverages

Nothing beats plain filtered water as a daily drink, but lemon water and fruit teas are also healthful options. It goes without saying that we need to drink water plentifully. Our bodies are 70% water and water hydrates our cells, eliminates toxins, aids digestion, regulates temperature, lubricates joints and helps support our liver and kidneys - two of the body's most important detox organs.

Choose these options over fruit juices and fizzy drinks. Juices are high in sugar, which we all get too much of anyway, and sodas often either have a lot of sugar in them or chemical/ artificial sweeteners that are linked to cancers in animal studies.

A note about oils

Despite what we have heard for years, vegetable oils are not healthy. Manufacturers have played on the word 'vegetable' to make us think these oils are a healthy option, but they are not. Throw them all out right now. During the 20th century, consumption of vegetable oils increased by 130% in the US, largely due to subsidies making them cheap and easy to produce. Unlike olive and coconut oil, vegetable and seed oils are often extracted from foods using solvents like hexane, which is a component of gasoline. In addition to being highly processed and damaged at high temperatures, they also promote inflammation because of their high omega 6 content. If you need to use an oil then use coconut oil, extra virgin olive oil or avocado oil.

Some foods do need an oil so use one of these three, but don't pour it on anything and everything. Try using stock or water as an oil substitute to keep things from sticking to the pan and if you need extra moisture in a dish then try delicious alternatives like blueberries, bananas, medjool dates, pineapple, avocado and prunes. These can all help maintain the moisture content of foods and prevent that 'stick to the roof of your mouth' kind of dryness!

CHAPTER 14: What to Aim For

The important thing to aim for is to reduce insulin resistance, reduce systemic inflammation, reduce oxidation, reduce cortisol (stress hormone), reduce toxin exposure, reduce processed foods and get moving!

If you have cancer then be even more vigilant and aim for at least 10 different superfoods servings per day. Diversity and variety is key. In order for cancer to be diagnosed there will already be trillions of cancer cells established. Anything that can help reduce the total cancer load and boost antioxidant capacity is going to be extremely helpful.

DIET

Eat organic - and avoid GMO's. Glyphosate is the most widely used agrochemical in the UK and the rest of the world. It is known to disrupt gut microbiota[301] and can cause certain cancers in cases of toxic exposure.[302] Unfortunately, in 2017 the EU extended the license for glyphosate for five years. 30% of UK breads have been shown to have glyphosate in them. [303] Glyphosate (one of the UK and USA's main agricultural herbicides) inhibits cytochrome P450 activity - enzymes that are produced by gut bacteria and are vital in our liver detoxification pathways. If the P450 pathway is significantly impaired, then we have a much higher risk of toxin accumulation. These chemicals irritate and excite the immune system. Don't forget to choose organic drinks as well - many beverages and wines are now heavily contaminated with pesticides and chemicals.

Eat low GI - excess sugar damages every tissue and organ in the body and drives insulin resistance.

Eat an abundance of local and seasonal plant foods - aim for 10 different varieties a day. Eat a colourful rainbow of fresh foods and berries (blueberries, strawberries, blackberries, gojis...). Eat a daily dose of greens like kale, broccoli, collards, leeks, spinach, onions and garlic.

Eat whole foods rather than processed foods. Processed foods are full hidden sugars, salt, chemicals, preservatives, transfats and more. In the UK currently 50% of the foods we eat are processed. This needs to change. We need to embrace whole foods in their natural state and move away from lab created toxin filled foods.

Eat gut healthy foods e.g. live yoghurt, kimchi, tempeh, miso - these help repopulate the gut with beneficial bacterial and help to repair the gut wall lining to reduce seepage of toxins causing inflammatory cascade (leaky gut syndrome). If you cannot stomach these then supplement with a high dose, high calibre probiotic.

Avoid fizzy drinks (even the diet variety) and juices. Studies have shown that sugary drinks are the single largest source of sugar and calories in the US diet. Avoid energy drinks too. They contain copious amounts of caffeine which interrupts your neuroendocrine-immune system.

Avoid trans fats - Trans fats (look for 'partially hydrogenated oil' on the label) - raise LDL (bad) cholesterol which causes inflammation. There is no safe amount of trans fats so steer clear.

Avoid processed, cured and BBQed meats. If you eat meat, eat only small amounts of organic grass-fed meats and wild-caught fish. Mass produced meat, poultry, dairy and farmed fish can bioaccumulate toxins in their tissue and fat. Humans, being at the top of the food chain, then consume these toxins in high concentrations. In short, we consume all the chemicals that have been used along the entire agricultural food chain. This can include antibiotics, pesticides, dioxins, hormones and GMOs. Incidentally, many of the studies proving GMOs to be safe for human consumption have been conducted by the very corporations that produce and sell them! Human studies have shown that IGF-1 is 13% lower in vegans and vegetarians than meat eaters. IGF-1 is related to inflammatory damage in tissues.[304] [305] Meat eaters also produce Trimethylamine-N-Oxide (TMAO), a metabolite that promotes heart disease.[306]

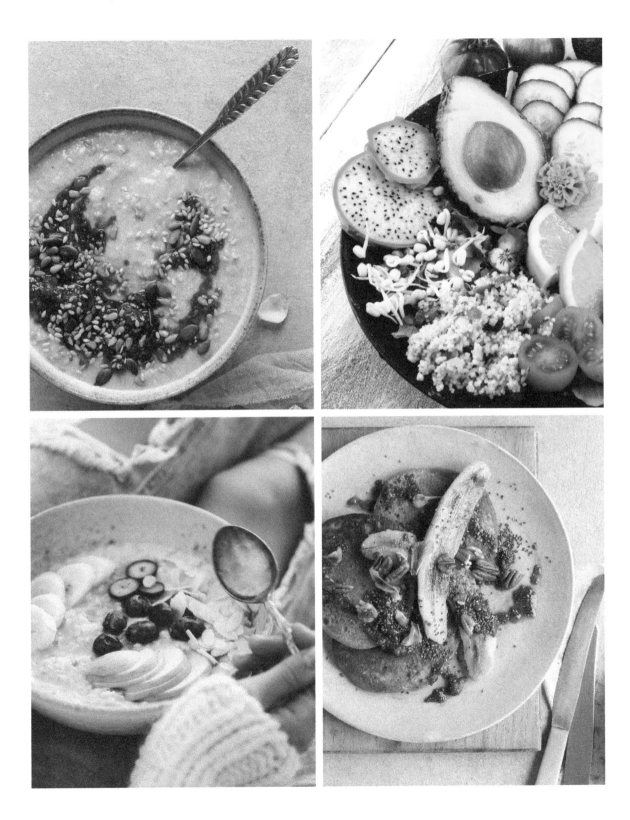

Drink organic green tea, hot lemon water and herbal teas as your hot beverage of choice. Green tea, black tea and coffee are all rich in polyphenols - drink these alongside water as your beverage of choice. Limit coffee to two cups a day. This seems to be the sweet spot where health benefits are gained (coffee protects against Alzheimer's & dementia)[307] without the negative effects of caffeine overstimulating the body's natural stress response and adrenal system.

Drink filtered water. Filtering water removes chlorine, arsenic, lead, hormones and pharmaceutic residues. Another option is water with lemon in it. Citric acid from lemons helps detoxify the body. I drink a hot lemon water every morning for this reason. Remember you can kill a goldfish (we've all done it) with tap water just because of its chlorine content. The Environmental Protection Agency (EPA) sets safe levels of chlorine at four parts per million but even this is harmful to our gut. The EPA has estimated that Americans now consume many times the safe level of chlorine in their tap water.[308] High levels of chlorine in drinking water can cause headaches, dizziness, increased risk of heart attack and cancer (gastrointestinal, bladder and rectal).[309] [310]

Reduce salt and use turmeric, garlic and other herbs and spices in your foods for taste. Herbs and spices are the most antioxidant-rich food category so use them to add flavour.

Avoid sugar in desserts, donuts, pastries. Refined carbohydrates (white bread, pastries, cereals, cakes, snack bars) - are high pre-sugar sugar and frequent consumption results in uncontrolled blood sugar, insulin resistance and cardio-metabolic syndrome.

Reduce dairy and use dairy alternatives. Dairy consumption for many is inflammatory.

Eat more omega 3-rich foods or supplement omega 3 (fish oil or algal oil).

Eat more fibre (aim for 30g per day). It protects against colon cancer and works as a prebiotic in the gut. Plant based foods are rich in fibre.

Ensure adequate intake of vitamins and minerals - vitamin B6, B12, vitamin C, vitamin D3, Vitamin E, iron, folate, zinc, selenium & magnesium.

Eat less rather than more. Try to calorie restrict. Get expert guidance from a Nutritionist if you are going down this route with cancer or any chronic disease.

Exclude growth promoters where possible - dairy, insulin, female sex hormones e.g. pill, HRT.

Do everything you can to avoid diabetes and getting fat. Obesity and diabetes carry an increased cancer risk. Insulin is a growth promoter too, so try and minimise your insulin doses by improving your diet. You will need your doctor's help and careful supervision for this but it will be well worth it.

Supplementing antioxidants

To boost co-enzyme Q10, take 250-500mg Q10 per day or as Ubiquinone.

To boost glutathione levels, take L Glutathione 250-500mg per day and selenium 150mcg at night.

To boost superoxide dismutase try SkinAx or consider taking copper 1mg AM, manganese 2mg lunch time, zinc 10mg PM.

To boost vitamin D, take D3 or cholecalciferol 2,000-5,000iu per day until blood levels of 75-150nmol/l. People with darker skin types and with higher body mass may need higher doses.

Other important antioxidants are vitamin C, vitamin E and vitamin A, all of which can be supplemented if low or sub-optimal.

Intelligent Supplementation

• • • • • • • • • • • • • • • • • • • •

Whole foods will always trump isolated nutrients but in some cases it is sensible & beneficial to supplement.

Vitamin D - beneficial to all, especially in the winter months when we cannot manufacture our own vitamin D from sunlight. Aim for Vitamin D3 1000iu.

Zinc - often low in plant based eaters. Zinc is required in an astounding number of cellular processes and is essential for cell division, growth, repair, immunity & skin health.

Omega 3 - universally beneficial. Vegetarians & vegans convert ALA to DHA & EPA weakly so it's important to supplement. Vital for brain, skin & cellular health. Try sustainable fish oil or algal oil.

Vitamin B12 - an essential supplement for plant based diets. Failing to take enough B12 in a plant based diet can be catastrophic for your health. Look for methylated B12 for better bioavailability.

LIFESTYLE

Exercise 5-7 hours per week

Maintain a BMI of less than 25 and keep waist circumference < 80cm for women and < 94cm for men. Carrying excess body weight results in higher levels of hormones like oestrogen (which is a growth promoter) and inflammation.

Practise daily stress management like meditation, yoga and massage. Stress is linked to higher inflammatory markers and cancer proliferation so it's important to learn to manage and control stress.

Sleep well - aim for eight hours. Sleep is healing and helps the body repair from molecular damage.

Ensure good antioxidant status. Antioxidants are your big protective players at the cellular level. They are vital for protection against oxidation, inflammation and tissue ageing.

Don't smoke/vape. Cigarettes contain thousands of chemicals and trigger all kinds of cancers because smoke is an irritant and a carcinogen. Vaping is just smoking reinvented. It contains many unknown chemicals that can irritate lung tissue.

Get a Fitbit and aim for a minimum of 10,000 steps each day.

Use a sauna and far-infrared (FIR) sauna for detoxification. Aim for little and often so 15-20 minutes several times a week. Most chemicals are sweated out in the first 20 minutes.[311] Sauna use is evidenced to help sweat out toxins and heavy metals such as mercury. Use Epsom salts in the bath if you cannot regularly use a sauna.

Avoid air pollution and toxic metals, volatile organic compounds (VOCs), pesticides and noxious gases.

Avoid known household and environmental toxins/carcinogens - numerous cleaning products, cosmetics, fragrances, antibacterial (triclosan) hand washes and many other household products contain toxins.

Practise safe sun. Use a daily SPF as UV radiation is a significant cause of cancer.

Take supplemental vitamin c, vitamin D3, omega 3, probiotics, Q10, zinc, magnesium, iron and multivitamins if needed.

Surround yourself with a positive network of people. We know that the mind and the body are inter-connected - there is no division between them. What you think has as much impact as what you do and what you are.

Nurture soulfulness or spirituality. Find moments of peace in your day - we live in a noisy world!

Take regular holidays from work. Rest and relaxation are vital.

Avoid unnecessary medications e.g. antibiotics, hormones (the pill, HRT). Female sex hormones have been classified as class one carcinogens by the World Health Organisation (WHO).

Avoid unnecessary radiation such as X-rays or CT scans. Radiation is an obvious cancer risk and the medical profession is responsible for huge doses. Ensure you are aware of the dose of radiation of any medical test you undergo (especially CT scans).

CHAPTER 15: What Else Can We Do to Super Boost Our Longevity?

Exercise is vitally important for your health and once you have readjusted your diet it is the next thing to optimise. Whilst you can't outrun a bad diet, exercise certainly complements a good diet and helps redirect your health destiny. Exercise is so important that if there were a way to prescribe exercise everyone would be prescribed it. The benefits of exercise are so wide-reaching and profound that it cannot be underestimated.

Humans were made to move but in the last hundred years our levels of movement have declined so much that many people's lives have become sedentary. That means they move little, spend long hours sitting at desks, drive everywhere, don't exercise and then sleep and repeat it all over again.

A hundred years ago, people got more than five times the exercise that the modern Brit or American gets in a day and movement was blended into daily life. My definition of a couch potato is doing less than thirty minutes of exercise five times a week. I suspect then that many people are couch potatoes. At times in my life I also have been a couch potato, but not anymore!

Professor Bauman from the University of Sydney makes an interesting comment about modern life: 'We don't expend energy doing anything anymore. We've actually engineered regular daily physical activity out of our lives'. This is highly worrying given that the health benefits of exercise are so profound and physical inactivity takes such a huge toll on our health.

Studies have shown that if you work full time in an office job, you sit an average of 13 hours a day. Add this to your 8 hours of sleep and you are sedentary for 21 hours a day! This has a negative impact on posture, cardiovascular health, bone health, mitochondrial health and brain health. We have to make exercise and movement a part of our daily life. With 25% of the UK adult population obese we have a huge crisis on our hands and we have to understand that we simply must move more.

Physical activity is one of the strongest predictors for successful ageing. Time and time again studies show that regular exercise improves long term cognitive and executive function, heart health, bone health, muscle health and mental health. It also reduces the risk of diabetes and cancer and improves cancer remission rates for those already diagnosed.[312] [313]

Much of modern life is spent sitting down - in cars, trains, planes, at desks, in cafes and restaurants. Sitting is really bad for our health so much so that it is becoming a public health problem. Humans were meant to move and be in a constant state of motion. Our sedentary lives totally contradict our body's design. When we engineer movement out of our lives we suffer a myriad of problems, both physical and mental, as a consequence - lower back pain, neck pain, arthritis, osteoporosis, heart disease, diabetes, obesity, low mood, depression and anxiety are all made worse by lack of movement.

Exercise also releases neurotransmitters - positive chemicals that condition our hearts, brains, psyche and other cognitive functions in positive ways. It helps us sleep better, function better and perform better and improves our mental health and wellbeing.[314]

Worldwide, nearly 31% of the world's population is physically inactive. The problem is that once you become physically inactive a sense of inertia sets in and it becomes incredibly difficult to return to physical activity. Our minds trick us into thinking that movement isn't what we were designed to do but it couldn't be further from the truth. If we look at Blue Zones, we see that the people who live the longest lives on this planet incorporate physical movement into their daily lives. Even those in their advanced years still move! They don't run around gyms or jog on treadmills, but they toil and work the land and walk many miles a day tending to their daily tasks. Physical activity is linked to vitality, metal clarity and longevity - ignore it at your peril.

Physical inactivity is linked to:

- Insulin resistance and type 2 diabetes[315]

- Higher rates of cardiovascular disease[316]

- Higher rates of breast, colon, endometrial and prostate cancer[317]

- Immune deficiency[318]

- Increased incidence of low mood and anxiety disorders[319]

- Reduction in bone health and increased rates of osteoporosis[320]

- Cognitive decline e.g. Alzheimer's and dementia[321]

- Accelerated ageing and increased organ deterioration[322]

EXERCISE AND CANCER

Exercise and cancer have long had an established link. Individuals who exercise have been found to have significantly lower rates of breast and colon cancer. Exercise also helps keep your weight down and this indirectly helps reduce cancer rates because we know now that obesity and carrying excess weight is the second most prevalent risk factor for cancer after smoking (WHO). Studies have shown that obesity accounts for over 20% of cancers in women and 14% of cancers in men. Regular movement is an essential part of an anti-cancer and wellness lifestyle. The positive benefits of exercise and how it relates to cancer cannot be ignored.

Several studies have now shown that even modest improvements in physical activity reduce the risk of developing cancer. In 2003, an epidemiological study found a link between physical activity of 30-60 minutes per day and a 30-40% reduced risk in colon cancer and 20-30% reduced risk for breast cancer.[323] This is massive. We don't even have any drugs that can do this. And if there was a drug, we would all be signing up for it. Ironically, exercise is free - but we fail to take advantage of it. Physical activity down-regulates and turns off genes that promote cancer growth and turns on genes that prevent cancer growth.[324] [325]

Karen Mustian, PhD and leader in the field of exercise oncology at the University of Rochester, notes that 80% of the cancer sufferers who enlist with her are sedentary at the outset. 'Nearly 15 years ago, when we started this work, a lot of people believed it wasn't even safe for most cancer patients to exercise,' she says.

'But now we know that exercise is a positive tool and can help survivors live longer, enjoy a better quality of life and avoid recurrence.'

The benefits of exercise if you have cancer are:

- Exercise reduces inflammation and protects against cognitive side effects of chemotherapy such as memory loss.[326]

- Exercise helps to improve the overall quality of life of cancer sufferers within four weeks.[327]

- Exercise helps to improve immunity in cancer patients.[328]

- Yoga[329]and Tai Chi[330] help to improve mental health, stress, fatigue and anxiety in cancer patients.

- Exercise improves all-cause survival rates for cancer.

- Exercise works better than medications to reduce cancer related fatigue, the most common side effect of any cancer treatment.[331]

Many things count as physical exercise including walking, gardening, dancing and yoga. They all bring huge benefits.

Lack of exercise is linked to obesity and linked particularly to colon cancer, post-menopausal breast cancer, oesophageal cancer, kidney cancer, gallbladder and uterine cancer. Women who gain weight or who are overweight during diagnosis and treatment of breast cancer are consistently shown to have poorer outcomes than those who maintain a healthy weight.[332] The proposed mechanism of poorer mortality rates is thought to be due to a combination of increased secretion of Insulin Like Growth Factor (IGF-1), elevated sex hormones and elevated pro-inflammatory cytokines.[333] These are all chemical messengers in the body that are adversely linked with breast cancer survival rates. Exercise is also a powerful systemic anti-inflammatory, so it helps lower total body inflammation - a known risk factor for all western diseases, including cancer. So now you know all this, isn't it time you start incorporating daily exercise into your routine? It could save your life.

EXERCISE AND HEART DISEASE

The 2015 British Heart Foundation Physical Activity campaign had a powerful punchline: 'Fight for every heartbeat'. They were trying to make the UK public understand just how important exercise is for our cardiovascular health. One of its key findings was that in the UK, 44% of adults never do any moderate physical activity. Alongside the significant health burden, this kind of regular physical inactivity costs the NHS more than £900 million.[334]

Vascular health depends on exercise. Exercise strengthens the muscles in your body, most importantly your heart. Exercise helps your heart muscle become more efficient and better able to pump blood throughout your body. An active, healthy heart pushes out more blood with each heartbeat, allowing it to beat slower and keep your blood pressure under control. Exercise also increases your levels of HDL cholesterol (the 'good' cholesterol) that lowers heart disease risk. Exercise also increase the body's production of nitric oxide, the magic molecule that protects endothelial health. Physical activity can be as beneficial to your heart as medication - and far safer. All it takes is 30 minutes per day. If you can take a 15-minute coffee break every day, then you can take a 15-minute exercise break. Start with this and then slowly increase over time.

MENTAL HEALTH AND EXERCISE

Without doubt, exercise is therapy. It is especially therapeutic for the brain. Exercise is one of the best natural anti-inflammatories that can help combat virtually every disease in the book. You are abandoning your body if you deprive it of daily physical activity. Such is the importance of movement to our mental and physical health.

It is fundamentally important if you are suffering from stress or low mood that you find time for movement in your day. If it's hard to do it initially then start slowly and make a 6-week plan that increases your activity gradually.

Get a pedometer and aim for a minimum of 10,000 steps a day. Grab a friend and exercise with them. Join a gym. Buy a cross trainer. Walk a dog. If you haven't got a dog, borrow a dog. Take the kids to the park. Borrow some kids to take to the park! Play tennis. Learn squash. Do some gardening. Walk to work. Cycle to work. Do walking meetings. Get up and walk around the office hourly. Get more active with your partner in the bedroom - that counts too! Do anything in your power to get moving daily because how long you live and how much you enjoy your later life depends on it.

Overhaul your lifestyle to make time to move. It feels good and it's so great for you:

- Aim for a minimum of 10,000 steps per day (a FitBit makes monitoring this easy).

- Aim for at least 30 minutes of aerobic exercise, five times per week.

- Run around in the park with your children, partner, family or friends.

- Walk to school / work or start a daily walk.

- Try a 'walking meeting' with colleagues.

- Walk rather than taking the car.

- Take the stairs, not the lift or escalator.

- Get a cross trainer or something in the home that you can use for movement on days you can't get to the park or gym.

- Do anything to get your heart rate up 4-5 times a week - housework counts!

- Try yoga and Pilates for core strengthening and resistance - they also help realign your thoughts and restore a sense of inner calm. Your body and mind are deeply connected.

THE DAILY 12

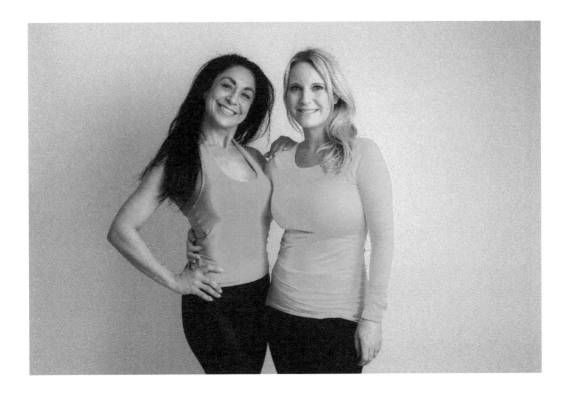

Dee Jones is my personal trainer, yogi and all-round muse. She has helped me get active and helped me find clever ways of getting exercise into my daily life. Her love of exercise is infectious and she is a testament to the incredible benefits of movement in life. Dee and I work together on my fitness and she designed some stretches for me to do every morning because once I turned 40, I found myself feeling incredibly stiff. I call them my Daily 12. Try them yourself. Hold each one for 30 seconds to a minute and see how much stronger, more supple and better you feel.

Ideally try and get a mixture of different kinds of exercise into your week. 2 -3 sessions of cardio a week, 1-2 weight training sessions and some restorative yoga or Pilates and long nature walks.

Daily 1 This neck stretch relieves a tight, sore neck. It's a great stretch if you sit at a desk or look at screens a lot.	**Daily 2** Pectoralis major, minor and anterior deltoid stretch. This will help to relieve tight chest muscles. This stretch also opens the rib cage and allows for freer breathing.
Daily 3 Known as 'triangle pose' in Pilates and yoga. It's a deep hip flexor stretch which relieves tight hips. A great stretch if you sit at a desk all day.	**Daily 4** This deep forward lunge stretches the hamstrings, calves, shoulders, chest and spine. Additionally, it strengthens the legs, knees, ankles and abdomen, obliques and back.
Daily 5 Known as 'child's pose' in Pilates and yoga. It helps to stretch the hips, thighs and ankles. It's also a pose you can hold during deep breathing and relaxation.	**Daily 6** 'Downward dog' yoga pose. This stretch targets the upper and lower body and works everything from the hands, arms, shoulders and upper back through to the legs, calves and feet. A full body stretch.

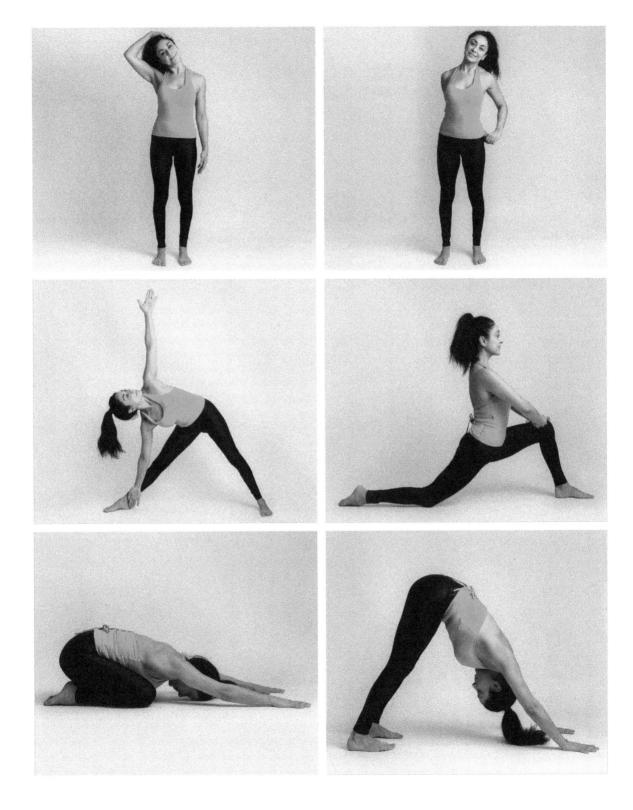

Daily 7	Daily 8
This stretches the entire front of the body, the abdomen and chest and also the thighs and groin. It also strengthens the muscles in the back and bottom.	The 'seated tree pose'. This stretches the hamstrings and relieves lower back pain.
Daily 9	**Daily 10**
Inner thigh or adductor stretch relieves tension in the inner thigh and improves groin flexibility. It is a lovely hip opening exercise and can relieve pressure in the lower back.	This is a 'wide leg forward fold stretch' and can be a progression from the seated tree pose. It targets the inner thighs and groin, as well as the lower back.
Daily 11	**Daily 12**
The 'supine abductor stretch' targets the muscles in your outer thigh and bottom and is also a hip opening exercise. It can help to relieve stress in the lower back.	The 'upward dog' yoga pose. This stretches the chest, abdomen and tops of the thighs as well as strengthening the back, shoulders, arms and wrists. Another great full body stretch.

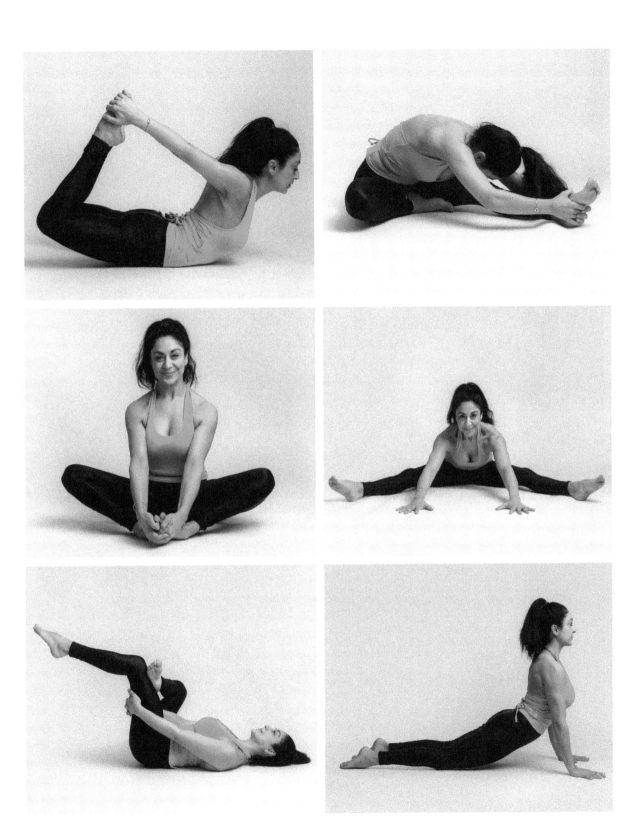

Exercise
is
Therapy

CHAPTER 16: Stress - The Great Saboteur

Stress can sabotage all healthy intentions. Whilst it is important to have enough tension or stress to have the get up and go to partake in life, it's also important for stress not to overwhelm and crush you. When stress becomes chronic or is sustained over a long period of time it can have deleterious effects on our health. Sustained stress lessens our healthspan and lifespan and is a major 21st century public health problem. It is therefore critical that you learn techniques to help you manage your daily stress.

The stress response has been hardwired into our systems through human evolution. It is the 'fight or flight' response. The stress response allows us to get out of imminent danger via the release of the body's main stress hormones, noradrenaline and adrenaline. When we face dangerous situations, the autonomic nervous system releases these stress hormones to help us get into flight mode and escape danger. Perceived danger kickstarts the process and the release of these hormones creates immediate physiological changes in our bodies. Our blood pressure and heart rate go up, our gut goes on 'shut down', our brain switches into hyperalert or 'combat' mode and our cells release sugar for energy. All these changes prep the body for a fast getaway. This stress response was helpful for primitive man, who had to avoid predators back in our hunter-gatherer days. However, in modern life we aren't normally required to run away from predators and this kind of response has instead become wired into the small micro-stresses that we face each and every day, like sitting in traffic or running late for work.

The vast majority of us subconsciously interpret micro-stresses in our lives in the same way that primitive man interpreted predator threats. That is, they link into the same system that releases noradrenaline and adrenaline and puts us into emergency mode. This is okay for short periods of time but if this happens every day in response to the normal stresses of daily life, we risk our long-term health.

Alongside the noradrenaline/adrenaline acute stress pathway works another complex pathway. It links to the brain and is called the Hypothalamic-Pituitary-Adrenal pathway. This is the chronic stress response pathway and is how the brain gets involved in the circuit.

Think of it as the brain eavesdropping on everything that is going on in your body. Nothing is private and everything is communicated back to the brain. From the poor food choices that you make (food stress) to feelings of low mood and anxiety (emotional stress) - it all loops back into the HPA system and stimulates a release of another stress hormone called cortisol. And - you guessed it - raised levels of cortisol cause widespread inflammation. Cortisol increases blood pressure, disturbs the digestive system, weakens the immune system and suppresses the reproductive and growth systems. Long term activation of the stress response system has serious sequelae and has an impact on every single bodily function. It is absolutely vital that you learn to manage your daily stress.

Chronically raised levels of cortisol are actually a normal finding in many people nowadays because we all multi-task and juggle so much. Whereas you would ordinarily expect cortisol to dip at night time and be at its lowest between 11pm and 4am, many people have such elevated levels that they are in ramped up, hyper-vigilant state and can't get to sleep. Ask any insomniac if they are tired and their answer will be 'utterly exhausted'. Insomnia is rife because disruptions in the sleep/wake cycle disturb the circadian rhythm and disturb the cortisol pathway so that lack of sleep can become a vicious cycle. Stress from lack of sleep elevates cortisol, which keeps you awake further, which causes more stress, which raises cortisol even higher… Insomniacs will tell you it's not that they aren't tired but that they just can't switch off. In reality, they are utterly exhausted because their stress levels are shot.

Living in a constant state of micro-stress can over-stimulate all three of the body's major stress hormones - noradrenaline, adrenaline and cortisol. Constant elevation of these hormones causes systemic inflammation and is pathogenic to virtually every single modern disease, from cancer to heart disease and dementia. Chronic stress also promotes cancer growth by release of proteins and hormones into the bloodstream and promotes heart disease via inflammatory atherosclerosis.[335]

So you see, stress is not only a part of modern life but is also a part of modern pathology. Unless we get on top of our stress and find a way to manage it, it can push us into an early grave. It really is that clear cut and getting on top of your stress is really _that_ important.

EVERY CELL IN
YOUR BODY IS
EAVESDROPPING
ON YOUR
THOUGHTS

MICRO-STRESS AND MACRO-STRESS

There are many different types of stress. Some people respond to small, daily stressors, such as being stuck in traffic, misplacing a mobile, arguing with a partner, being faced with an unexpected bill etc. We can all relate to these kinds of micro-stresses because modern lives are jam-packed with them. There are also many major stresses in life such as divorce, separation, a cancer diagnosis and bereavement. These kinds of stress are not momentary or transient and can take significant periods of time to heal and recover from. For those dealing with massive stress such as bereavement and divorce the smaller stresses can be the last straw and push individuals perilously close to the edge. We fall over the edge when we reach the limits of our personal stress threshold and have no capacity left. Macro-stress can often bring people to this point and that's why most professionals advise people to seek professional help in times of macro-stress. It can be positively life-saving.

The levels of stress that we see in society today cannot be underestimated. Studies suggest that over 80% of GP consultations these days are in some way related to complaints of low mood and stress. We know from studying the world's Blue Zones (where people live the longest) that minimal stress is part of the explanation for their longevity. If we want to live long, happy, healthy lives then we all need to recognise and address the levels of stress that envelop our lives. It starts with addressing the small stresses that we can mitigate and prevent, which helps to redefine our own personal stress level. Obviously, some life events are out of our control, but basic levels of micro-stress resilience can help shield us from the impact of some of the larger stresses. Controlling the smaller stuff helps brace us for the bigger stuff and will allow a kind of 'ceasefire' from our stress response for times of recovery in between.

Sadly, we see a lot of stress in the lives of children and young people from social media, pressure of exams, substance abuse, low mood and bullying. Whilst technology has put convenience at the epicentre of life, it has also brought its own set of baggage. Our children are bombarded with messages from social media, advertising, school etc. and it's not surprising that they find it overwhelming. We also live in an age of more frequent divorce and broken families, which has a huge impact on childhood stress levels.

Like adults, children also benefit from stress management techniques and mindfulness. In fact, many schools are beginning to introduce things like yoga and mindfulness in recognition of the changing emotional and psychological landscape facing our young people. Taking regular time out from technology and doing a 'digital detox' can help distance yourself and your child from the stresses of social media and information overload. This can help reduce some of the relentless micro-stresses in young people's lives.

When stress exceeds our ability to cope with it, when it is overwhelming or cannot be resolved, it becomes chronic. Chronic stress has significant long-term physical effects as well as psychological and neuroendocrine effects. Post-mortem studies of depressed people have shown that chronic stress induces changes in the brain, such as volume shrinkage, grey matter reduction, neuronal death and atrophy of basal ganglia in the pre-frontal cortex of the brain.[336] These all cause mental blunting, low mood, reduced cognition and reduced levels of engagement. Stress also impacts our immune system and has been shown to have similar immune-stimulating effects as a bacterial infection, with elevated levels of inflammation and circulating cytokines (chemical messengers that communicate within the immune system). When the stress is overwhelming the neuro-immune communication axis can become overwhelmed, causing imbalances and a low-grade chronic inflammation that is a prelude to many chronic diseases.[337]

It is helpful to make a list of the micro-stresses and macro-stresses in your life. Identifying what triggers stress for you is an important part of learning how to deal with it.

Here is my micro-stress list - it may look familiar to some of you of your parents!

- Getting my three children ready for school every morning

- The school run - in itself a stressful event!

- Keeping on top of a constant barrage of emails

- Managing my diary and meetings for work

- Getting children to do their homework

- Dealing with children bickering

- Losing bits of school uniform

- Not enough hours in the day

- Bedtime and bath time routine

You can see from my list that it is the responsibilities that come with being a parent that are creating most of my daily stress. Measures to deal with that could be finding some help with the children, getting someone to help with admin duties or cooking batch meals so dinner is a much easier affair. Some things I cannot change, like bickering children(!) but with time these sources of stress should improve. I know I am not alone as a parent enduring this repeated stress and I often exchange my stories of school run distress with other parents who are going through the very same thing. No matter what your age or what your source of stress, one thing seems to run through the very fabric of our lives. We all seem to have more and more things that we need to do with less available time and support.

One of the best ways of dealing with micro-stresses in your day is to improve your organisational skills. I find 'to do' lists really helpful so I can see things visibly getting ticked off. Whilst it might not feel like I have had a productive day, a series of ticks on my list makes me realise I have been productive with my time and that I actually have achieved something. This sends a small dopamine boost to my brain that sets off my reward system.

Another great way of dealing with the small stuff is to change your frame of mind or perspective. Many people around the world live happy lives with half the material possessions and technology that we do. 'Things' don't equate to happiness. When you realise this, you start realising that much of what we stress about simply doesn't matter. Simplifying your life and your routine can help take the pressure off.

Another great way of managing micro-stress is through moments of meditation and mindfulness. I find these two therapies really helpful and use them regularly myself and with my patients to help achieve a better sense of balance and inner calm. If you can manage to wake up even ten minutes earlier than you normally do, a great practice is to sit or lie alone somewhere quiet and meditate. My mind used to wander terribly when I first tried to meditate and I often would wonder what on earth I was doing. But once you master it meditation can bring great benefits to your life, even 5 a minute meditation can help.

I generally do gratitude meditation, which means I think of one thing I am grateful for in my life and I hold onto that thought and relive it in my mind. It might be a beautiful moment between me and my child that I had the day before or a rewarding consultation spent with one of my patients. You can focus on anything at all as long as you feel grateful for it and spend time just holding the thought of it. This kind of practice helps you start the day in a positive and grateful mindset and helps shape the way your day will unfold. My children do this at night time before bed. We do a gratitude prayer, where we think of all the amazing things in our life and say thank you for them.

You don't have to be religious or spiritual to get great benefit from this kind of practice and it's amazing how powerful it is at calming and quietening the mind. We live in a noisy world where peace is at a premium. The mind needs quiet and solitude to thrive so it's important to cultivate the right conditions for stillness of the mind. Against the backdrop of modern living, with its constant stimulation, it's important for the mind to find some rest and peace. Before bedtime it's great to get into a quiet mode, switch off, practise gratitude and get the body and brain ready for some quality rest and relaxation.

STRESS AND CANCER

For many people nothing can bring on stress more quickly than a cancer diagnosis. Very few things in life are more stressful than realising your own mortality and that you may not have much time.

We know it is really important to find a sense of calm and purpose in the midst of a cancer battle. Managing stress and finding a positive mindset is extremely beneficial and can help build a wall of resilience that even cancer and chronic disease find hard to penetrate.

Anil Sood, a gynaecology oncology researcher from MD Anderson, has shown that stress creates a micro-environment triggered by noradrenaline, in which cancer cells can proliferate and grow. His research shows us that the whole body is connected and there is multi-directional communication between the brain, hormones, gut, cytokines and everything in between. From his work (and the work of others) we now know categorically that cancer cells respond to stress and that stress helps cancer develop and grow.[338]

These findings were confirmed in 2008 by a meta-analysis of 165 published studies by psychologists at University College London which confirmed the link between stress and cancer and confirmed how stress reduction can boost survival in people who have cancer.[339] In these studies, stress included anything from stressful events such as bereavement and divorce to individual feelings like low mood and helplessness. Prolonged negative mental states and inability to find a place of mental peace makes us vulnerable to all kinds of disease, but especially cancer. The mechanism for this is thought to be the fact that stress puts the body into emergency or inflammatory mode. This shuts down the digestive, reparative and immune systems in favour of the emergency combat 'fight or flight' systems. The stress hormones then exert the dominating effect, promoting tumour proliferation. When stress becomes chronic it can damage our body's defences against cancer.

The University of Helsinki in Finland has conducted some profound studies that show a significant link between separations and divorce and increased risk of breast cancer. One study tracked more than ten thousand women who had experienced a break up or separation and showed that this more than doubled their risk of breast cancer.[340] Some studies have even shown that the risk of developing breast cancer is up to nine times more following the stress of separation and divorce.[341]

David Servan-Schreiber, one of my favourite medical authors on the issue of cancer and himself a cancer sufferer, explored the relationship between stress and cancer exquisitely in his phenomenal book, *Anti-Cancer Living.* If you or a loved one has cancer, this book should not be missed. In his memoirs, *Not the Last Goodbye* David wrote that 'one of the best defences against cancer is finding a place of inner calm'. His approach to defeating cancer was fourfold - David believed that four fundamental things need to be optimised to reduce cancer risk and help sequester existing cancer cells.

These four things are:

1. Optimising your diet to reduce cancer promoters and intake a greater number of phytochemicals.

2. Avoiding environmental carcinogens.

3. Creating a mind-body relationship that stimulates the immune system and nurtures immune resilience.

4. Mental calm and reducing psychological wounds that feed the biological mechanisms at work in cancer.

David's research formed the basis of many books that followed on holistic cancer prevention and survival and much of what I know is due to his teachings.

STRESS REDUCTION

Some of the best ways to cope with stress are free of charge, easy to implement and make you feel great. Meditation, mindfulness, exercise and yoga are some of the most under-rated stress management strategies available and can deliver profound therapeutic benefit. Couple this with good restorative sleep and good social support and love and much of the smaller stresses in life can be dissipated and calmed.

Meditation

Starting a mind-body practice such as meditation can have profound health and wellness benefits. Meditation is not about getting rid of your thoughts but finding peace with them. The practice of meditation has been found to help improve brain function, reduce inflammation, change gene expression, reduce anxiety, improve gut health and reduce stress hormones in the blood.[342] Meditation can also help us modulate the experience of pain. Researchers have found that those trained in meditation can reduce their perception of pain by up to 40%.[343] In comparison, opioids like morphine are thought to reduce it by only 25%.

When practised regularly, meditation can free you from toxic stress, cut your risk of illness, improve wellbeing and help to rewire the brain into a positive mindset. The effects of meditation are not just limited to adults; children as young as nine have been found to benefit from meditation practice with improved thinking and learning and improved mood.[344] This has significance because early symptoms of distress in childhood can signal later risk for mental health problems and major depressive illness. Giving children robust coping mechanisms can help them cope with the stresses of adolescence. Given that current estimates suggest almost 25% of US children have some kind of mental disorder, these tools may be just what the next generation needs to cope with the demands of modern living.[345]

We know that meditation can help cancer sufferers too. Daily 20-minute meditation practice has been shown to reduce chemotherapy side effects, lower cortisol levels and reduce systemic inflammation. By calming your mind, you can experience significant downstream calming effects.

I am a firm believer that meditation and mindfulness could have great potential in our current medical system. In the last 25 years we have tried unsuccessfully to medicate away most of our mental health problems. This kind of approach often fails because it fails to address the root cause of the problem and the relentless and eroding nature of stress. Medication doesn't take away heartbreak, bereavement, stress, anxiety, post traumatic stress disorder, social isolation, fear of death or the many other things in modern life that tip people over the edge.

One of my main frustrations working as a GP has always been the limited resources allocated for Cognitive Behavioural Therapy (CBT), counselling, talking therapy and stress management for people who are defeated mentally. When a referral to counselling or bereavement services takes over three months it becomes easier for doctors to prescribe medication than it is to give real, tangible human help.

We seem to medicate changes in mood and anxiety very quickly but medicines fail to address the lives we are all living that create the problems in the first place. To put this into perspective, more than 64.7 million prescriptions for anti-depressant drugs were written in the UK in 2016 - this represents a massive 108% increase on the 31 million anti-depressants dispensed in 2006.[346]

There are ways to reprogram and remap the brain and medicines aren't the only option. At the very least we should be using these kinds of therapies alongside medical therapy because they too have a growing evidence body. The problem with the medical industry is that we are so focused on pharmaceutic-type medicine that we largely ignore the mountain of evidence that exists in favour of complimentary therapies. Complimentary therapies can happily sit alongside western medicines if we just open our minds to it. I use everything from reflexology and acupuncture to meditation and mindfulness in my own life because I find them so effective. I cannot scientifically explain why some of them work but that doesn't always matter to me. If it makes me feel better, it's achieved more than some drugs can and that is enough to have a huge impact on my internal inflammatory markers.

Acknowledging that highs and lows are a normal part of life is important - it makes us human. If we medicate away all our lows, then we may not experience the highs and live life to the fullest. It reminds me of the words of the poet Khalil Gibran: 'The deeper that sorrow carves into your being the more joy you can contain'.

When I was 14, I was involved in an armed robbery with four other members of my family. The experience left me with PTSD (post-traumatic stress disorder) and a constant fear of gun crime and massacres and traumatic nightmares that still persist. No amount of CCTV or security takes away the irrational fear that someone might break in and hold me at gunpoint again. Twenty minutes of trauma can create a lifetime of managed anxiety. I share this only to make the point that the mind is an incredibly complex beast and the shortest of traumas can have lasting and deeply powerful effects.

Meditation and mindfulness have helped me deal with the PTSD and helped me find context for the experience and my reactions to it. There is also another successful therapy for PTSD called EMDR - Eye Movement Desensitising and Reprocessing - which is very effective in helping sufferers.

If you like apps, then meditation apps like Calm and Headspace are great. I often use them to help me realign and reconnect with my inner self after particularly stressful days.

Mindfulness

Mindfulness is another great and undervalued practice. It's about letting go of all distracting thoughts and just being in the here and now, going with the flow. Not thinking or planning forward, not reflecting on the past but actually being here in the present moment - in the flow zone. Amazingly, few of us really live in the here and now. Our minds are always so busy planning the next thing that we often forget to enjoy the moment. If you do this your whole life you may find yourself on your death bed feeling like you didn't really live. Trust me, it happens.

One of the biggest distractions of our generation is phones and technology. It's scary how many people are staring into their phones when you get on the tube or train in any major city. The constant fear of missing out means we are failing to make connections in our real lives. Connection is what life is about and true happiness comes from our real lives, not our virtual ones... Your phone can't make you feel loved the way another person can. Technology severs our vital inter-connectedness and creates a chasm where we fail to truly connect with each other. Look up from your screen for a moment and you will see how many opportunities to connect are being lost because of the massive hold that technology has on society. Humans need connection. Connection makes us feel alive.

It's becoming more obvious that we all need to look after our mental health and that one of the first casualties of a high-tech society is mental health and wellbeing.

Yoga

Yoga is an ancient form of mind-body exercise that has been passed down from Tibetan Monks and continues to thrive all over the world. In Eastern traditions, yoga is deeply connected to the act of worship and seen as a communion between the individual and the higher being. In Sanskrit, the term 'yoga' denotes the merging of the mind and body in the pursuit of inner peace. Whether you are religious or not, yoga is a great way of connecting the physical body with the inner self and helps to keep the body supple.

Yoga is an effective stress management tool and workplaces are starting to embrace it as an effective way of preventing things like lower back pain, headaches, repetitive strain injury and even 'executive burnout'. Corporations are starting to realise that if their workers aren't happy, balanced and in great physical shape, levels of absenteeism skyrocket. Yoga is also a great tool for keeping us all connected. Modern life has severed many of us from any sense of higher purpose and spirituality and yoga can help restore this. It is also a great tool for recovery and repair of tissues.

Clinically evidenced benefits of yoga

Reduces pain[347]

Reduces tension[348]

Reduces risk of injury[349]

Improves posture[350]

Improves communication

Increases energy

Increases attention span[351]

Enhances feelings of wellbeing and mental health[352]

Research shows that we all need to take time out of each and every day to reflect and relax. In an increasingly 24/7 world this seems harder and harder to achieve.

Yoga can be particularly beneficial for those suffering from chronic diseases like cancer, arthritis and heart disease. A Randomised Control Trial at the University of Rochester in the USA took 400 cancer survivors who were having problems with their sleep and advised them to attend two one-hour yoga sessions a week. Within the space of four weeks they reported that their subjective sleep quality was better, and this was backed up with objective measures of their sleep.[353]

Another RCT on the efficacy of yoga conducted at MD Anderson in America took women with breast cancer undergoing radiotherapy and split them into two different groups. The first group did yoga three times per week and the other group did light stretching. What they found was incredible and is testament to the potential health benefits of yoga for everyone. The yoga group experienced significant improvements in their cortisol hormone regulation compared to the group that only did light stretching. The lower cortisol levels had implications not only for their sleep quality but also for control of their cancer. In the study these cortisol improvements lasted one month after the cessation of yoga, which is simply phenomenal and speaks volumes about the benefit of mind body yoga.[354]

I practise yoga and have found that it has helped guide and steer my life in a positive direction. The combination of physical exercise with the practice of mindfulness is unique and exquisite. Just one session can help reduce stress and refocus the mind. As I do my sun salutations I welcome in the new day with positive energy and optimism and use the time to set a positive mental landscape for the day ahead. I also use the time to do my own kind of inner prayer.

I am not amazing at yoga - I can't crow or stand on my head - but that really isn't the point. For me it's just a way of switching off, stretching and connecting with something higher, bigger and more profound than myself. I am not religious but there are moments in my practice where I feel enlightened. It's like a daily conversation with the Universe. In my busy life, with three children and a demanding career, this can be a real lifeline. I strongly encourage you to try yoga and to find a place for it in your life. You don't need an expensive gym membership to do it. You can do it in your own home following videos on the internet. I often use 5ParksYoga and GayatriYoga on YouTube and YogaGlo is a great app for when you are on the move. For amazing visual yoga inspiration follow @bikini_yogini_ on Instagram. She is a dream.

Try some of these yoga moves with Dee to test your balance, suppleness and core strength and to get started on the restoration path.

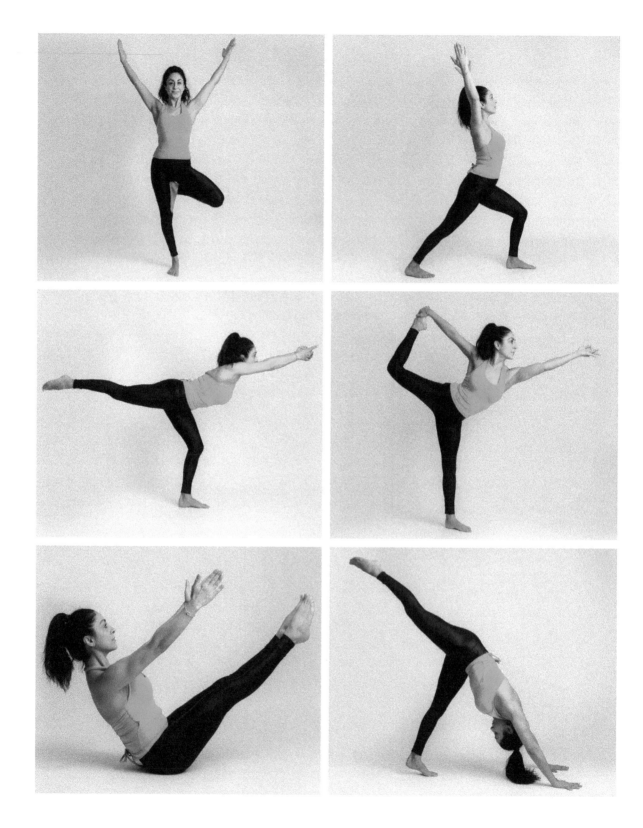

SLEEP

Humans spend nearly a third of their lives asleep. Sleep is one of the body's great reparative processes and all living creatures take time to rest. It is during this time of rest that the body undergoes significant recovery and repair and good quality sleep is a vital part of any health plan. Sleep reduces and relieves all kinds of physical, emotional and mental stress. The vast majority of adults need 7-9 hours' sleep - neuroscientist Matthew Walker puts it bluntly: 'The shorter your sleep, the shorter you live'.[355]

Sleep disorders are becoming increasingly common, with the Centre for Disease Control estimating that up to 70 million Americans suffer from chronic sleep disorders and a third of working adults get less than six hours sleep a night. In studies, rats totally deprived of sleep die within a few weeks. It is thought that if humans tried to go without sleep, they would die within two weeks. A 2014 study published in the *Journal of Neuroscience* found that a mere 24 hours of sleep deprivation was enough to make healthy people have hallucinations and schizophrenia-type symptoms.

People who don't get enough sleep often have reduced immune function, reduced cognitive (brain) function, reduced reflexes and find it harder to resist poor quality foods, alcohol and addictions. Hormonal imbalances can also result from sleep deprivation. For example, too little sleep stimulates the stress hormone cortisol, which can then start a vicious cycle of inability to get to sleep and insomnia. When we sleep the pituitary gland in the brain secretes growth hormone, which is vital for growth. In children whose sleep is impaired due to chronic pain, itching from eczema, difficulty breathing from asthma etc. this can affect normal growth and development.

When we sleep (in the non-REM stage) the pineal gland in the brain secretes melatonin which is a hormone that has anti-inflammatory, antioxidant and anti-coagulant properties all around the body. It is also thought that the brain uses sleep time to clear out metabolic and toxic waste.[356] Neuroscientists have linked disturbed or shortened sleep patterns to beta-amyloid protein build-up in the brain - a hallmark of Alzheimer's. Poor sleep quality is associated with a reduction in the production of melatonin, which is linked to increased breast cancer rates in shift workers.[357]

Poor sleep wreaks havoc on your short-term memory and cognitive capacity. If you are tired it is much harder to learn new things and retain them and sleep-deprived people tend to talk in short, monotone sentences with less expression, reflecting the stunted ability of the fatigued mind.

When researchers forced subjects to stay awake for 88 hours their blood pressure went up (a predictable stress response), their heart rates increased, and their CRP inflammatory markers also raised. Chronic sleep deprivation is a pathway to irritability, poor mood, poor memory, erroneous vision, poor skin healing, reduced immunity, increased blood pressure, increased heart rate, increased isolation and long-term inflammation. So you can see that good quality sleep is vital for combatting and reducing the effects of stress.

I remember vividly the effects of sleep deprivation when I had my third child. After three weeks of being up all night and then trying to look after all my other duties in the daytime hours (including school drops and homework for my other two kids) I just hit a wall. And when I mean hit a wall, I mean I slammed into it face first. My body had nothing left to give - I felt like a zombie, I was nauseous, disconnected, disorientated, emotional, tearful and a total mess. Sleep deprivation has got to be the hardest part of having children and has left many a parent feeling broken. Once you have experienced extreme sleep deprivation it's easy to understand why it's used as a form of torture.

Sleep requires a good routine and is all about developing good sleep habits. Throughout the day our brains make a million new connections a second. This phenomenal brain activity can be hard to slow down when it comes to sleep time and it's very easy to have lots of thoughts flying around your head when you are trying to get to sleep. I certainly did whilst trying to write this book! Half of it was written in my head as I lay in bed at night and then (frustratingly) lost to the ether by the time it was morning. A good sleep routine will help your brain switch into relaxation mode. Changing one simple habit at a time is powerful. Over time the benefits accumulate.

If you have trouble getting to sleep there are lots of great sleep aids available. Apps like Calm and Headspace have sleep meditations and stories and there is some superb REM-inducing sleep music on Spotify and YouTube.

For those insomniacs out there, it's important to think of the sleep routine as a sort of self-hypnosis. Start the routine and then be ready to ride the sleep wave. One wave comes every 90 minutes or so, so be ready.

Sleep Tips

- Make your bedroom a calm and loving space. Take out any televisions and technology and create a sense of peace.

- Invest in a great posture-supporting mattress and pillow. Comfort is vital for good sleep.

- Ban all screens and technology one hour before bedtime. They stimulate your brain. The bedroom should be a calm space.

- Invest in a soft eye mask to block out any environmental light. Sleep requires darkness. Even a streak of light can disturb sleep.

- Invest in blackout blinds if early waking is the problem.

- Charge all devices in another room so technology cannot wake you from your deep sleep. An email notification coming in at night can ruin your sleep.

- Reduce disturbing sounds. Use earplugs if a household member snores or if there is lots of outside noise.

- Try a sleep meditation or sleep story if getting to sleep is the problem.

- Exercise in the daytime to physically tire yourself out ready for the night.

- Eat dinner before 6pm if your bedtime is 10pm. Four hours is enough time to digest your meal and prepare for sleep mode. It is important that your gut has time to rest and repair too.

- Limit coffee/tea to morning time and don't drink it after 2pm. Caffeine has a long half-life and believe it or not, your lunchtime coffee can still be in your system at 8pm. The same applies for dark chocolate, green tea, black tea and anything else with caffeine in it.

- Track your sleep with a tracker to see what your patterns are.

If you are really struggling to get to sleep then melatonin supplements in a dose of 1-3 mg can be helpful. As we age our melatonin levels deplete, so replenishing them can be helpful if sleep deprivation is becoming a problem. Valerian root 400mg can also be helpful if you wake in the middle of the night and cannot get back to sleep. Nytol can also help but don't take it halfway through the night if you wake up and can't get back to sleep as it can leave you feeling very groggy as if you have a red wine hangover.

SOCIAL SUPPORT

To have support and feel loved are two of the most important things in life. When people have meaning and purpose in their lives, they tend to cope with all kinds of stress better and they tend to live longer. Love can shield you from stress and acts as a reflector to some degree. People who have the strongest sense of love and purpose in their lives are much more resilient to stress that those who don't. When it comes to suffering a chronic disease, love and social support can be as effective as medicine in the process of healing and recovery. If you have low levels of stress and are surrounded by love and support, you are statistically more likely to fare better after a cancer diagnosis than those who don't.

In 2005, researchers at the George Washington University performed a study on women with Grade 2 and 3 breast cancer and found that those who were well supported from sources in their community were 60% less likely to die from their cancer even a decade after their initial diagnosis.[358] We have studies that support the opposite too. People who have limited social or familial connections during a cancer diagnosis are more likely to feel depressed and report higher levels of pain.

A 2014 breast cancer study from Ohio State University College studied 164 women and showed higher levels of depression, pain and inflammatory markers in those who had low levels of social support.[359]

What we can take from these kinds of studies is that social support helps create a positive mindset, which reduces internal stress. Stress raises the levels of stress hormones (cortisol, adrenaline and noradrenaline) which in turn raises whole body inflammation. This is important because we know that inflammation promotes cancer growth and proliferation and virtually every other disease too.[360]

Another study by American researchers reproduces these results, but with significant numbers. In fact, theirs is the largest study to date and followed breast cancer sufferers in the US and China for over 20 years. It showed that building an anti-cancer support network is an incredibly important part of any cancer journey. What they found was that women with fewer social connections were 43% more likely to have a cancer recurrence and 64% more likely to die from breast cancer.[361] This is astonishing and is testament to the huge importance that love, and loving people, have in our lives. Humans were made to connect.

One of the biggest challenges for the next generation will be how to maintain a sense of connectedness and support in a digital world. We know that technology is a double-edged sword: although it brings convenience and efficiency, it also brings isolation and loss of connection. With more people working from home than ever it is important that we never lose ourselves in technology so much that we lose our sense of community, belonging and support. These are the very things that humans need and crave and they cannot be replaced by technology. If you want to read a great book on this, try *Lost Connections* by Johann Hari. It's a fascinating exploration of our collective mental health decline in the technological age.

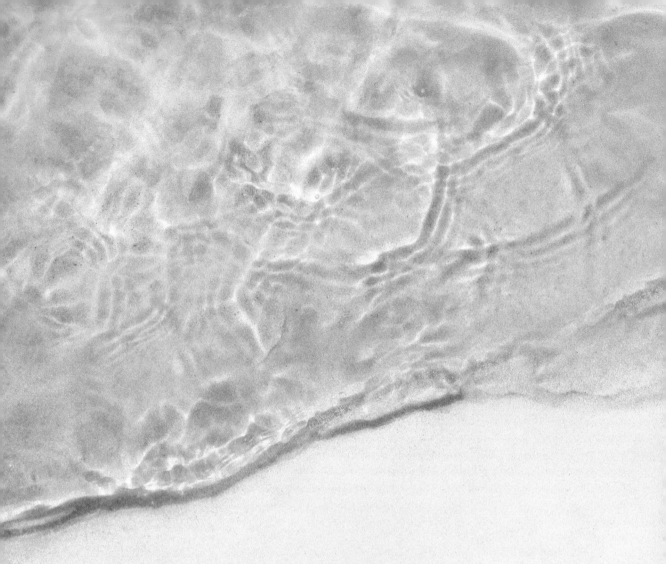

I find being by water healing and uplifting and this phenomenon is reinforced by science. The ebb and flow of water and visualising water scenes are scientifically shown to change our brain waves and put us into a mild meditative state, switch off and relax. Ocean time and sun exposure have been suggested as treatments for seasonal affective disorder and can help us survive dark times in our lives, literally and metaphorically.

If you are feeling down or low, try and find a place where you can get some mental peace. If you cannot get to the beach or near water, take a walk in nature, breathe deeply and let go of your thoughts. Or simply find a comfortable place and do a brief meditation or mindfulness session. You don't need to travel anywhere to physically benefit from the practice.

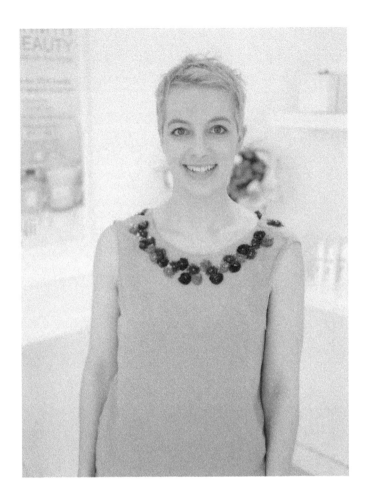

Sam Burton

Sam is my mindfulness therapist. She has helped me find meaning and clarity in my life and helped me work through my PTSD issues. I asked her to create a meditation exercise just for you. You can do it anywhere you go in the world and at any time in your life. Daily meditation can help you take more from life and brings a sense of gratitude and calm to life that helps underpin good health.

Start by either lying or sitting down in a safe and comfortable space.

~~~

Close your eyes so you are not distracted by your surroundings.

~~~

Bring attention to the breath. The inhale and exhale of the breath.

~~~

Where do you feel the breath the most? Through the nose and throat?
In the chest or abdomen? The flow of breath through the whole body?

~~~

Bring attention to the sensations of the breath

as it moves in and out of the body.

~~~

Notice when the mind has wandered away from the breath, as it will, and gently bring

focus back to the breath.

~~~

There is no judgement of these thoughts or the wandering of the mind, just acceptance

that it has happened.

~~~

Return to focus on the breath.

~~~

After a few minutes begin to focus attention on the different parts of the body, one at a

time. What are the physical sensations here? Is there any tension or pain? Don't try to

change the sensation; accept it and notice it with curiosity.

~~~

Move through the body as though you are having a scan - starting with the toes, then

the feet, moving up the legs, hips, abdomen, lower back, upper back,

chest, shoulders, arms, palms, fingers, neck,

face (chin, cheeks, eyes, forehead, top of the head).

~~~

With each body part, linger for a few moments.

There is no need to rush any focus of attention.

~~~

Notice the sensations occurring.

~~~

When the mind wanders, return to the breath

and then bring attention back to the body part.

~~~

Once the scan has covered the whole body, return to focus attention on the breath,

then inhale and exhale and enjoy the movement of the breath - spend a few moments

here.

~~~

Notice any sensations?

~~~

Come to the end of your body scan meditation. Open your eyes and gently stretch.

~~~

PART THREE
There is no Planet B

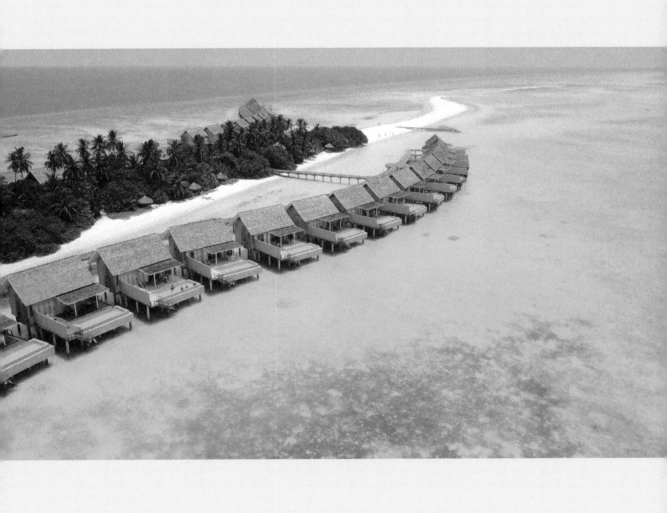

CHAPTER 17: Healthy Choices Can Save Our Planet

The healthiest choices for our body are also the healthiest choices for our planet. It often turns out that when we begin taking care of ourselves we also begin to take care of our surroundings and the places and people who matter.

Eating a whole food, plant-based diet is by far the healthiest diet for our planet. There is overwhelming evidence that now correlates plant-based diets with the most environmentally friendly diets. The very same foods that reduce our risk of heart disease, cancer and stroke have the least impact on our planet and are the most compassionate foods for our fellow creatures.

What we have forgotten in our race to develop and advance technologically is that all living things are connected. It is easy to lose appreciation of this interconnectedness when you live in an urbanised world, but the fact is we are all dependent on our biosphere for life. We are connected to the earth, the sea, the sun, the clouds, the rain, the land, the water, to animals and to other human beings. If we relentlessly pollute our air, water, land and soil then we pollute ourselves and undermine our own ability to survive. We are perilously close to this point.

Most people are now aware that our planet is under tremendous strain. We face the possibility of ecological ruin and we are the last generation that can potentially do something about it. We need to stop subsidising polluting industries and start taxing industries and countries that pollute our world. We also need to stop thinking about revenue and start thinking about what we can 'gift' or give back to the earth. It can no longer be a one-way deal. The choices we make as individuals, as consumers and as a society will dictate the destiny of Planet Earth.

More so than at any time in human history, our individual choices really matter. So much is at stake. In the space of a few generations we have caused extinction, deforestation and terrifying global warming. We have also introduced technologies like genetic engineering, which dangerously alters the very blueprint of life and has the potential to wipe out everything.

With 7.2 billion people in this world, the 'dream' of unlimited consumption is totally unsustainable. By 2050, the global population is expected to reach 9.6 billion. With food poverty a very real threat we need to rethink the way we eat and live in the west to help reduce the poverty and hunger of the developing world. We can no longer turn a blind eye.

Developing countries suffer enormously from our excessive consumption - the real costs of our excess are felt in countries far removed. Famine, droughts and floods affect the world's poorest people and the consequence of global warming will be enormous for them. The World Bank estimates that climate change has the power to push more than 100 million of the world's poorest people into food poverty in the next ten years. To make matters worse, one third of all the food produced in the world (over 1.3 billion tons) is never consumed but wasted.[362] To produce this food waste adds 3.3 billion tons of greenhouses gases to the world's atmosphere and costs over $1 trillion per year.[363] Clearly, something needs to change. And, my friend, it starts with me and it starts with you.

Experts are predicting that by the end of the century we will experience a two to five degree increase in temperature that will have catastrophic effects. The clock is ticking dangerously close to midnight for humankind. In October 2018, leading climate experts warned that we have until 2030 to change our ways. If we don't, then we can expect more flooding, famine, hurricanes, tsunamis, earthquakes, forest fires and freak catastrophes. All bring with them incredible displacement, disease and human suffering - not to mention death. The hidden costs of climate change are running into billions every year already. We have to stop it.

Natural disasters are happening with far more frequency already and are set to continue at lightning pace if we don't do something drastic now. The abstract has to become personal. We all need to play a role in this battle to save our world. We must refuse to let ourselves become overwhelmed by the enormity of the task ahead. The IPCC predicts that the earth will warm by another two degrees by 2050 if we don't reduce our greenhouse gas emissions by a whopping 50-80%. Humans have effectively broken the planet in a very short space of time. The Industrial Revolution brought us convenience and abundance - but has ultimately cost us our world.

Human innovation and motivation are our only hopes now. We have to find a way to halt that predicted two-degree temperature rise or face disasters of epic proportions. We need to stand up to our politicians and make them act now. They need to untangle themselves from corporate and industry pressure and start making policies that actually move us in the direction of sustainability and recovery. Any politician who doesn't understand the enormity of the situation is doing us a disservice and is not fit to be a leader in my mind.

Carbon taxes, clean energy and getting rid of fossil fuel subsidies on a national level would be a great start. On a personal level we can all change what we eat, what we drink and reduce our incessant food waste. We know you can't really throw anything away these days because there is no such place as 'away'. Everything finds its way back into landfill, the soil, the ocean, into our drinking water and back into our foods. So we need to take a serious look at the things we consume and decide if they are sustainable. It's not someone else's problem any more. It's our collective problem.

"What most people don't know is that changing what we eat can have the single biggest impact of all on our ecological footprint."

By 2050 we will need to feed more than two billion more people in the world, so the question of WHICH DIET takes on a fierce and new urgency. This population increase represents a 34% rise in the world population compared to today. The foods we choose to eat will ultimately shape the future of our planet. A diet reliant on meat and dairy has huge planetary ramifications and takes a greater toll on our planet's finite resources than a plant-based diet. It is my belief that if people knew how damaging their food choices were, they would want a chance to change them. Surely we all see the value in aligning our lifestyles and diets with a sustainable future? And surely all of us can see that something is wrong when, in the space of a generation, our planet and all the life it holds has come under serious threat? Profits and capitalistic gain cannot trump our collective planetary mission.

LIVESTOCK

Livestock is one of the most significant factors in global warming. Meat production is one of the largest contributors to our environmental problems at every level. Livestock rearing creates enormous volumes of toxic greenhouse gases, air pollution, water pollution, land pollution and land degradation and significantly contributes to climate change. In fact, livestock farming is thought to cause more damage to our planet than the global transport sector does. Add to this the potential disease impact of animal-based foods and a strong case can be made for vegetarianism for global and personal health improvement.

Since the 1970s, cows have been farmed intensively and switched to cheap GMO soya and corn feeds because these have been heavily subsidised by governments. Because many cows no longer eat grass (their native food) they create significantly more amounts of methane gas - and methane is 23 times more potent than carbon dioxide. In the US alone, cows create more environmentally-damaging gases per year than 22 million cars.

Methane comes from both ends of a cow and from cow manure and is one of the greatest threats to the future of our planet. Methane is a greenhouse gas that is 23 times stronger than carbon dioxide and warms the planet about 200 times more than carbon dioxide.[463] It is estimated that about 25% of the global warming we are experiencing now is due to methane emissions.[464] Methane gas acts like a blanket over the earth, trapping the sun's heat and causing global warming. Add to this the toxic nitrous oxide emitted from 500 million tonnes of cow dung per year, which accounts for two thirds of the world's nitrous oxide pollution, and we are in serious trouble. Nitrous oxide is 300 times more damaging to the environment than carbon dioxide. We need to ditch our toxic hamburger habits fast.

Worldwide, there are an estimated 1.5 billion ruminant cows and bulls and millions of other ruminant animals such as sheep. Bacterial microbes in their stomachs create the toxic methane gas. Cows emit the most methane gas through their belching and flatulence. Experts estimate that the average livestock or dairy cow emits between 200-500 litres of methane a day, directly comparable to the amount of pollution caused by one car per day.[364] The 10 million cows in the UK are thought to contribute about 3% of our greenhouse gases and up to 30% of our methane. Since the beginning of the century methane gas is estimated to have gone up by over 150%. Livestock now uses 30% of the world's land surface, so it's important that we look into alternative cow feeds that might reduce methane emissions; we also need to look at reducing global meat consumption.[365] Scientists have suggested adding garlic and tannins to cow feed and changing the foods they feed on to try and reduce methane emission. As Professor Dave Reay from the University of Edinburgh elegantly puts it, 'Cows belching less methane may not be as eye catching as wind turbines and solar panels but they are just as vital for addressing climate change.'

OUR BROKEN FOOD SYSTEM

Did you know...?

- Global meat production has increased over the last 50 years by 4-5 times since 1961.[366]

- In Asia meat production has increased a staggering 15-fold since 1961.[367]

- Per capita meat consumption has increased approximately 20kg since 1961. The average person consumed 43kg of meat in 2014.[368]

- Globally, cattle meat production has doubled since 1961, increasing from 28 million tonnes annually to approximately 68 million tonnes in 2014.[369]

- In 2012 the world produced and consumed 290 million tonnes of beef, pork, sheep and goat meat and poultry.[370]

- Beef is the most environmentally consequential meat that we eat.

- The United States is the world's largest beef, producer producing 12 million tonnes of beef and buffalo meats in 2014.[371]

- The American beef industry is a powerhouse worth $74 billion per year.

- The United States is also the world's largest poultry producer, accounting for more than 20 million tonnes of poultry in 2014. China and Brazil are second and third, with 18 million and 13 million tonnes outputs respectively.[372]

- Beef production requires seven times more land and emits seven times more greenhouses gases than poultry production.[373]

- Beef production is 20 times as land- and greenhouse gas-intensive as bean production.

- US beef consumption is four times as high as the world average.

- A 17% decline in beef consumption between 2005-2014 resulted in a total US diet-related greenhouse gas reduction of 10%.[374]

A United Nations report showed that livestock and animal farming are responsible for 14.5% of greenhouse gases and more recent studies from the Worldwatch Institute claim that half of all human-caused greenhouse gases come from rearing animal product for foods. A 2006 Chicago study showed that following a vegan diet reduces your carbon footprint far more than driving a hybrid car does[375] and a 2014 Oxford University study found that the carbon footprint of a vegan diet was 60% smaller than that of a meat-based diet and 24% smaller than a vegetarian diet.[376]

What's the solution? Most experts agree that we need to work to reduce global meat consumption and create more sustainable and regenerative ways of farming. This doesn't mean that you cannot eat meat but that you should reduce your consumption and make mindful food choices. Choose local and pasture reared meats rather than factory, mass produced meats - every choice you make has a ripple effect and constitutes an agricultural, social and environmental act.

Every small reduction has an incremental effect. Every ecosystem needs animals in it because there is a complex interplay between the animal and plant kingdoms. The answer doesn't have to be no meat whatsoever ever again. The best option is to reduce our collective meat consumption and invest in farmed products that are sustainable, local, pasture raised and raised according to the laws of nature. We need to invest in regenerative farming and adopt humane farming methods that work in synergy with the natural world. We need to regenerate, replenish, sequester, nurture and support biodiversity. It's the only way we can move forward with our world intact.

- Gram for gram, beef and lamb have about 250 the emissions of legumes.

- Pork, chicken and fish have much lower emissions than beef.

- Fish caught by trawling is three times as destructive as fish caught by traditional methods.

- Rice has five times the emissions per gram of protein as wheat.

A number of studies that look at the trilemma of diet, health and environment show that vegetarian and pescatarian diets are the most environmentally low impact. A study conducted by Professor of Ecology G. David Tilman of the University of Minnesota examining almost 50 years' worth of data from the world's hundred most populous countries showed that pescatarian, vegetarian and vegan diets are the most environmentally friendly.[377]

The Vegan Society claims that 600,000 people in the UK now identify as vegan and three million class themselves as vegetarian. This is a huge increase from the 150,000 vegans that were estimated back in 2014. When surveyed, most of these vegans have changed the foods they eat for ecological and animal compassion reasons. A large number of these are the younger generation and their efforts need to be applauded. What vegans need to know is that certain things need to be supplemented in the vegan diet, these include Omega 3, B12, zinc, magnesium & vitamin D3.

'The most important thing we extract from the ocean is our existence'

Dr Sylvia Earle

Despite many people making the change to plant-based eating, global meat and dairy production is worryingly projected to more than double by 2050. Why? Because our population is constantly expanding. We currently consume 229 million tonnes of meat and 580 million tonnes of milk but by 2050 it will rise to 465 million tonnes and 1,043 million tonnes respectively.[378] Japanese scientists have figured out that eating a kilogram of beef is equivalent to the amount of carbon dioxide emitted from driving a car 250km or burning a 100-watt bulb for 20 consecutive days.[379] Imagine the electricity savings we could make if all 9.6 billion of us (in the future) reduced meat?

If all Americans would consume 10% less meat the amount of economised corn could feed in excess of one billion of the world's people.

What I have noticed from speaking to friends, colleagues, patients and the general public is that very few people are aware of how powerfully connected to the plight of this planet our eating choices really are. I suspect if more people knew how damaging our eating habits were, they would want to do something positive to realign them.

According to Professor Carolyn Roberts from Gresham College, 'food accounts for about 20% of all our greenhouse emissions ... If all of our meat eaters switched to a vegan diet it would roughly halve total greenhouse gas emissions associated with food'.[380] Isn't this a powerful thought? If I haven't convinced you to reduce meat and dairy for the sake of your health, then maybe you will consider it for the sake of our beautiful planet?

It's not all doom and gloom. In 2018 we started to make a BIG difference!![381]

- 19% of the UK population are actively reducing dairy consumption

- 29% are eating locally sourced produce

- 31% are eating less meat

- 47% are boycotting plastic bags

- 9% have switched their cars to hybrid or electric

- 43% are using recyclable plastic bottles and coffee cups

- 43% are using LED lights

- 28% are cutting down the amount they drive

- 48% have made their homes more energy efficient

- 50% are reducing plastic packaging

- 53% are taking power showers instead of baths

A 2018 Oxford University study concluded that:

'A vegan diet is probably the single biggest way to reduce your impact on Planet Earth, not just greenhouse gases, but global acidification, eutrophication, land use and water use'.[382]

Replacing all animal-based products in the US diet with plant alternatives will create enough food to feed 350 million additional people.[383]

Even if you don't want to cut out all meat and dairy then simply making efforts to reduce your animal protein intake will help. For example, it has been estimated that if everyone in the USA swapped one chicken meal per week for a vegetarian meal it would be the carbon equivalent of taking half a million cars off the road. Imagine if the whole world did this? Just one meal a week. Meatless Mondays? Sustainable Sundays? Surely we can all manage that, knowing that the planetary impact would be so huge. In the UK alone, chicken accounts for 50% of the meat we consume - and we eat an estimated 900 million chickens per year. We can get the same or better nourishment from eating chickpeas!

We can end world hunger if we all choose to eat sustainably. Reducing meat and dairy would significantly help redistribute the world's foods.

As ForksOverKnives points out, in 2011 we had a record grain harvest, enough to feed the world twice over, but instead we chose to use half of it to feed the livestock and dairy industries. In parts of Africa they have poverty and food hunger levels of up to 40%, yet have millions of cattle, chickens, goats and sheep eating their food, using their land and drinking their precious water. Instead of feeding themselves with the foods they grow locally, they feed animals and then export them to fat, rich Americans and Europeans!

If we keep demanding it, the developing world will keep sacrificing their local resources to produce it. Instead, we need to teach developing nations how to grow sustainable crops so they can achieve a level of self-sufficiency. 82% of the worlds hungriest children live in countries where food is fed to animals that are killed and exported halfway across the world. The way I see it is that if we don't start embracing sustainable diets we are actively colluding with the demise of our planet. It is an act of incredible selfishness not to eat and live in a way that will benefit future generations.

We all find it hard to see the impact our food choices have on others, particularly on those in other parts of the world that feel distant and removed. We tend to live in our own small microcosm and we forget that it's all linked. If the problem and suffering is not directly in sight, many of us assume it's not real or we find a way to ignore it. The abstract needs to become real.

Sustainable foods need to take into account ecological footprint, food miles, biodiversity, soil quality, waste and embedded energy. A sustainable diet needs to be affordable for all and have a low impact environmentally. Greenhouse gas emissions are an international benchmark for sustainability and emissions in a sustainable diet would be low. When we look at meat-heavy diets we can see that they wouldn't qualify as sustainable because of their high ecological footprint.

In 2012, the world produced and consumed 290 million tonnes of beef, pork, sheep, goat meat and poultry and 154 million tonnes of fish (United Nations Report 2012). This translates into a staggering number of animals raised solely to be slaughtered for meat.

Sustainable diets should use low amounts of water and energy. The World Water Council has tried to educate us about the direct and indirect impact of water in our diets by raising awareness of the vast amounts of water consumed by meat-rich diets. A meat-rich diet accounts for 5,400 litres of water per day whilst a vegetarian diet uses 2,600 litres per day.[384] The water footprint of EU diets could be reduced by one third if we consumed vegetarian rather than meat-based diets.

Sustainable diets need to have the following:

- Low ecological footprint

- Low carbon footprint

- Low food miles

- Low water use

- Low energy use

- Low wastage

- Maintain soil quality

- Maintain biodiversity

- Maintain animal welfare

- Maintain human welfare

- Be nutritious and optimise human health

As a mother of three, nothing gives me more joy than knowing that the positive food choices I make each and every day have a major impact on my children's (and an entire generation's) future. We cannot shrug it off anymore. Something has to be done right now. We are slowly killing off our oceans and our land - the very lungs of the earth are being drowned and it is not good enough anymore to turn a blind eye. There is a price that has to be paid for unlimited consumption.

That price is now becoming abundantly clear. If we do not stop polluting and depleting our planet THERE WILL BE NO PLANET.

What can we do?

- Eat less dairy and meat

- Choose sustainable foods

- Eat local and seasonal foods

- Compost our food waste

- Start organic urban farms, allotments and home grow

- Apply hefty carbon taxes to discourage polluters

- Stop deforestation

- Plant more trees

- Reduce fossil fuel consumption

- Use more wind and solar power

- Invest in alternative energies

- Change the way we farm

- Close down coal plants

- Enforce electric cars

- Reduce plastic

- Recycle everything

- **Elect Politicians and Leaders Who Take Climate Change Seriously**

OCEANIC POLLUTION

The oceans are the lungs of the earth. The oceans have the capacity to capture carbon, generate oxygen, maintain the air and maintain a planetary 'steady state'. 70% of the Earth's surface is water but we are rapidly contaminating and polluting our oceans such that we are threatening marine life and the entire oceanic ecosystem. The oceans are the end point for most of the rubbish and toxic waste we generate on land. We are killing our oceans at a lightning pace and if it continues, not only do we threaten our sea and marine life, but we also threaten our very own existence.

Just because we have vast expanses of water doesn't mean that chemicals and toxins get diluted away. They don't. Instead, what happens is the small animals at the bottom of the food chain absorb and eat them and then the larger fish and marine life eat them and effectively concentrate the contaminants. By the time humans eat the fish or seafood the chemical and toxic contaminants have become significantly bio-concentrated. This poses a risk to human health via toxicity, cancer, endocrine disruption and immune dysfunction.

Seafood sustainability

Humans need omega fats for brain, heart, skin and cellular health. How do we fulfil this basic physiological need, considering the duress our oceans and marine life are currently under? Is there a way of consuming seafood that is sustainable? Are there plenty of fish in the sea? Can we all switch to eating algae so eat the omega source directly?

Sustainable fishing is possible but we still all need to reduce our reliance on fish. Sustainable fishing involves the practice of fishing that leaves habitats intact, works in harmony with the environment and doesn't deplete fish numbers. It's very important that we choose sustainable options given the damage we have already done to the world's oceans.

Our oceans are in trouble.

Plastic does not break down.

Small fish and animals eat the plastic.

The biggest pollutants of the ocean are from the land.

More than one million birds are killed each year by our toxic oceans.

300,000 dolphins and porpoise die each year
from entangling in fishing nets.

Oil spills suffocate marine life; oil is a big contaminant of our oceans.

Toxins and chemicals interfere with marine life,
their behaviour, reproduction and growth.

If you choose to eat seafood for its omega 3 benefits, then choose fish that have been sustainably sourced. Every year we kill 1-2 trillion fish. One way is to try and eat fatty fish that reproduce quickly, like sardines and anchovies. Salmon is less sustainable because its reproductive time is longer and in the wild it comes from far flung places. Salmon have been overfished in the wild and in fish farms suffer some significant disease. Ironically farmed salmon is a solution that presents its own problems. Fish farms often have high levels of toxins and disease and need active measures to control viral spread, excrement and feed issues. Seafood Watch recently gave Scottish Salmon a bad score on the basis of contaminations.

Many fish farms have huge issues with sea lice (literally eats the fish alive) and other diseases such as Infectious Salmon Anaemia (ISA) and Heart and Skeletal Muscle Inflammation (HSMI) and Pancreatic Disease (PD). No one knows the true impact on humans of these diseases but common sense would tell us that diseased fish are not a good source of nutrition - whatever the PR might say.

Another issue with farmed fish is that they are fed fish. UN data shows that factory farmed fish, pigs and poultry are fed 28 million tons of fish each year, six times the amount of seafood eaten by Americans themselves! Crazy, I hear you say - I totally agree.

Genetic engineering of salmon is another concern. Advocates of genetic engineering often claim that engineering offers advantages and sustainability but quite often it's the opposite. When we play God and manipulate salmon growth and size by genetic splicing or borrowing from other species (including human growth genes), we risk wiping out the whole wild population. Each year millions of farmed fish escape through damaged nets and mate with the wild population. Whilst they may have an advantage of growth and size, often the new genes don't afford longevity and the salmon die prematurely.

Genetic engineering represents a bio-hazard. Playing God is never a good idea. We won't know for years if these new transgenic supersized engineered fish are a threat or not. By then it could be too late. We should exercise a certain level of mistrust at genetic engineering and adopt more sustainable practices rather than splitting genes when we have no real understanding of how it might impact the planet in the long term. For example, engineered Chinook super salmon were able to grow to twice their size in experimental breeding programmes. This was celebrated at first until many were found to have deformed heads and severe genetic abnormalities.[385] Is this really an acceptable alternative?

Fishing techniques are really important. Indigenous cultures have eaten fish for thousands of years but with the world's population growing, increasing demand is taking its toll. Taking marine life from the sea faster than populations can reproduce is known as overfishing. International agencies and governments set safe limits for catch numbers, but illegal practice goes on all the time and is thought to have caused the dwindling numbers of Chilean Seabass, Beluga Sturgeons and Bluefin Tuna, amongst thousands of other species.

Trawler fishing is another problem. Trawler fishing involves huge machinery dragging along the ocean floor, depleting the seabed and coral reef - a practice that's not too dissimilar to land deforestation in its indiscriminate damage.

Trawler fishing catches tonnes of fish in its nets and the fish it doesn't intend to catch normally come up dead or fatally injured. This is called by-catch. Fishers remove more than 77 billion kilograms of wildlife from the sea each year and some coral reefs in Florida and New Zealand have been 95% destroyed by the practice of trawling.[386]

We need to set clear guidelines for fishing and fish in harmony with our planet. Sustainable practices need to allow fish stocks to replenish themselves. The only way to stop this is to actively manage the oceans and fisheries and designate protected and trawl-free areas. And fishing practices themselves need to show regard for the marine eco-system and catch only what they need.

Seafood Watch is a great app that tells you when fish numbers are down and when to abstain. And the Environmental Working Groups have a great seafood calculator that will help you select the right fish and the right time to eat those fish. To maintain fish stocks, we need to reduce overfishing and by-catch through proper management practices. This requires co-operation at all levels of government and involves an intellectual and sustained commitment from all nations of global community. Until we learn how to fish more sustainably, we all need to take a serious look at how much we eat and what the planetary cost is. Some people would argue that there actually is no way to sustainably fish right now given the depleted state of our oceans.

So, what do we do if we need to supplement omega 3? Krill oil is a no no - if we reduce krill biomass, we reduce everything. It's that fundamental to all marine life and there really is no compromise on this one. Fish oil supplementation looks to be a low mercury option, but it has to be from sustainable fisheries using small fish like sardines and anchovies that reproduce rapidly and have low risk of contaminations otherwise it doesn't help us get our oceans sorted. Studies of fish oil supplements show that concentrations of mercury and other contaminants are very low compared to actual fish.[387] Consumer Labs tests of fish oils sold in the US found none with more than 0.01 parts per million mercury - in other words, significantly less mercury than a single serving of fish.[388]

Another option is algal oil, but with algal oil you mainly get DHA which is great for the brain and eyes but you tend to miss out on the anti-inflammatory EPA and they work best synergistically. Algae are some of the most abundant organisms in the ocean and are the base of the food chain.

Algal oil is clean (in that it doesn't bio-accumulate contaminants like fish do) and sustainable because it can be grown in factories without devastating our marine environment, so it's a good option for vegetarians and vegans - but maybe not as beneficial to our health as fish oil.

I regard Omega 3 as another universally beneficial supplement. I tend to advise a daily amount of 1000mg of EPA and DHA combined.

In the wise words of renowned marine scientist Dr Sylvia Earle, 'If we value the ocean and the ocean's health at all, we have to understand that fish are critical to maintaining the integrity of ocean systems, which in turn make the planet work'.

SUSTAINABLE PLANT FOODS

Kilo for kilo, litre for litre, plant-based foods use vastly less water and carbon to produce than animal-sourced foods. They are full of healthful nutrients and as we have seen in the preceding chapters are positively great for your health.

There are some problems, however, even with plant-based diets that we cannot simply gloss over. Because we haven't geared up or planned for the huge boom in vegetarianism and plant-based eating (this would require years of planning and planting), purchases of avocado, soya, almonds, cashews, acai, goji (and the rest) are causing depletions and price wars in other parts of the world. Sustainability is about managing foods and not causing food crises in developing countries where the food so often originates. It's always better to eat locally grown and seasonal plant-based foods than it is to eat foods transported halfway across the world. In 2013 - dubbed 'the year of quinoa' by the UN - quinoa prices skyrocketed and locals, who eat quinoa as a staple, were priced out of the market. The price of quinoa has trebled since 2006 to £5/kilo. Not all plant-based foods are currently sustainable.

Mexico is a good example. It provides 45% of the world's avocados yet the price per kilo of avocados is more than a day's wage for the locals. Clearly this is not sustainable. Sustainable foods have to be affordable, attainable and nutritious.

The same has happened in California with almonds. We now consume ten times as many almonds compared to forty years ago. Almond production is water intensive, so much so that the increased demand has resulted in water being depleted in the nearby water systems, causing problems with the local salmon.

It takes over 6,000 litres of water to produce one litre of almond milk so, whilst it's better than cow's milk for your health it's not better for the planet. The almond milk craze has caused havoc to land in California, which has been in drought for most of the last ten years. Cashew milk has also boomed in popularity in both Europe and America but that boom places huge strains on local rural populations in India (where 60% of cashews come from) who work for the equivalent of about £2 a day and suffer skin burns due to the cardol and anacardic acid in cashew shells. Oat milk is much more sustainable.

Rice is also water intensive and is a daily staple, feeding over 3.5 billion people worldwide. Being mindful of our food choices is really important. Don't just follow fads but find out what foods are low impact and sustainable.

Better still we can correct some of this by buying local and seasonal plant-based foods. If the UK were to plant more protein and bean crops, we would reduce our dependence on imports and create a more sustainable and home-grown food crop. The UK currently assigns only 16% of its agricultural land to growing protein crops and instead imports beans, quinoa, lentils, chickpeas etc. from far flung places like Brazil, Canada and the USA. If we were to reorganise and reallocate the land, we could grow these crops locally to achieve a better food self-sufficiency level and therefore reduce imports. A company already exists that grows lentils, fava beans and quinoa in Essex so anything is possible.

We can also start our own herb and vegetable gardens or encourage people to grow their own in allotments. Many varieties of vegetable grow well in domestic gardens. All you need is a bucket of soil, some sunshine and the will to do it.

Ask yourself this question - if supermarkets stopped selling you food how would you survive? Most people wouldn't know what to do and would have no back up plan whatsoever other than a few days of freezer foods. This should make you realise that the very foods we rely on depend on an entire chain of events to run smoothly. In the modern world we face the very real issue of unsustainable growth that can no longer be met by natural resources. It's time to wise up - we are at the point now where being sustainable isn't just a nice idea, it's SURVIVAL.

If we all stopped eating meat today, then everyone currently engaged in the livestock industry would find themselves without a livelihood.

This would be a massive disaster, both locally and in developing nations. The transition needs to be managed and planned well at local, national and international level to reduce mass social upheaval and consequent economic impact.

One Green Earth

"On the one acre of land needed to produce 250 pounds of beef, we could grow 50,000 pounds of tomatoes, 53,000 pounds of potatoes or 30,000 pounds of carrots. The average person who eats plant-based can save 162,486 gallons of water a year and cut their carbon footprint in half. But the icing on the plant-based cake is the fact we could redirect enough grain from the livestock system to feed 1.4 BILLION people if every American stopped eating meat."

WHAT ELSE CAN WE DO TO LIVE SUSTAINABLY?

Plastic

Plastic can <u>never</u> be thrown away. AWAY DOESN'T EXIST. It goes either to landfill or into our oceans - it doesn't bio-degrade for hundreds of years. All those plastic shopping bags, straws, cups, forks and containers accumulate in our oceans along with other contaminants like oil, chemicals, agricultural waste, fertiliser run off, radioactive waste, sewage and residential waste. We need to recycle all our plastic and also stop producing plastic and use alternatives.

We need to use paper bags and cardboard boxes again instead of plastic for our shopping. We need to refuse plastic straws and cutlery at our local cafe or eatery. Use reusable coffee and beverage cups. Avoid buying our children plastic toys. We should filter our water and reuse water bottles rather than buying water in plastic bottles. To put this into context, every day in the UK we use 35 million plastic bottles a day – 23 million of which don't get recycled. Let's end our reliance on plastic and bring back the good old water fountain. If we all make an effort, that collective effort will be huge. For example, the enforced 5p plastic bag charge has been a huge success; we now use 6.5 billion fewer bags annually. This is progress.

"Your bag-for-life [needs to be used] 8 times before its carbon footprint is lower than an ordinary carrier bag. An organic cotton tote must be used 149 times to be in credit." Tony Naylor, The Guardian

35m

plastic bottles per day

Sustainable fashion

We are a disposable society. When we don't want something any more we just throw it away. There are two victims of our global obsession with cheap and disposable clothing - the environment and the textile workers. The environmental cost of our love of cheap fashion is water pollution, toxic chemicals and textile waste. Textile dyeing is the second largest polluter of clean water globally after agriculture. And polyester sheds microfibres that end up polluting our oceans and represent a non-biodegradable threat to our marine life. As with all things, they end up polluting us because micro plankton eat the microfibres, which get eaten by fish, which get eaten by us - and before you know it, we are full of microfibre. Cotton is another problem. It requires high levels of water and pesticides to prevent crop failure. Most cotton grown worldwide is genetically modified to be resistant to pests, but toxic pesticides are harmful to livestock and humans.

The rise of supermarket fashion, our busy lives and our lack of textile skills means it's easier to buy a constant slew of new clothes than repair the old ones. This has made fashion disposable in a way it never used to be. If we all choose sustainable fashion, organic fabrics, quality over quantity we will make a big difference. Alongside sensible food choices, banning plastic and using sustainable fuels, we might stand a chance at saving ourselves and this beautiful planet.

We must never forget the bigger picture. We are all connected to the land, the ocean, the air, the water, to animals and to other human beings. Our very existence depends on them - as does the future of our planet. The issues are global but the solutions are local. Let's work collectively to save ourselves and our beautiful planet.

"Water and air, the two essential fluids on which all life depends, have become global garbage cans."
Jacques Cousteau

CHAPTER 18: Plant-based Recipe Inspiration

"The Aim: Living to a ripe old age and feeling young when you get there."
Dr James Duke

In this final section I have collaborated with Charlotte Kjaer, a UK plant-based chef. Who better to work with than someone who spends their life creating nutritious foods with sustainable, seasonal and whole food ingredients?

Our collaboration will hopefully inspire you to get back into the kitchen and start enjoying whole foods again. Our recipes showcase the diverse and delicious foods you can make using plant based whole foods. You can add to them or change them as you need to accommodate different family member's dietary preferences but they will give you a lovely plant-based focus for your food that is healthy and nutritious.

Too many of us have allowed labs to create our foods when the better and healthier option is to cook for ourselves… The art of cooking nutritious foods is dying in a tidal wave of fast and convenience foods. We owe it to future generations to invest the time and energy into recapturing and reprioritising our health. If we leave it to the food industry to feed us, they will end up killing us! Diabetes, heart disease and cancer are all collaterals from eating too much processed food.

Creating your own food is the only way to take back control of what you are eating. It's also incredibly satisfying, fun and can help protect our wonderful planet.

CHARLOTTE KJAER, PLANT-BASED CHEF

Charlotte's love of food and nutrition started in her youth, when she would watch her father Larry create incredible family meals. As a young teenager Charlotte was diagnosed with leukaemia and underwent three years of gruelling chemotherapy. She spent a lot of time at home with her father, immersing herself in the culturally diverse meals that dinner time provided. After dealing with the harsh side effects of chemotherapy, Charlotte began a more natural journey focusing on a plant-based approach to health.

This directed her food journey and her cooking is nothing less than an exquisite celebration of all the wonders this earth provides to help heal and nourish.

Charlotte works in harmony with nature, using seasonal ingredients underpinned by a deep understanding of the nutrients in food. With incredible precision and attention to detail, each meal is created to be perfectly balanced. Expect fresh vibrant flavours, local seasonal produce, fermented and mood boosting food that harnesses the healing properties of the natural world.

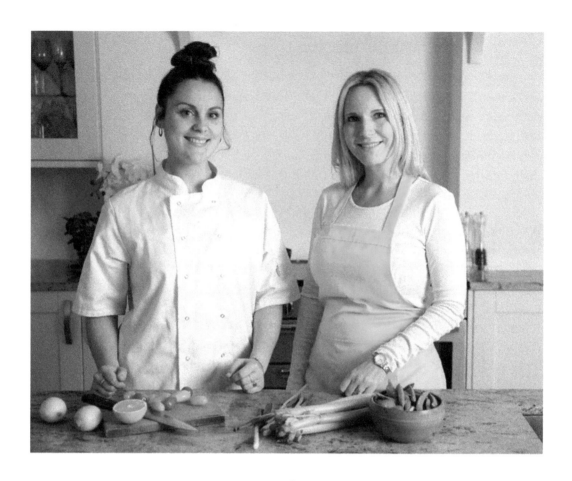

Charlotte Kjaer (left) with Dr Johanna Ward

BREAKFAST

Commercial breakfast cereals and bars are full of sugar so please avoid these at all costs.

A healthier way to start the day is with berries, rolled or steel cut oats or with a superfood smoothie. Fruit juices should be avoided as they contain high amounts of sugar (in the form of fructose) and are missing the fibre. Since phytonutrients are bound to fibre, you miss out on a lot when just juicing. When you consume fruit juices you get an intense sugar hit because the fibre that would have slowed the sugar spike has been removed. It's much better to consume the whole piece of fruit than just the juice or juice vegetables instead of fruit. Harvard University researchers found that consumption of whole fruits was associated with a lower risk of type 2 diabetes and that fruit juice consumption was associated with increased risk. Smoothie blending is a much better alternative to juicing because the fibre and phytonutrients are retained.

Berries contain much less sugar than many other fruits and are packed with phytonutrients and beneficial antioxidants. These antioxidants and phytonutrients are not destroyed by the freezing process, so when berries are out of season it is fine to use frozen berries instead. Use berries liberally with your breakfasts. They are some of the most powerful anti-cancer foods.

Sprinkle some cinnamon or seeds on your oats or smoothie. Just adding cinnamon to oats has been shown to increase its antioxidant capacity by 400%. Nuts and seeds are a great addition too. Walnuts, for example, are a great source of healthy fat and can be delicious sprinkled over breakfast. Countless studies have shown that people who eat nuts tend to live longer and suffer fewer cancer and heart disease deaths.[389] Flaxseeds and chia seeds are also great to sprinkle on oats and smoothies and are a great source of omega 3. Given that brain needs a constant supply of omega 3 to make new connections, it's a great idea to start your day by giving your brain the fuel it needs.

Commercial smoothies often contain a lot of sugar. Innocent smoothies, for example, have 30% more sugar than a can of coke - not so innocent after all! Instead of supermarket smoothies, make home-made ones and choose ingredients like greens (spinach, kale) and bases like sustainable avocado to end your reliance on banana. Choose frozen berries rather than high fructose fruits so you can enjoy them all year around. Add some unsweetened non-dairy milk, flaxseeds and portion control and that way your smoothie isn't a sugar bomb.

Studies have shown that half our fruit and vegetable consumption comes from the same five fruits - apples, bananas, grapes, oranges and watermelon [390] - and that most of our vegetable consumption is in the form of potatoes, lettuce and tomatoes. It's important to consume a great variety and diversity of fruits and vegetables because each piece offers different antioxidant and phytonutrient benefits, not to mention a different vitamin and mineral profile. Try not to get into the habit of eating the same foods over and over again but mix it up and use these recipes to experiment with new foods, creating new tastes and new healthful habits.

SCRAMBLED TOFU, RED ONION AND ROAST TOMATO BREAKFAST

Serves 4. GF, NF

300g organic tofu
1 red onion
8 tomatoes on the vine
Handful of fresh basil
1 tsp oregano or mixed herbs
1 tsp turmeric
1 tsp black pepper

Method

Heat the oven to 180 degrees Celsius.

Place the vine tomatoes on a baking tray, drizzle with olive oil, season and roast for 7-10 minutes until soft.

Crumble the tofu with your hands into small pieces into a mixing bowl. Add the turmeric, black pepper, herbs and mix well.

Dice the onion and fry in coconut oil until soft and translucent. Add the tofu and fry until the tofu is slightly crisp and golden brown, around 3-5 minutes in total.

Serve on rye bread with vine tomatoes and freshly torn basil.

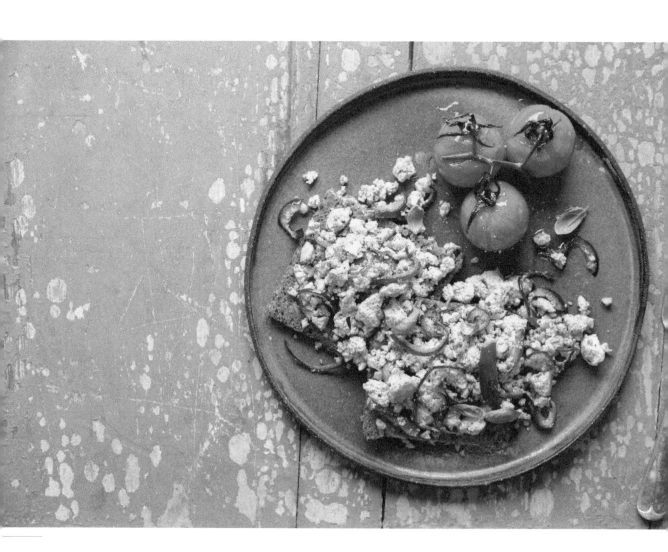

BANANA & BUCKWHEAT PANCAKES

Serves 2. GF, NF

1 banana
1 cup buckwheat flour
1 tbsp baking powder
1 tbsp apple cider vinegar
1 cup plant milk
1 tsp cinnamon
1 tsp vanilla
1 tbsp melted coconut oil

Method

Place all ingredients into a jug blender or food processor and blend well.

Melt coconut oil in a frying pan on medium heat.

Using a ¼ cup measure per pancake, pour the mixture into the pan and fry the pancakes until small bubbles appear on the surface - about 3 minutes.

Flip the pancake and cook on the other side for 1 minute or so.

Serve immediately with any combination of Chia Berry Jam, blueberries, oat cream or caramelised bananas. Enjoy!

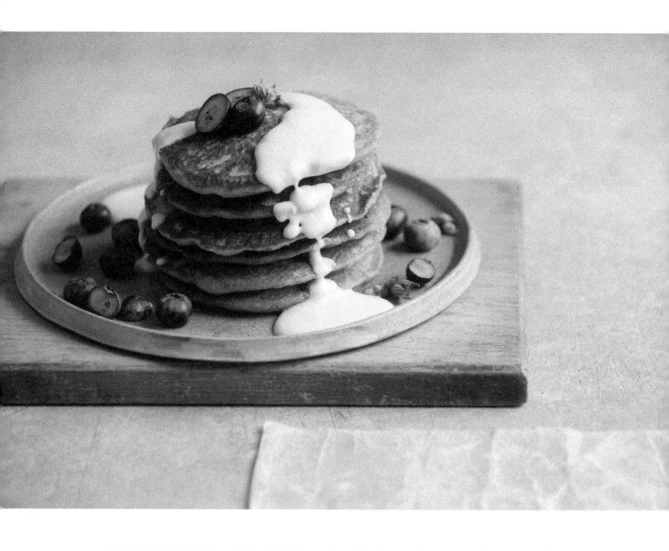

These pancakes are divine and perfect for families with children because they taste great and are fun to make. Buckwheat is actually a seed, not a grain and is not related to wheat (despite its name!). It's gluten free and high in protein. Best of all, buckwheat is non-GMO - it's never been genetically modified. Buckwheat has a low glycaemic index and is a good source of fibre, magnesium, manganese and copper.

CHIA BERRY JAM

Serves 4-6. GF, NF

2 tbsp chia seeds
2 cups frozen berries

Method

Place the frozen berries in a pan and simmer gently until softened and the juices released.

Take off the heat and add the chia seeds, mix well.

Leave to cool and thicken; if not thick enough add 1 tsp more chia seeds.

This jam goes well with the Multi-Grain Porridge and the Buckwheat Pancakes but can add taste to any dish and is a great alternative to sugar-loaded commercial jam.

~~~

CARAMELISED BANANAS

Serves 4

2 bananas
1 tbsp coconut oil
1 tbsp maple syrup

Method

Slice the bananas lengthways down the centre. Heat the coconut oil in a frying pan and place the maple syrup and banana, cut side down into the pan and gently fry for 1-2 minutes until softened but not falling apart. Serve with Banana and Buckwheat Pancakes.

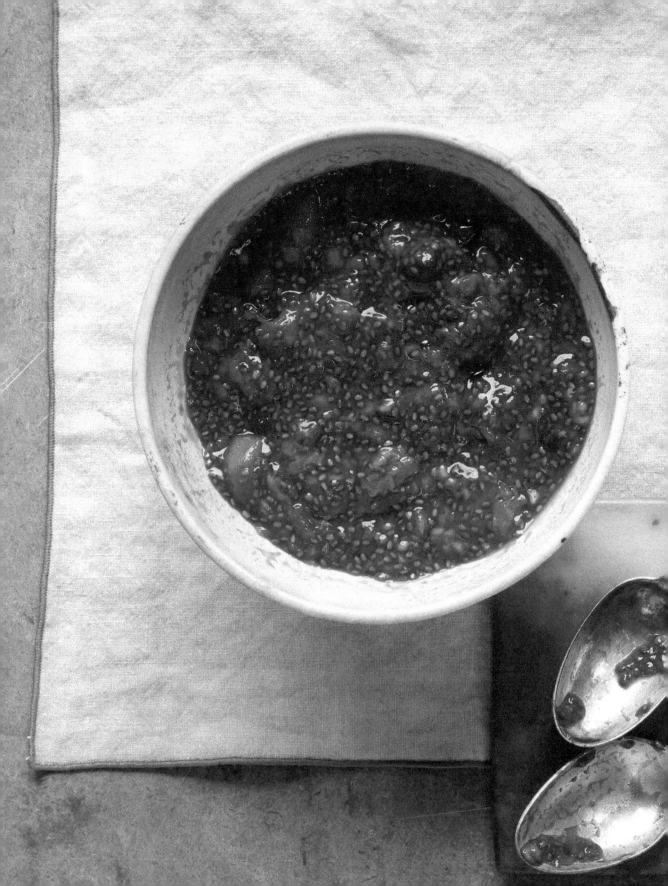

MULTI-GRAIN PORRIDGE

Serves 2. GF, NF

½ cup wholegrain oats
¼ quinoa flakes
¼ buckwheat flakes
1 tbsp flaxseeds
½ tbsp pumpkin seeds
1 tsp cinnamon
1½ cups plant milk

METHOD

Add the oats, quinoa, buckwheat flakes, flaxseeds and plant milk to a pan.

Simmer gently on a medium heat until thickened, about 3-5 minutes.

Once cooked, add the cinnamon, serve with the pumpkin seeds and chia berry jam.

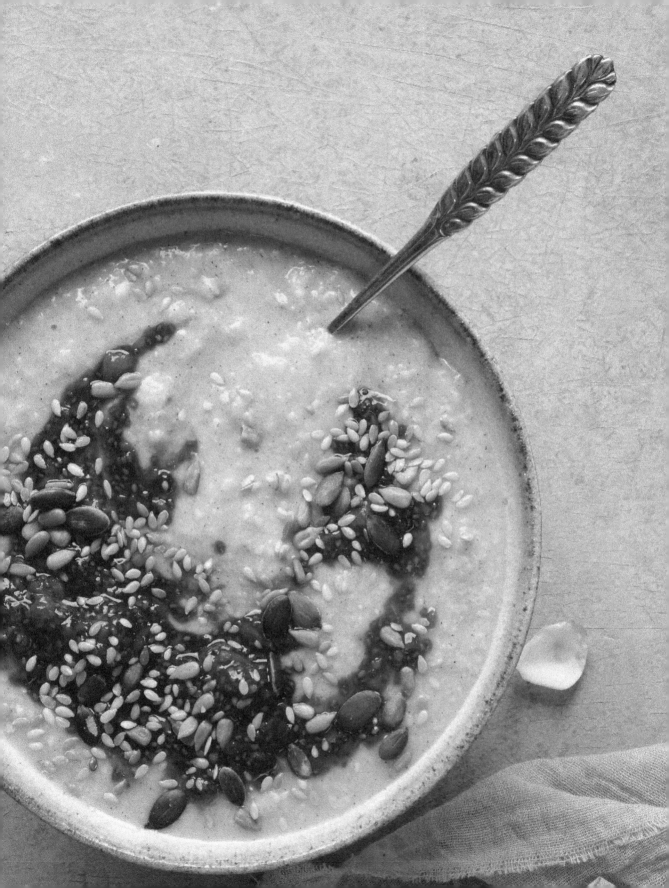

SUPERFOOD 'SUPERBUG' SMOOTHIE

Serves 2. GF.

250ml coconut water
1 cup frozen mixed berries
1 banana
1 tsp flaxseed
½ lemon, squeezed
Coconut kefir

Optional extras:

Probiotic powder
Acai powder
Chlorella powder

METHOD

Place all ingredients into a jug blender.

Blend on high until smooth.

Kefir is a fermented food rich in probiotics. Coconut kefir is a wonderful dairy-free way of repopulating the gut with beneficial bacteria and it can be added to any smoothie for extra gut health benefits. I like to add probiotics, prebiotics and spirulina powders to my smoothies. Did you know your gut has more bugs in it than humans have ever populated this planet? It pays to look after your bugs.

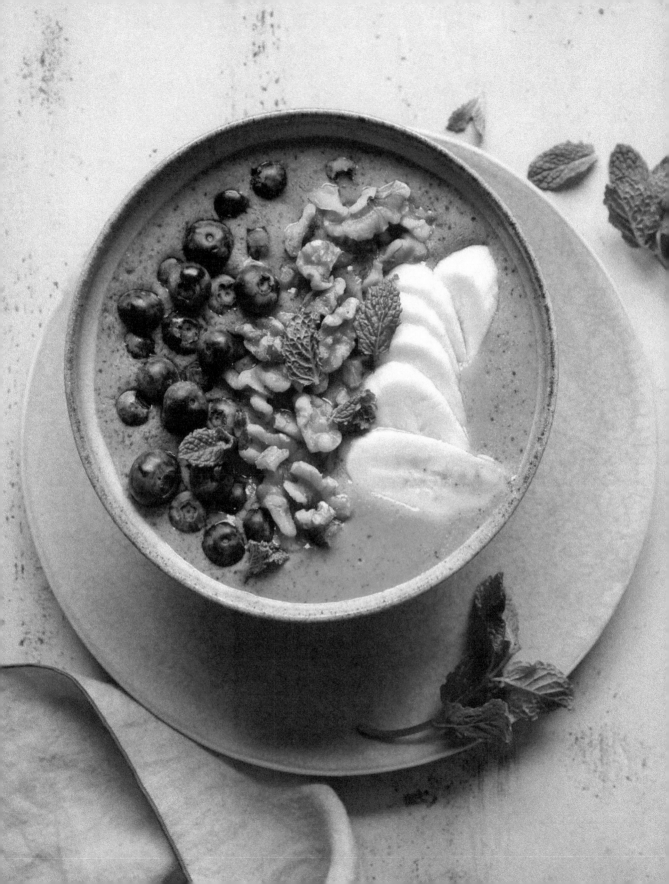

VITALITY SMOOTHIE

Serves 2. GF

250ml plant milk
½ avocado
Large handful spinach
Small handful kale
Handful of blueberries
1 tsp flaxseed
1 tbsp cashew butter
1 tbsp spirulina
½ lemon, squeezed

Optional extras:

Probiotic powder
Coconut kefir
Acai powder
Pomegranates

METHOD

Place all ingredients into a jug blender.

Blend on high until smooth.

Commercial smoothies are often loaded with sugar, but home-made ones are a wonderful way of getting a powerful mix of superfoods and super nutrients into a single meal. I recommend a smoothie a day. To ensure your smoothie isn't a sugar bomb, try avocado as a base. Smoothies are a great way of getting health foods like spirulina, probiotics and acai into your daily diet because you can simply add them in as powders and the smoothie conceals the taste. Add some unsweetened non-dairy milk, flaxseeds and portion control.

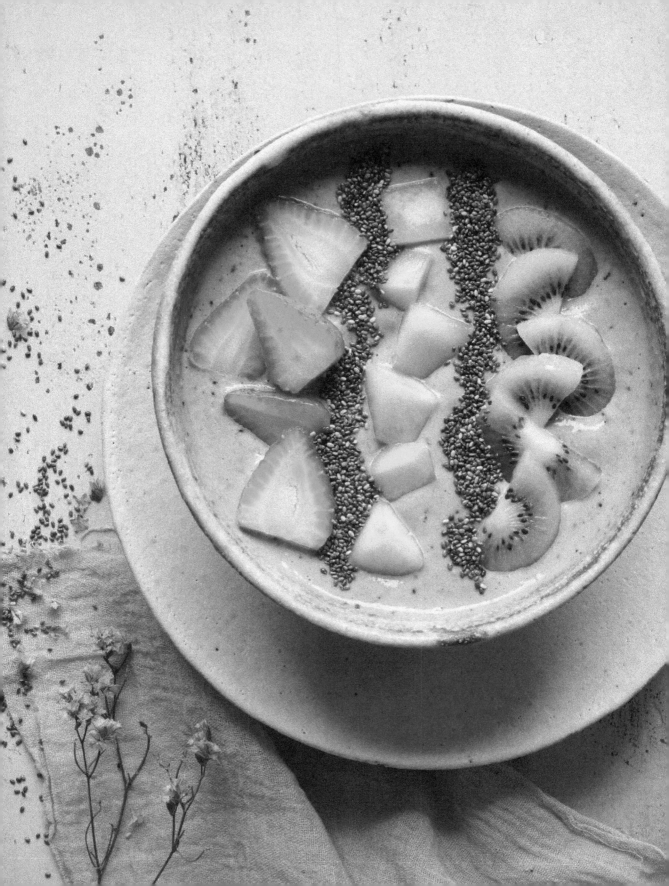

HOME-MADE GOJI GRANOLA

Serves 4.

1 cup organic rolled oats
¼ cup organic chopped almonds
¼ cup organic chopped pecans
3 tbsp mixed seeds (ideally pumpkin, flax & sunflower seeds)
3 tbsp goji berries
2 tbsp melted coconut oil or macadamia nut oil

Optional extras:

Organic manuka honey.

METHOD

Preheat the oven to 160 degrees Celsius.

Add the oats, nuts, seeds and melted coconut/macadamia nut oil to a bowl and mix well.

Line a baking tray with greaseproof paper, place oat mixture on the tray and bake for 5-7 minutes until toasted and golden brown.

Take out of the oven and add the cinnamon and goji berries.

Mix well, allow to cool.

Granola will keep for 2 weeks in an airtight jar.

Serve with coconut yoghurt, plant milk or fruits of your choice.

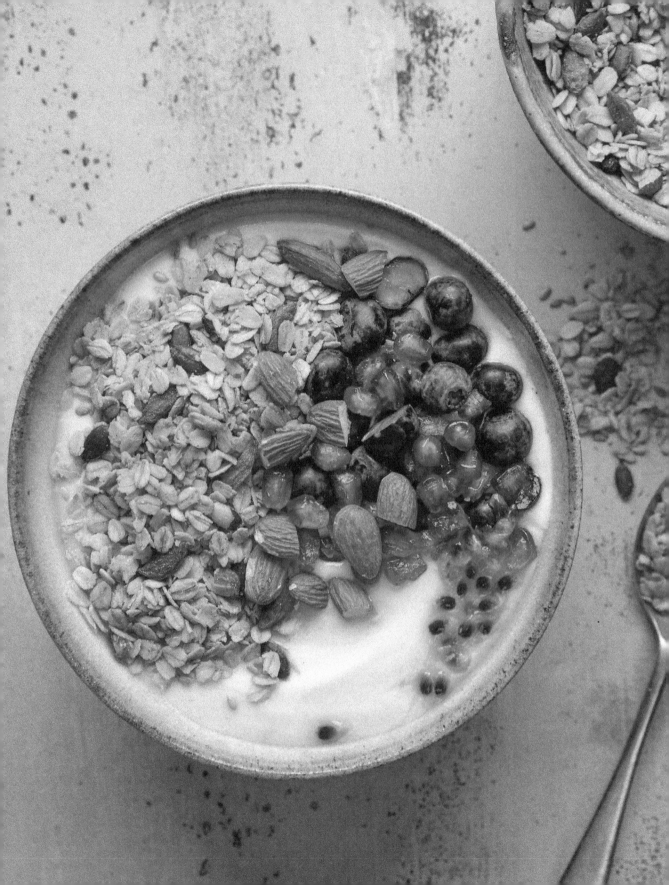

LUNCH

Lunch is possibly the most important meal to consider when first trying to improve your eating because for many people lunch is eaten outside the home. It is often the lunchtime meal that takes a day that started healthy on a grand detour. It is always worth pre-preparing lunch in the early days to ensure you have something nutritious and delicious close to hand. This will allow you to stay focused on healthy eating without giving in to the temptations of convenience foods.

The best thing to have for lunch each day is an abundant, big green salad. Pile it high with leafy greens (broccoli sprouts, rocket, kale, collards, spinach) and mixed vegetables so it is filling. Dark greens are the healthiest foods on the planet and come top of the superfood list. The only caution is if you are on the medicine Warfarin which thins the blood: you may need to get your doctor to adjust your dose as greens have an abundance of vitamin K.

Add some flaxseeds (rich in omega 3) or nuts and avocado (sustainable) to your salads. Or be adventurous and try mint, parsley and oregano. Mint is the highest antioxidant-containing common herb! Healthy salad dressings are possible if you use ground nuts and seeds. You just need to know a few recipes and you will soon learn to enjoy the taste of healthy, home-made salad dressings rather than commercial dressings.

If you need some other lunch options then seasonal soups are great and are extremely filling. You can make a huge soup batch at the weekend and then eat it slowly for your lunches over the week. Sprinkle soups with different seeds and nuts for extra texture and flavour.

'You should eat more fruit and vegetables as if your life depended on it, because it probably does.'
Dr Michael Greger, Author 'How Not to Die'

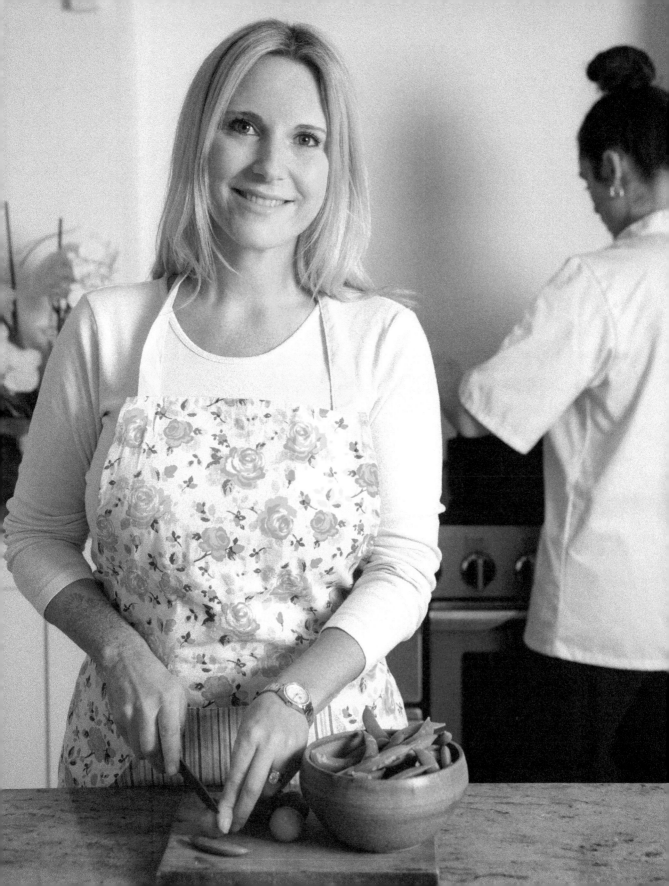

WINTER BOWL – ROOT VEGETABLES WITH TAHINI DRESSING

Serves 2. GF, NF

100g quinoa	½ cauliflower	**Dressing:**
1 carrot	Handful salad leaves	3 tbsp tahini
½ squash	Handful spinach	1 lemon, juiced
1 red onion	2 rosemary sprigs	2 tbsp olive oil
1 parsnip	5 cloves garlic	1-2 tbsp water to thin

METHOD

Preheat the oven to 180 degrees Celsius.

Chop the carrot, squash, onion, parsnip and cauliflower into similar sized chunks and place onto a baking tray.

Add the garlic cloves in their skins and rosemary, pour over 2 tbsp melted coconut oil, pepper and then mix well.

Roast in a hot oven for 30-40 mins until cooked and golden brown.

While the vegetables are roasting, cook the quinoa in vegetable stock and prepare the dressing by whisking all ingredients together into a small bowl.

To serve, place the quinoa and salad leaves into a shallow bowl, add the roast vegetables and pour over the dressing.

Quinoa is a dream to cook with because it cooks quickly (15 mins), is highly nutritious and contains all 9 essential amino acids, which is rare in plant-based foods. It provides 5 more grams of fibre and double the protein of rice and is just as versatile. It has a lovely nutty taste, holds spice well and is gluten free. Quinoa flour is a great option for gluten free baking too.

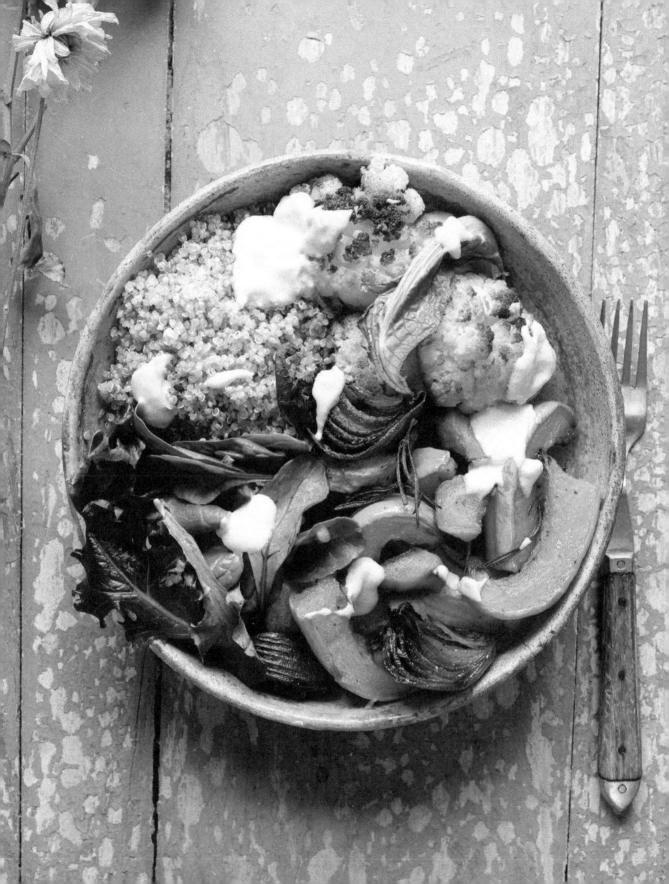

SUMMER BUDDHA BOWL - COURGETTE, EDAMAME, PEAS & MINT WITH LEMON VINAIGRETTE

Serves 2. GF, NF

100g quinoa
1 avocado
½ courgette
75g edamame beans
50g peas
Handful of mint
Handful of salad leaves

Dressing:
1 lemon, juiced
2 tbsp olive oil
1 tsp Dijon mustard
1 garlic clove, crushed

METHOD

Cook the quinoa in stock according to packet instructions.

Use a peeler to cut thin slices of the courgette.

Defrost peas in warm water.

Make the dressing by whisking all ingredients in a bowl.

Edamame beans are young soy beans that have been harvested early. They are a complete protein and a highly nutritious plant-based food. Loaded with vitamins and minerals and high in polyunsaturated ALA fats, edamame beans are also high in folate which reduces homocysteine levels and genistein, the predominant isoflavone in soy which is known to inhibit the growth of cancer cells. They are soft beans unlike the mature beans used to make soy milk and tofu.

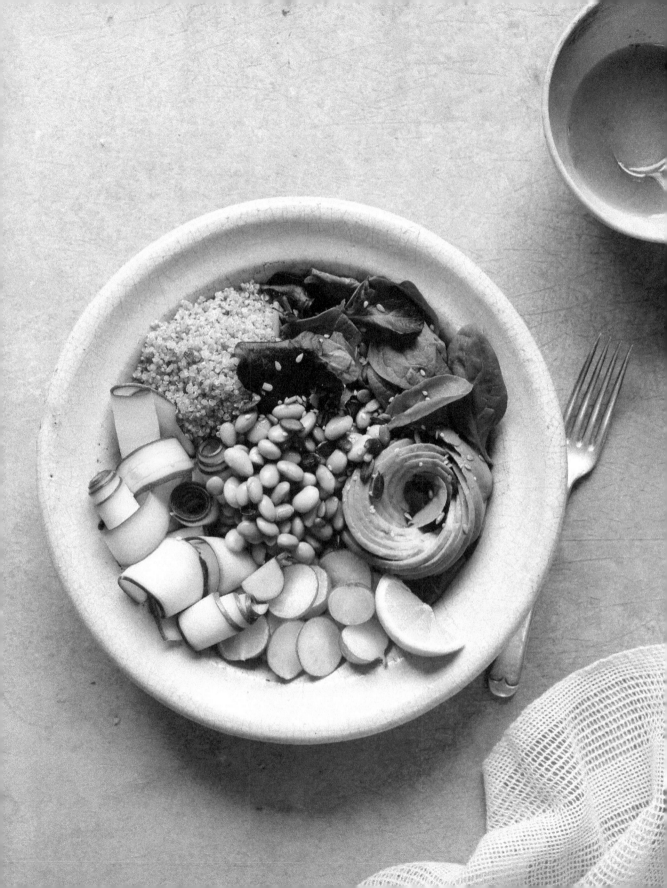

MILLET TABBOULEH SALAD WITH ROASTED CHICKPEAS AND POMEGRANATE

Serves 2.

100g millet	1 tin chickpeas	**Dressing:**
2 bunches parsley	1 tsp turmeric	3 tbsp olive oil
1 bunch mint	1 tsp cumin	1 tsp all spice
½ cucumber	½ tub	1 lemon, juiced
3 spring onions	pomegranate	1 orange, juiced
200g cherry	seeds	
tomatoes		

METHOD

Preheat the oven to 180 degrees Celsius.

Drain and rinse the chickpeas, place on a baking tray and season with turmeric, cumin, pepper and 1 tbsp coconut oil.

Roast for 7-10 minutes until golden brown and crunchy.

Rinse the millet and cook in vegetable stock according to packet instructions.

Once cooked, rinse the millet under cold water, drain and place in a mixing bowl.

Chop the cucumber, parsley, mint, cherry tomatoes and spring onions and add to the millet.

Make the dressing by whisking all ingredients into a bowl. Pour over millet tabbouleh and mix well.

Serve with pomegranate seeds and roast chickpeas scattered on top.

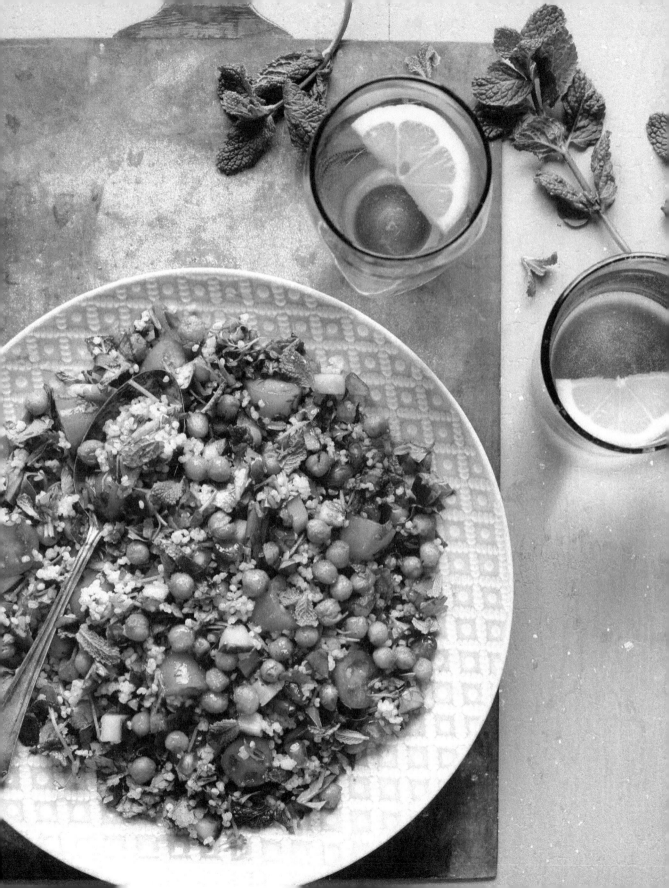

LENTIL & SWEET POTATO SOUP

Serves 4. GF, NF

200g red lentils
750g (3 medium) sweet
potatoes, diced
2 celery stalks
1 carrot
1 red onion
1 tin coconut milk
4 garlic cloves

1 tsp turmeric
1 tsp ground coriander
1 tsp paprika
1 tsp smoked paprika
1 tsp ground coriander
1 tsp black pepper
1 tsp cayenne pepper
1l vegetable stock

METHOD

Cover lentils with water and soak while you prepare the other ingredients.

Dice the onion, celery and carrot and fry in coconut oil until lightly browned.

Add the garlic and spices and fry for 1 minute until fragrant.

Add the sweet potato, lentils, coconut milk and stock.

Simmer gently for 30 minutes or until the lentils and sweet potato are cooked.

Blend until smooth and serve with plant milk cream and Seed Crackers (recipe on next page).

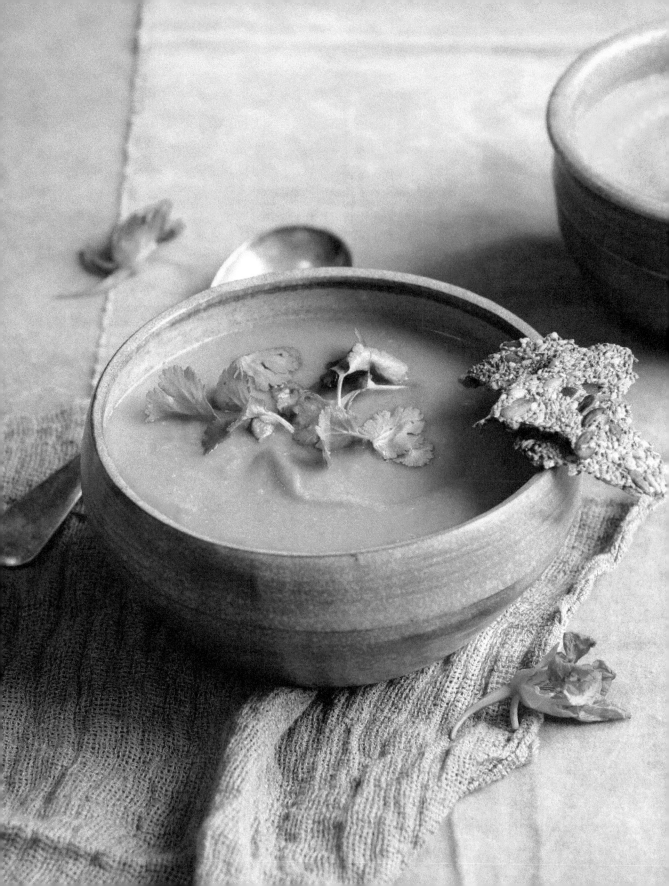

SEED CRACKERS

Serves 4 – 6. GF

1/4 cup flax seeds
¼ cup pumpkin seeds
½ cup chia seeds
1 tsp fennel seeds
1 tsp nigella seeds
1 tbsp nutritional yeast
1 tsp black pepper
1 cup water
1 tbsp coconut oil, melted

METHOD

Place all the dry ingredients in a bowl and mix well.

Add the water and allow to thicken for 30 minutes.

Preheat the oven to 180 degrees Celsius.

Place a lightly oiled sheet of greaseproof paper on a baking tray and thinly spread out the seed mixture.

Place in the oven for 30 minutes or until dried. Let cool and break into rough shapes.

Keep in an air tight container.

Serve with Sweet Potato and Red Lentil Soup.

SUPERFOOD SUPER SALAD

Serves 2.

100g kale	**Dressing:**
100g broccoli sprouts	1 avocado
150g green beans	1 lemon, juiced
Handful coriander	1 tbsp olive oil
Handful mint	1 garlic clove, crushed
3 spring onions	2 tbsp apple cider vinegar
Handful rocket	
2 tbsp Tamari roast seeds	

METHOD

Place the kale in a large bowl and cover with 1 tbsp olive oil. Using your hands, 'massage' the kale by squeezing and kneading it. It's ready when it has softened and reduced in volume.

Blanch the broccoli and green beans in boiling water until still crisp, refresh under cold water.

For the dressing, place all the ingredients into a jug blender with a splash of water to thin and blend until smooth.

To serve, place the kale and rocket in a bowl. Add the broccoli, green beans, spring onion, coriander and mint (reserving a few leaves for garnish).

Pour over the dressing, mix well and scatter the tamari roast seeds (recipe in the snack section), coriander and mint leaves on top.

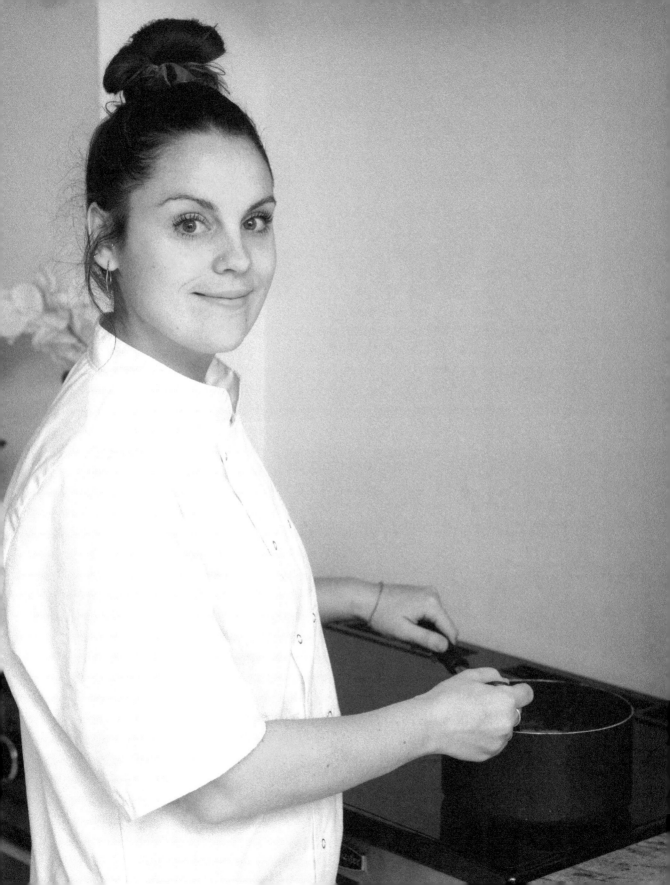

DINNER

Dinner should be eaten early, ideally before 6pm if you go to bed at 10 or 11pm. It's important for the body to have time overnight to reset so an early dinner allows for digestion while you are still awake. Night time can then be reserved for really important functions, such as cellular renewal and repair.

Dinner should always include a salad or greens; place your dinner on a bed of greens if you aren't having a salad. Salads are great because they allow you to eat more raw superfoods such as lettuce, rocket, peas, tomatoes and increase the diversity of your vegetable intake. Try and incorporate herbs and spices into your lunch and dinners too. They are the most antioxidant-rich food group and confer significant health benefits. The body needs to be flooded at every meal with antioxidants and anti-inflammatories because oxidative stress is happening all the time. Plant-based food is super tasty when you know how to use herbs and spices well. If you think vegetables are boring then you have never had them cooked well. Our dishes will certainly get you using lots of different vegetables with lots of beneficial herbs and spices. Use these to taste and season your food rather than salt.

If you want to try some intermittent fasting, then eating an early dinner is a great way of kicking it off. Eat your dinner at 6pm and then simply don't eat until you are hungry the next morning or until after 10am. In other words, you just eat between the hours of 10am and 6pm. A great tip is to brush your teeth after dinner to stop you from the risk of grazing. Many people underestimate their calories when they allow themselves to graze. If you have a medical condition, double check with your doctor that this is safe for you.

Intermittent fasting is a great way to kick-start your metabolism and ensure that you don't overeat. Fasting is used by many cultures and primitive man certainly didn't eat 3-5 meals per day. Another way of fasting is to eat only 600-800 calories on two non-consecutive days of the week and then eat normally on the other five. This regime is called the 5:2 diet.

COCONUT RICE NOODLE SOUP

Serves 4. GF

This recipe is a great one because it encourages you to use lots of healthy herbs and spices, which are loaded with antioxidants and have significant health benefits - plus they add great texture and depth to a dish.

Paste
1 onion
4 garlic cloves
2-inch piece ginger
2 chilli
2 lemongrass stalks
1 bunch coriander stalks, reserve leaves for garnish
1 tsp cumin
0.5 tsp cinnamon
1 tsp turmeric
1 tsp ground coriander
1 tsp paprika
1 tsp black pepper
2 tbsp cashew nuts (& garnish)
1 lime, juice

Soup
3 star anise
3 cardamom pods
1 tin coconut milk
500ml veg stock
1 tbsp miso paste
200g rice noodles
2 handfuls seasonal veg

Method

Place the paste ingredients into blender with a splash of water and blend until a smooth paste forms.

Heat 2 tbsp coconut oil in large saucepan and fry the paste for 1-2 minutes until fragrant, be careful not to burn it.

Add the coconut milk, veg stock, star anise, cardamom and miso paste and bring to a gentle simmer for 10 minutes.

Add the seasonal veg to the soup (try broccoli, spinach, red pepper and courgette) for 5 minutes until cooked but with a bite.

Cook the rice noodles according to packet instructions and divide between 4 deep bowls. Ladle over the soup and vegetables and garnish with coriander leaves, cashew nuts and lime wedges.

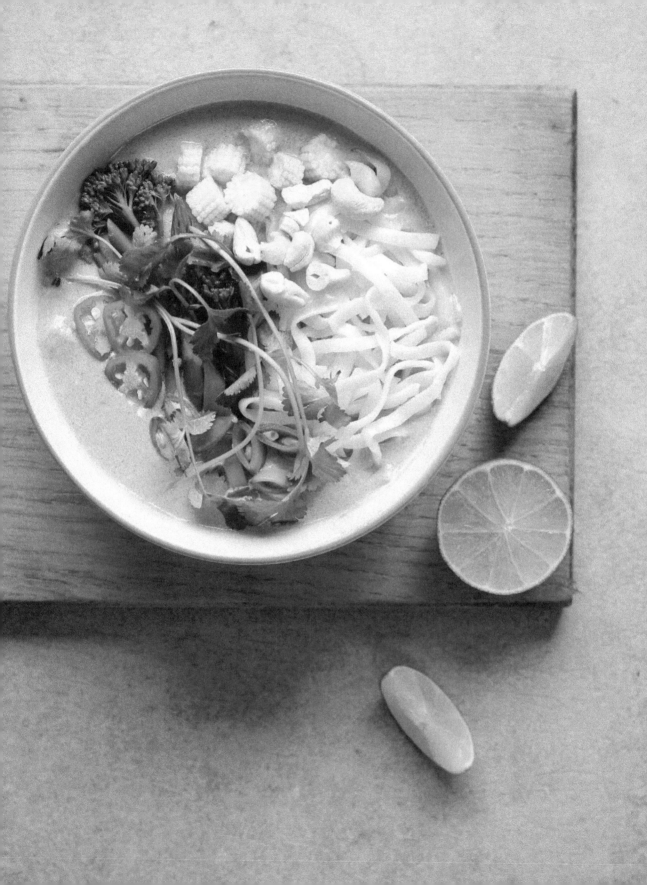

MUSHROOM, CANNELLINI BEAN AND SPINACH WELLINGTON

Serves 6

1 ready rolled puff pastry sheet	4 garlic cloves
8 field / portobello mushrooms, chopped	100g walnuts
	50g dried cranberries
1 tin cannellini beans	4 sprigs rosemary
500g spinach	2 tbsp mixed seeds

Method

Preheat the oven to 180 degrees Celsius.

Place the mushrooms, rosemary sprigs and garlic in skins onto a baking tray with a pinch of pepper and a drizzle of oil. Roast for 10-15 minutes until the mushrooms are soft and juicy.

Wilt the spinach by placing it in a colander and pouring freshly boiled water over it into the sink. Leave to cool slightly and use your hands to squeeze out the excess water.

Place the cannellini beans in a bowl and roughly mash with a fork. Add the wilted spinach, walnuts, cranberries, pepper to taste and squeeze out the roasted garlic from their skins. Mix well.

Lay out the pastry sheet flat in front of you and spread the bean mixture horizontally along the centre of the sheet. Lay the mushrooms on top of the bean mixture and gently fold up the two outer edges to overlap in the centre.

Place the Wellington (seam side down) onto a greaseproof lined baking tray.

Make a few small slits on the top of the Wellington for steam to escape, glaze with plant milk and sprinkle over 2 tbsp of mixed seeds for decoration.

Roast for 25-30 minutes until the pastry has risen and is golden brown. Serve for Sunday lunch with mushroom gravy.

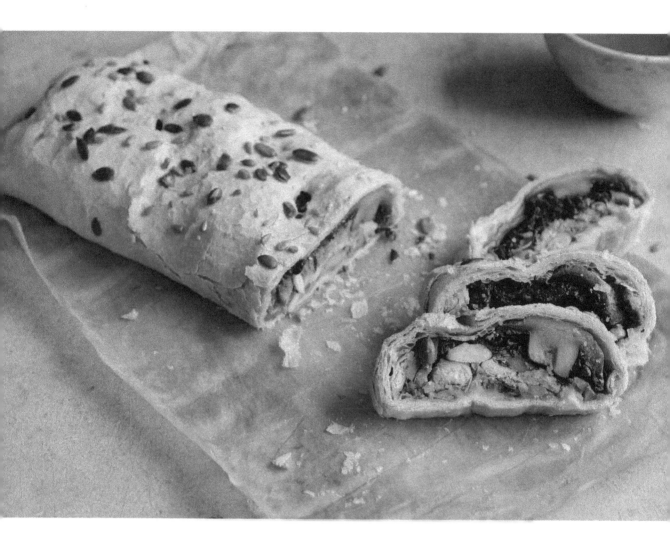

Cannellini beans are a great source of protein and fibre and are an inexpensive way of giving yourself a health boost. You can buy them canned and they retain their nutritional value well. A 200g serving of beans contains 50% of your daily fibre requirement. Most Brits consume less than 50% of the daily recommended dose of fibre. Fibre is important because it protects against colon cancer.

CREAMY CASHEW SPAGHETTI

Serves 4. GF

150g (1½ cups) cashew nuts
4 tbsp nutritional yeast
2-3 garlic cloves
½ lemon juice
1 tsp bouillon stock powder
1 cup plant milk

300g brown spaghetti

300g mushrooms

Method

Soak the cashews for 2-3 hours (or quick soak in boiling water for 1 hour).

Drain and rinse the cashews and place in a blender with the remaining ingredients.

Blend until smooth and creamy.

Serve with spaghetti and garlic fried mushrooms.

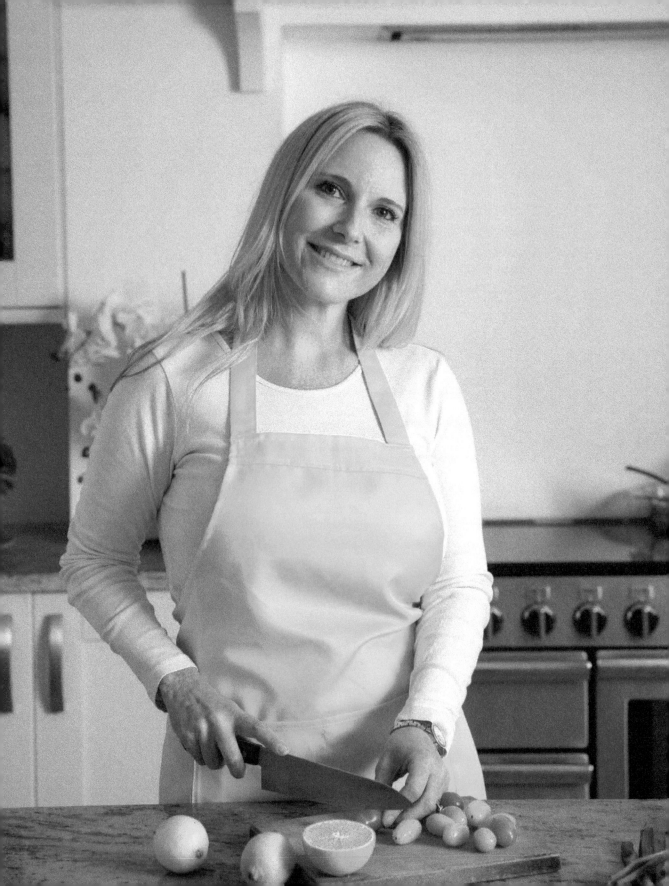

MISO ROAST AUBERGINE WITH TEMPEH & STIR FRY VEGETABLES

Serves 2. GF, NF

Aubergine	Tempeh	Vegetables
1 aubergine	1 pack (300g) tempeh	1 carrot
2 tbsp miso paste	2 tbsp tamari soy sauce	1 celery stalk
1 garlic clove, crushed	1 tbsp rice wine vinegar	100g mange tout
1 tsp sesame seeds	3 garlic cloves, crushed	100g bean sprouts
1 tsp nigella seeds	1-inch ginger, grated	1 red onion
		1 broccoli head

Method

Preheat the oven to 180 degrees Celsius.

Start by making the tempeh marinade by adding the tempeh ingredients to a bowl and mixing well. Cut the tempeh into 1cm cubes and add to the marinade - set aside while you prepare the other ingredients.

Place the miso, garlic and 1 tbsp water into a bowl and whisk until combined. Cut the aubergine lengthways down the centre and diagonally score the flesh of each half, being careful not to cut all the way through. Brush over the miso marinade and place onto a baking tray. Cover the aubergine lightly with foil and roast for 15 minutes until the aubergine is soft. Remove the foil and roast for 5 minutes more to caramelise.

Heat 2 tbsp coconut oil in a large frying pan, remove the tempeh from the marinade and fry it for 5 minutes.

Add the vegetables and fry for another 5 minutes until softened but still crisp, pour over the remaining marinade and mix well.

Serve with rice or noodles.

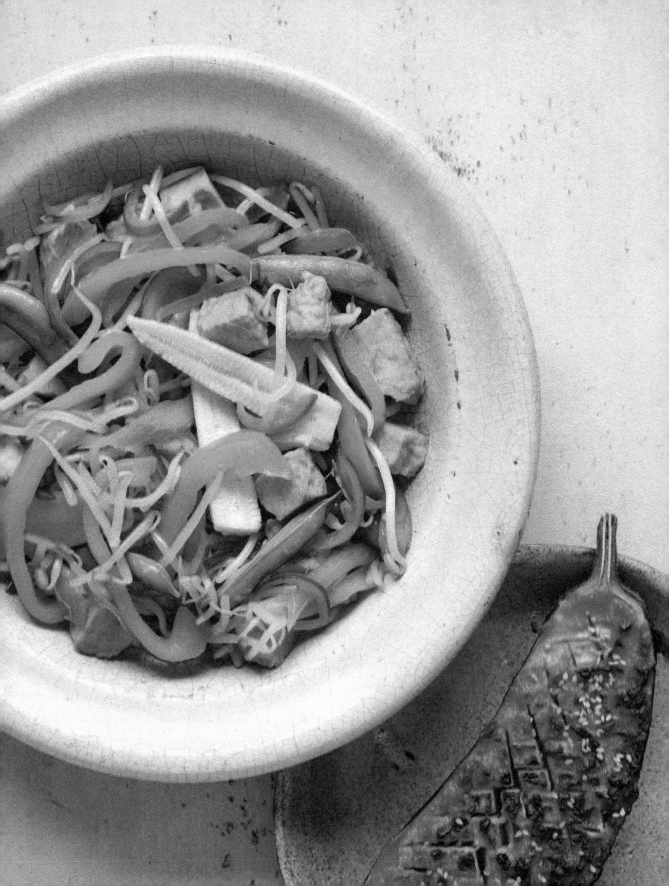

SWEET POTATO, SMOKY BLACK BEANS, PICKLED RED ONION, TOMATO SALSA AND AVOCADO

Serves 4. GF, NF

4 medium sweet
potatoes
1 tin black beans
1 tin of tomatoes
1 white onion
1 leek
1 carrot
1 red pepper

1 chilli
1.5 tbsp smoked
paprika
1 tsp all spice
1 tsp cumin
1 tsp turmeric
1 tsp black pepper

To serve
1 red onion
300g cherry
tomatoes
1 avocado
1 bunch coriander
3 tbsp apple cider
vinegar

Method

Preheat the oven to 180 degrees Celsius and roast the sweet potatoes for 30-40 minutes until soft.

Start by pickling the red onion by slicing thinly and placing in a bowl with 3 tbsp of apple cider vinegar.

Heat 1 tbsp coconut oil and fry the onion until soft and translucent. Add the spices, sliced leek, carrot and red pepper and fry for a further 2 minutes.

Add the black beans and tomatoes, fill the tomato can half full with water and add the water to the pot.

Simmer for 20-30 minutes while the potatoes are cooking until thickened and the flavours have developed.

To serve, cut open the sweet potatoes and spoon over the black beans. Top with the pickled red onion, cherry tomatoes, avocado and coriander.

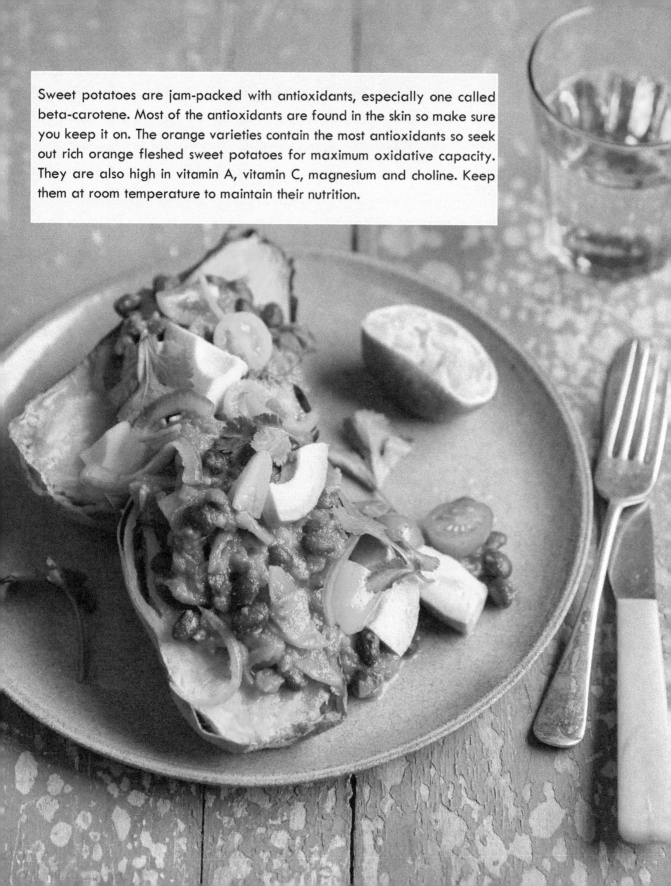

Sweet potatoes are jam-packed with antioxidants, especially one called beta-carotene. Most of the antioxidants are found in the skin so make sure you keep it on. The orange varieties contain the most antioxidants so seek out rich orange fleshed sweet potatoes for maximum oxidative capacity. They are also high in vitamin A, vitamin C, magnesium and choline. Keep them at room temperature to maintain their nutrition.

DESSERT AND SNACK INSPIRATION

I don't recommend that you eat desserts or snacks every single day, but these recipes are for those occasions in life when you want to enjoy good, tasty food with family and friends and indulge a little. These recipes are all low in sugar and can and should be enjoyed guilt free. They have been created with healthful, superfood ingredients and with simple preparation techniques that preserve the nutritional value of the foods.

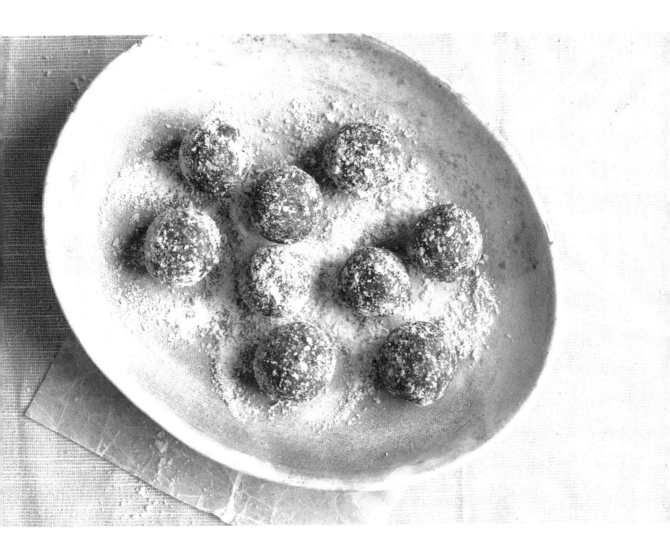

RAW CACAO & ORANGE BLISS BALLS

1 cup medjool dates
1 cup almonds
2 tbsp raw cacao
1 orange, juiced

Desiccated coconut for garnish

Method

Place the dates in a food processor and blend until broken up and they form a ball in the bowl. Remove from the food processor and add the almonds. Whizz the almonds until they are finely chopped. Add the dates, orange juice and cacao to the food processor and blend until mixed well.

Remove the mixture and place in a bowl. Using your hands, roll into even-sized balls.

Scatter desiccated coconut onto a plate and gently roll the bliss balls on the coconut to coat them.

Keep in the fridge.

CINNAMON POACHED PEARS

Serves 4. GF, NF

4 pears
2 cinnamon sticks
1 tbsp ground cinnamon
2 bay leaves
1 unwaxed orange – juice and peel
1 tbsp maple syrup
Oat cream & toasted hazelnuts to serve

Method

Peel the pears and place in a saucepan. Add the cinnamon sticks, bay leaves, maple syrup and orange juice and peel to the pan.

Pour in cold water to cover the pears by 1 inch.

Gently heat the pears until simmering and cook for 5-7 minutes until the pears are cooked through but not mushy.

Serve warm drizzled with oat cream and toasted hazelnuts.

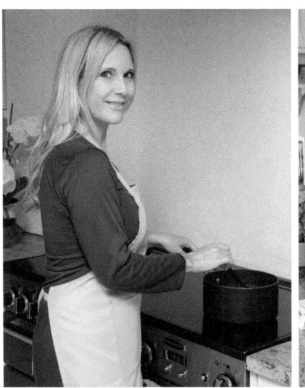
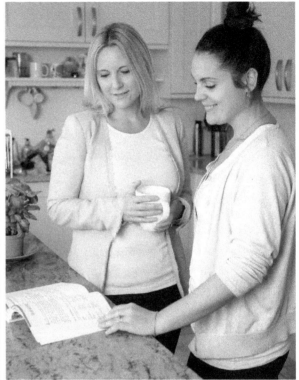
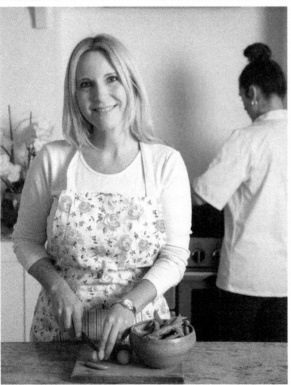
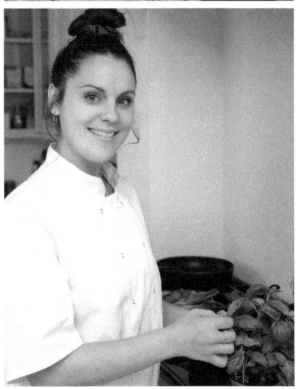

CREAMY COCONUT MANGO CHIA PUDDING WITH BLUEBERRIES AND TOASTED COCONUT CHIPS

Serves 4- 6. GF, NF

1 ripe mango
3 tbsp chia seeds
400ml tin coconut milk
1 lime, juice and zest
1 tbsp vanilla or vanilla pod
Blueberries & coconut chips to serve

Method

Peel and dice the mango, place in a jug blender with the lime juice and blend until smooth.

Add the coconut milk to the mango and vanilla and blend together.

Place the mango coconut mixture in a bowl, add the chia seeds and mix well.

Cover and place in the fridge for around 30mins to set. If the mixture feels too loose, add 1 tbsp more of chia seeds and leave to thicken.

Serve in bowls decorated with blueberries and coconut chips.

Chia seeds are one of my favourite superfoods. They have been eaten for centuries in South America and have become popular here in the UK. Chias have so much to offer nutritionally. They are rich in tryptophan - an essential amino acid that is a precursor to the neurotransmitter serotonin and the hormone melatonin. Both help us feel happy, calm and content. Chias are also high in ALA omega 3 fatty acids, fibre, calcium, zinc and phosphorous.

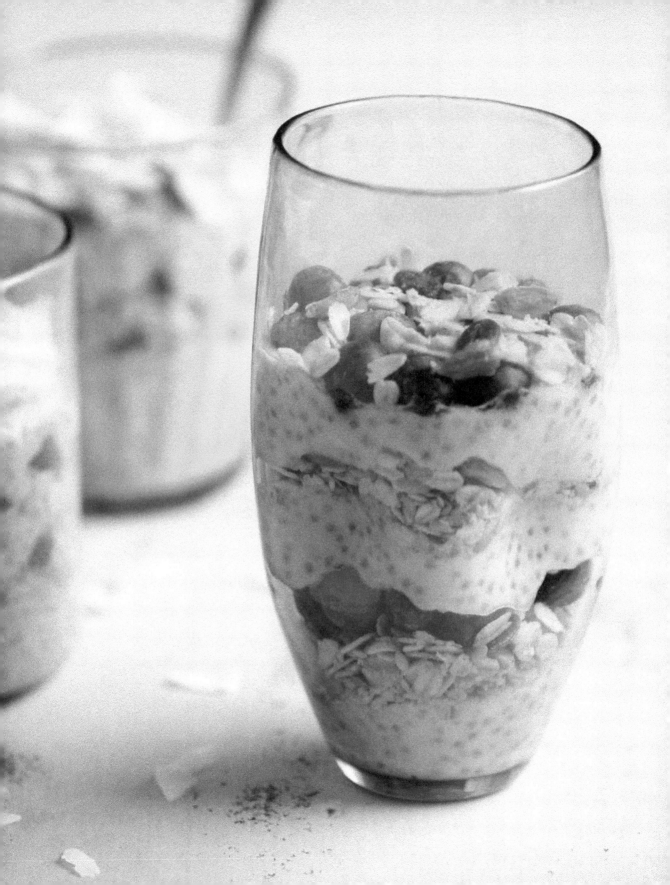

BANANA & GOJI LOAF
WITH WALNUT BANANA N'ICE CREAM

Serves 4 – 6. GF

2 ripe bananas + 1 to decorate
2 tbsp goji berries
200g buckwheat flour
50g coconut oil
150ml plant milk
1 tbsp ground flaxseed
2 tsp ground cinnamon
1 tbsp mixed spice
1 tbsp baking powder
1 tbsp vanilla
0.5 tbsp apple cider vinegar

Method

Preheat the oven to 180 degrees Celsius.

Start by making the flax egg – add 1 tbsp ground flax seeds to a bowl and add 2.5 tbsp cold water, leave to thicken.

In a separate bowl, mash the bananas with a fork, add the oil, plant milk, flax egg, vanilla and vinegar.

Add the buckwheat flour, cinnamon, goji berries and baking powder to the wet ingredients and mix until incorporated.

Grease a loaf tin and pour in the cake batter, decorate with sliced banana and bake for 20-25 minutes until a knife comes out clean.

Serve with Banana N'ice cream

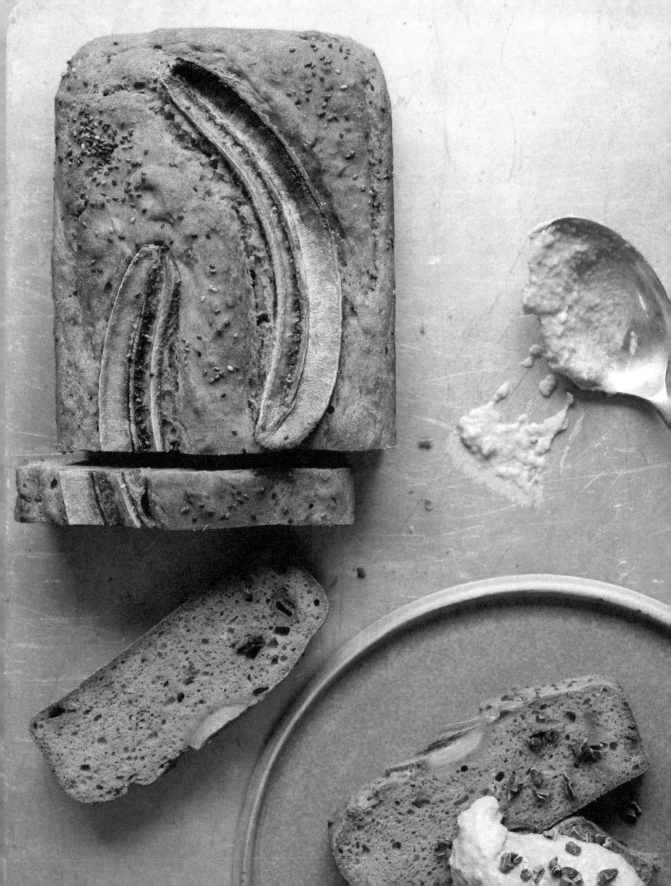

HAMMI'S NUTTY APPLE CRUMBLE

2 cooking apples unpeeled
200 ml water
1 tbsp Xylitol natural sweetener
1 tsp of cinnamon
120g soft butter
2 heaped tbsp of brown sugar
or Xylitol

2 heaped tbsp of ground
almonds
2 heaped tbsp of mixed seeds
2 heaped tbsp of chopped
hazel nuts
2 heaped tbsp of crushed
walnuts or mixed nuts
1 1/2 - 2 cups of mixed flour
(plain flour, buck wheat flour
and spelt flour)

Method

Cut the apples into thin slices and simmer them in 200ml of water with xylitol and cinnamon for ten minutes until all the pieces are soft. Make sure that you don't let all the water evaporate, just add a little bit more if needed.

Leave to cool before spooning onto the bottom of a medium size pie dish.

For the crumble: Mix the soft butter, xylitol and ground almonds in a large mixing bowl.

Grind the seeds and nuts into small pieces or place in food processor briefly and add them into the bowl.

Add the flour and use your fingers to pinch the flour and butter and all the ingredients together into nice crumble mix.

Sprinkle the crumble gently over the apples.

Place in the oven at 180C for 20-30 mins.

Serve hot with oat cream or Banana N'ice Cream

TAMARI ROAST SEEDS

1 cup mixed seeds
2 tbsp tamari soy sauce
1 tbsp smoked paprika

Method

Preheat the oven to 180 degrees Celsius.

Place the seeds in a bowl and mix in the tamari and smoked paprika.

Line a baking tray with greaseproof paper and lay out the seeds in a thin layer.

Bake for 10 minutes until toasted and fragrant.

Remove from the oven and mix well to break up any seeds that have stuck together. Leave to cool completely and transfer to a glass jar to use when needed.

BEETROOT & BUTTER BEAN DIP

1 tin butterbeans
100g cooked beetroot
2 cloves garlic
Handful mint leaves
2 tbsp olive oil
1 lemon, juiced
½ tbsp tahini

Method

Place all ingredients in a food processor.

Blend until smooth and serve with a drizzle of olive oil.

AVOCADO HUMOUS

1 tin chickpeas
1 medium, ripe avocado
1 tbsp tahini
1 lemon, juiced
2 tbsp olive oil
2 garlic cloves

Method

Peel the avocado and place in a food processor with all the other ingredients.

Blend until smooth.

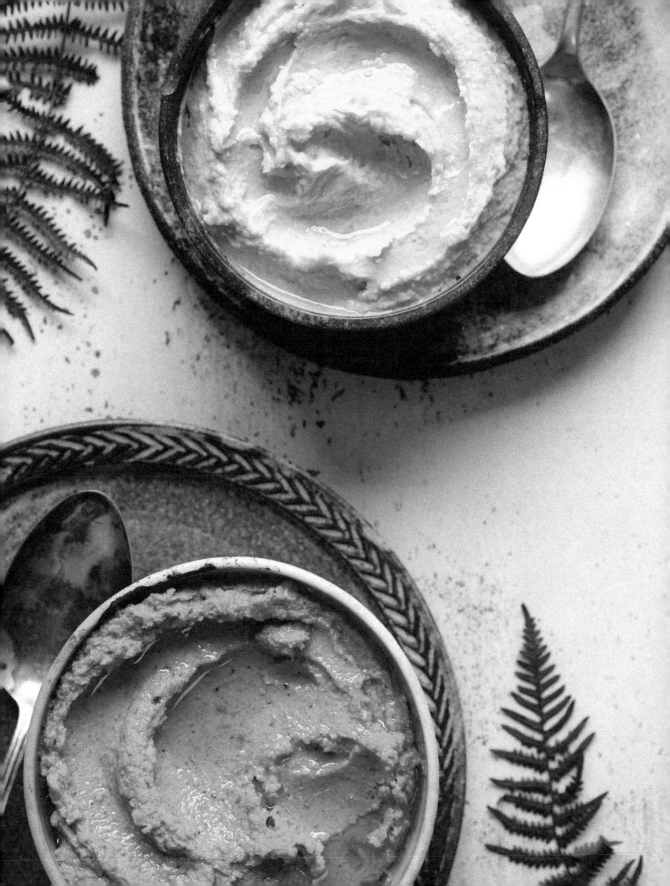

FINAL WORD

Thank you for taking this journey with me. I truly hope that this book leaves you feeling inspired and ready to put into action all that you have learned.

Remember, health is a lifelong commitment and journey – a marathon, not a sprint.

Wishing you all the happiness and health in the world.

Dr Johanna Ward

REFERENCES

[1] Tukker A, Huppes G, Guinee J et al 'Environmental Impact of Products (EIPRO) Analysis of the Life Cycle Environmental Impacts Related to the Final Consumption of the EU-25: EUR 22284 EN Brussels: European Commission Joint Research Centre 2006

[2] https://www.forksoverknives.com/animal-agriculture-hunger-and-how-to-feed-a-growing-global-population-part-one-of-two

[3] Omran AR, 'The Epidemiological Transition. A Theory of Epidemiology of Population Change', Milbank Mem Fund Q 1971: 49: (4): 509-38

[4] Strange KC, Zyzanski SJ, 'Illuminating the black box - a description of 4454 patient visits to 138 family physicians', J Fam Prac 1998:46(5): 377-398

[5] Honolulu study

[6] White L Petrovich H "Prevalence of dementia in older Japanese American men in Hawaii: The Honolulu Asia raging study. JAMA 1996:276: (12): 955-60

[7] Grant WB 'Dietary links to Alzheimers disease' Alzheimer Dis Rev 1997:2:42-55

[8] Barbara Starfield 'Is US health really the best in the World?' JAMA 284:4 Jul 2000: 483-85

[9] Michael Schroeder 'Death by Prescription' US News and World Report Sept 2016

[10] US Department of Agriculture Economic research
http://www.ers.usda.gov/datafiles/Food_Availability_Per_Capita_Data_System

[11] Diabetes UK 2017 Survey https://www.google.co.uk/amp/s/www.diabetes.org.uk/abous_us/news/brits-failing-to-meet-the-recommended-daily-allowance-of-fruit-and-veg%3famp

[12] Dobbs R, Sawyers C, Thompson F et al 'Overcoming Obesity: An Initial economic Analysis' Discussion Paper www.mckinsey.com/industries/healthcaresystems-and-services/our-insights/how-the-world-could-better-fight-obesity (accessed Nov 10 2014) New York:McKinsey & Company 2014

[13] BBC New Feb 2018 'Millennials set to be the fattest generation' http://www.bbc.com/news/health-43195977

[14] Young LR, Nestle M 'The contribution of expanding portion sizes to the US obesity epidemic' The American Journal of Public Health 2002: 92 (2): 246-9

[15] International Journey of Epidemiology

[16] Michael Pollan 'In Defense of Foods'

[17]NATIONAL INSTITUTE FOR HEALTH AND CARE EXCELLENCE SCOPE 2017 https://www.nice.org.uk/guidance/gid-mt516/documents/final-scope

[18]2017 Centres for Disease, Control & Protection

[19] WHO Fact Sheet http://www.who.int/news-room/fact-sheets/detail/cardiovascular-diseases-(cvds)

[20] Campbell TC, Parpia B, Chen J 'Diet, Lifetsyle and the Etiology of coronary artery disease : The Cornell China Study' Am Journal Cardiology 1998:82:18-21

[21] Voller Rd, Strong WB 'Paediatric aspects of atherosclerosis' Am Heart Journal 1981:101(6):815-36

[22] Strong JP 'Landmark perspective: Coronary atherosclerosis in soldiers. A clue to the natural history of atherosclerosis in the young' JAMA 1986: 256(@)):2863-66

[23] https://heartuk.org.uk/press/press-kit/key-facts-figures

[24] British Heart Foundation https://www.bhf.org.uk/-/medial/files/research

[25] https://heartuk.org.uk/press/press-kit/key-facts-figures

[26] ShikanyJM, Stanford MM et al 'Southern dietary pattern is associated with hazard of acute coronary heart disease in the Reasons for Geographic and Racial Differences in Stroke (REGARDS) study. Circulation 2015: 132: 801-14

[27] Chiuve SE, McCullough ML, Sacks FM 'Healthy lifestyle factors in the primary prevention of coronary heart disease among men: benefits among users and non-users of lipid lowering and anti-hypertensive medications' Circulation 2006 : 114(2):160-167

[28] Earl Stadtman 'Protein oxidation in aging and age-related diseases' Ann NY Acad Sci 2001 Apr;928:22-38

[29] Murray CJ, Atkinson C 'The state of US health 1990-2010: Burden of diseases, injuries and risk factors' JAMA 2013:310:591-608

[30] Bromfield S, Munter P 'High blood pressure: The leading global burden of disease risk factor and the need for worldwide prevention programs' Curr Hypertens Rep 2013:15(3): 134-6

[31] Campbell TC, Parpia B and Chen J "Diet, Lifetsyle and the eithiology of coronary artery diseases: The Cornell China Study' Am J Cardiology 82 (1998): 18T-21T

[32] Machilha-Carvalho J, Crewe DE 'The Yanomamo Indians in the INTERSALT Study' Arq Bras Cardiology 2003:80(3):289-300

[33] Go AS, Bauman MA Coleman SM, 'An effective approach to high blood pressure control; a Science advisory committee from the American Heart Association, the American College of Cardiology and the Centres for Disease Control and Prevention (CDC) J Am College Cardiol 2014; 63(12):1230-8

[34] Obarzanek E, Sacks FM, Moore TJ 'Dietary approaches to stop hypertension - sodium trial'Annual meeting of American Society of Hypertension 2000, New York

[35] 'Urinary sodium excretion and cardiovascular mortality in Finland: a prospective study' Lancet 2001(9259):848-51

[36] Business Insider https://www.BusinessInsider.com foods-most-salt-sodium-in-diet

[37] Michael Greger MD 'How Not To Die'
[38] Public Health England National Diet and Nutrition Survey 2014

[39] Sacks FM, Rosner B 'Blood Pressure in Vegetarians' Am J Epidemiol 1926:1000(5):390-8

[40] Sacks FM, Rosner B, Kaas EH 'Blood pressure in vegetarians' Am J Epidemiol 1974 100 (5): 390-8

[41] Fraser GE 'Vegetarian diets: what do we know of their effects on common chronic diseases?' Am J Clin Nutr 2009:89(%): 1607S-1612S

[42] Physical Inactivity and Sedentary Behaviour Report 2017 British Heart Foundation 2017

[43] Michael Greger MD 'How Not To Die'

[44] William H Goodson et al 'Assessing the Carcinogenic potential of low dose exposures to chemical mixtures in the environment: The Challenge Ahead' Carcinogenesis 36.1 Jun 2015:S254-96

[45] Travis Christofferson 'Tripping over the Truth - How the Metabolic Theory of Cancer Is Overturning one of Medicines Most Entrenched Paradigms'

[46] World Health Organisation 'Cancer' 2017 www.who.int/mediacentre/factsheetd/fs297/en

[47] World Cancer Day Global Press Release 2013

[48] Seyfried 'Cancer as a Metabolic Disease' 2012

[49] 'The anti-proliferative and antioxidant activities of common vegetables: a Comparative study Food Chemistry January 2009

[50] Y Fan, X Jin, C Man, Z Goa, X Wang 'Meta-analysis of the association between the inflammatory potential of the diet and colorectal cancer risk' Oncotarget 8 no 35 (August 2017):59592-600

[51] S J D O'Keefe, J Vi, L Lahti et al 'Fat, Fibre and Cancer Risk in African Americans and rural Africans' Nature Communications 6 April 2015:6342

[52] ibid

[53] GC Kabat, MY Kim, HD Strickler et al 'A longitudinal study of serum insulin and glucose levels in relation to colorectal cancer risk among post menopausal women' British Journal of Cancer 106 no 1 (Jan 2012):227-32

[54] I Drake , E Sonestedt, B Gullberg et al 'Dietary intakes of carbohydrates on relation to prostate cancer risk: A prospective study in the Malmo diet and cancer cohort American Journal of Clinical Nutrition' 96 no 6 Dec 2012 1409:18

[55] Centre for Disease Control and Prevention 'Cancer and Obesity' October 3 2017

[56] G M Massetti, WH Dietz 'Excessive weight gain, obesity and cancer: opportunities for clinical intervention' Journal of the American Medical Association 318 no 20 (November 2017): 1975-76

[57] Jie Sun et al Antioxidant and anti-proliferative activities of common fruits' Journal of Agriculture and Food Chemistry Dec 2002:7449-54

[58] Lisa S McAnulty et al 'Effect of Blueberry Ingestion on Natural Killer cell counts, Oxidative Stress and Inflammation prior to and after 2.5h running' Applied Physiology, Nutrition and Metabolism' 36.6 Nov 2011

[59] Cancer Research UK 2015

[60] D Romaguera, E Gracia-Lavedan et al 'Adherence to nutrition based cancer prevention guidelines and breast, prostate and colorectal cancer risk in the MCC Spain case control study' Int Jour of Cancer 141 no 1 July 2017:83-93

[61] European Journal of Cancer 2005 May: 41(8): 1164-9

[62] Menopause September 17 2018

[63] BMJ 2018:360:K671

[64] American Journal of Clinical Nutrition June 2007: 85(6): 1586-1591

[65] Anticancer Research February 2011:31(2):607-611

[66] Cancer Therapy Advisor March 23 2016

[67] American Journal of Clinical Nutrition June 2007 : 85(6): 1586-1591

[68] Dr Zahid Naeem 'Vitamin D Deficiency - An Ignored Epidemic' Int J Health Sci 2010 Jan:4(1): V-VI

[69] Ed Yong Cancer Research UK & Nice Guidelines and Hypponen and Power Am J Clinic Nutrition 85:(3): 860-8 2007

[70] Marilyn A Kwan, C Kroenke April 2015 Journal of National Cancer Institute

[71] Michaels KB, Rosner BA et al 'Preschool diet and adult risk of breast cancer' Int J Cancer 2006: 118(3):749-54

[72] ibid

[73] Stripp C, Overvad K, Christensen J 'Fish intake is positively associated with breast cancer incidence rate' J Nutr 2003: 133(11): 3664-69

[74] Chen WY, Rosner B, Hankinson SE 'Moderate alcohol consumption during adult life,drinking patters and breast cancer risk' JAMA 2011:306:1884—90. Allen NE, Beral V, Casabonne D 'Moderate alcohol intake and cancer incidence in women' J Natl Cancer Institute 2009:101(5):296-305

[75] IM Lee 'Physical Activity and Cancer Prevention Data from Epidemiological Studies' Med Sci Sports Exerc Nov 2003 35 (11) 1823-1827

[76] American Association of Endocrine Surgeons: Beyond Surgery Caldwell Esselstyn, San Jose, CA, April 15 1991

[77] Singh PN et al 'Dietary risk factors for colon cancer in low risk population' American Journal of Epidemiology 148 (1998) 761-74

[78] Ibid

[79] Ibid

[80] Ibid

[81] Zaynah Abid, Amanda Cross, Rashmi Sinha 'Meat, dairy and cancer' The American Journal of Clinical Nutrition 2014 Jule: 100(1) 386S-393S

[82] Daniel CR, Cross AJ, Koebnick C, Sinha R, 'Trends in meat consumption in the USA' Public Health Nutrition 2011:14:575-83

[83] Lee JE, McLerran DF, Rolland B, Chen Y et al 'Meat intake and cause specific mortality: a pooled analysis of Asian prospective cohort studies' American Journal of Clinical Nutrition 2013:98(4):1032-41

[84] Daniel CR, Cross AJ, Graubard BI, Park Y et al 'Large prospective investigation of meat intake, related mutagens and risk of renal cell carcinoma' American Journal of Clinical Nutrition 2012:95:155-62

[85] Sinha R, Park Y, Graubard B et al 'Meat and meat related compounds and risk of prostate cancer in a large prospective cohort study in the United States' American Journal of Epidemiology 2009:170 :1165-77

[86] Cross AJ, Freedman ND, Ren J, Ward MH et al 'Meat consumption and risk of oesophageal cancer in a large prospective study' Am J Gastroenterol 2011:106: 432-42

[87] Freedman ND, Cross AJ, McGlynn KA et al 'Association of meat and fat intake with liver disease and hepatocelluar carcinoma in the NH-AARP cohort' J Natl Cancer Inst 2010:102:1354-65

[88] Tasevksa N, Sinha R, Kipnis V et al 'A prospective study of meat, cooking methods, meat mutagens, heme iron and lung cancer risks' Am J Clinical Nutr 2009:89:1884-94

[89] Stolzenberg-Solomon RZ, Cross AJ, Silverman DT et al 'Meat and meat mutagen intake and pancreatic cancer risk in NIH-AARP cohort' Cancer Epidemiol Biomarkers Prev 2007: 16: 2664-75

[90] Sinha R, Cross AJ, Graubard BI et al 'Meat intake and mortaility: a prospective study of over half a million people' Arch Intern Med 2009:169:562-71

[91] Favero A, Franceschi S, La Vecchio et al 'Meal frequency and coffee intake in colon cancer' Nutr Cancer 1998: 30(3): 182-5

[92] Grosse Y, Baan R 'Carcinogenicity of nitrite, nitrate and cyanobacterial peptide toxins' Lancet Oncol 2006:7: 628-9

[93] Balter Michael 'Scientific Cross Claims fly in Continuing Beef War' Science May 28 1999 ppb1453-5

[94] Health Professionals Follow Up Study 'Dairy products linked to prostate cancer' Associated Press 2000 April 5

[95] Harvard's Health Professionals Follow-Up Study

[96] P Anand, A B Kunnumakara C Sundaram et al 'Cancer is a preventable disease that requires major lifestyle changes' Pharmaceutical Research 25 No 9 (September 200*0: 2097-116

[97] Giovanni de Pergola 'Obesity as a major risk factor for cancer' J Obes 2013: 291546

[98] Holly Harris, Shelley Tworoger et al 'Plasma leptin levels and increased risk of breast cancer in premenopausal women' Cancer Prev Res 2011 sept 4(9): 1449-1456

[99] Langunova Z et al 'Obesity and increased risk of cancer: does decrease of serum 25 Hydroxyvitamin D level with increasing body mass explain some of the association?' Nutr Food Res August 2010: 54(8): 1277-33

[100] Q Dai, YT Gao, XO Shu 'Oxidative stress, obesity and breast cancer risk: Results from Shanghai Womens Health Study' Journal of Clinical Oncology 27 no 15 May 2009: 2482-88

[101] Bagnardi V, Rota M 'Light alcohol drinking and breast cancer risk: A meta-analysis' Ann Oncol 2013:24(2):301

[102] Anand S T, Ebell M H "circadian disrupting exposuers and breastcancer risk: A meta-analysis' Int Arch Occup Environ Health 2015 July: 88(5): 533-47

[103] World Cancer Research Fund International 'Our cancer prevention recommendations'.

[104] Orlich MJ, Singh PN, Sabate J 'Vegetraian dietary patterns and mortality in Adventist Health Study 2 AMA Intern Med 2013: 173: (13): 1230-38i

[105] Cummings J et al, 'Low meat high vegetable diets cut cancer risk' British Medical Journal 317:1998 1636-40.

[106] World Health Organisation 2014 'Diabetes mellitus, fasting blood glucose concentration and risk of vascular diseases: a collaborative meta-analysis of 102 prospective studies' Emerging Risk Factors Collaboration'

[107] Diabetes UK

[108] Karve H, Hayward RA 'Prevalence, diagnosis and treatment impaired fasting glucose and impaired glucose tolerance in non-diabetic US adults' Diabetes Care 2010:33(11)2355-9

[109] Jancin B 'Fitness sharply cut death in high BMI diabetics' Family Practice News 2008 Oct 1: 19

[110] The United States of Diabetes: Challenges and opportunities in the decade ahead. United Health Centre for Health Reform and Modernization. Working Paper 5 Nov 2010

[111] Larsson SC, Orsini N, Wolk A 'Diabetes Mellitus and risk of colorectal cancer: a meta-analysis' J Natl Cancer Inst 2005:97(22): 1679-87

[112] Pollack M, Russell Jones D 'Insulin analogues and cancer risk'int J Clin Pract 2010 April 64(5):628-36

[113] Joel Fuhrman 'The End of Diabetes' pp 8 2013

[114] A Pan et al 'Bidirectional Association between Depression and Type 2 Diabetes Mellitus in Women Arch Int Med 170 no 21 Nov 22 2010

[115] Canhada S et al 'Omega 3 fatty acids supplementation inAlzheimers disease: A systematic Review' Nutr Neuroscie 2018 Oct: 21(8):529-538

[116] M Smith, L Riby, J Reay 'B Vitamins and Cognitive Performance in Older Adults: Review' ISRN Nutr 2013; 2013: 650983.

[117] Giorgio La Fata et al 'Effects of Vitamin E on Cognitive Performance during Ageing and in Alzheimer's Disease' Nutrients. 2014 Dec; 6(12): 5453–5472.

[118] C Geroldi et al 'Insulin Resistance and Cognitive Impairment' The InCHiANTI Study, Archives of Neurology 62, No 7 2005: 1067-72

[119] https://www.theguardian.com/science/2018/feb/02/ultra-processed-products-now-half-of-all-uk-family-food-purchases

[120] Journal of American Medical Association 2008

[121] EM Shulte NM Avena, AN Gearhardt 'Which foods might be addictive? the role of processing fat content and glycemic load' PloS One 10 no 2 Feb 2015:e0117959

[122] D BUettner 'The Blue Zones; 9 lessons for Living Longer from the People who Who've Lived the Longest' Washington DC; National Geographic 2012

[123] Q Yang 'Gain weight by going diet? Artificial sweeteners and the neurobiology of sugar cravings: Neuroscience 2010' Yale Journal of Biology and Medicine 83 no 2 (June 2010):101-8

[124] SD Anton, CK Martin, H Han 'Effects of stevia, aspartame and sucrose on food intake, satiety and postprandial glucose and insulin levels' Appetite 55 no 1 March 2010:37-43

[125]'Evidence that intermittent, excessive sugar intake causes endogenous opioid dependence' Rada P et al, Obes Res. 2002 Jun;10(6):478-88.

[126] Dr Sarah Myhill 'Sustainable Medicine' pp xxii 2015

[127] Michael Pollan 'In Defense of Food'

[128] PM Kris Etherton et al 'Polyunsaturated fatty acids in the food chain in the United States' Am J Clin Nutr 71 Suppl 1 (January 2000);179S-88S

[129] Canhada S et al 'Omega 3 fatty acids supplementation inAlzheimers disease: A systematic Review' Nutr Neuroscie 2018 Oct: 21(8):529-538

[130] H Hiza, L Bente 'A Summary Report' Nutrient Content of the US Food Supply 1909-2004

[131] Sidney Smith Jr, eerily Allen, Steven N Blair 'AHA/ACC Guidelines for Secondary Prevention for Patients with Coronary and other Atherosclerotic Vascular Disease 2006 Update' Journal of American College of Cardiology Volume 47 Issue 10 May 2006

[132] 'Differentiation of ALA (plant sources) from DHA & EPA (marine sources) https://www.DHAomega3.org

[133] Anahad O'Connor 'What's in your fish oil supplement?' The New York Times, Jan 22nd 2014

[134] Rouhani MH, Salehi-Abargouei A et al 'Is there a relationship between red or processed meat intake and obesity? A systematic review and meta-analysis of observational studies Obesity Reviews 2014: 15(9): 740-8

[135] Dr Maryam Farvid et Al 'Adolescent meat intake and breast cancer risk' International Journal of Cancer Sept 2014

[136] Huer OE,Kruse H, Grave K et al 'Human health consequences of use of antimicrobial agents in aquaculture. Clinical Infectious Diseases 2009 49 (8): 1248-53

[137] 'Stepping off the Toxic Treadmill' Worldwatch paper 153 Nov 30 2000

[138] 'FDA launches study on dioxin in fish and dairy foods' Food Chemical News Feb 27 1995

[139] 'Milk intake and risk of hip fracture in men and women: A meta-analysis of prospective cohort studies' Journal of Bone and Mineral Research 14th Oct 2010

[140] 'Food Allergies: Reducing the Risks' FDA Consumer Updates

[141] Rogers I, Emmett P et al 'Milk as a food for growth? The insulin-like growth factors link.' Public Health Nutr. 2006 May: 9(3):359-68.

[142] Levine ME, Suarez JA et al 'Low protein intake is associated with a major reduction in IGF1 , cancer and overall mortality in the 65 and younger but not older population' Cell Metab 2014; 19(3):407-17

[143] US Department of Health and Human Services '14th Report on carcinogens' 2016

[144] American Cancer Society "Alcohol use and cancer risk' April 5 2017 www.caner.org/cancer/about-cancer/causes-prevention/diet-pyhsical-activity/alcohol/alcohol-use-and-canecr.html

[145] G Tetsino 'The burden of cancer attributable to alcohol consumption' Maedica 6 no 4 (October 2011): 313-20

[146] D E Nelson, D W Jarman, J Rehm et al 'Alcohol attributable cancer deaths and years of potential life lost in the United States' American Journal of Public Health 103, no 4 (April 2013): 641-48

[147] Bagnardi V, Rota M 'Light alcohol drinking and cancer: A Meta-analysis' Ann Oncol 2013:24(2):301

[148] Lim SS, Vos T, Flaxman AD et al 'A comparative risk assessment of burden of diseases and injury attributable to 67 risk factor clusters in 21 regions 1990-2010; a systematic analysis for the Global Burden of Disease Study 2010 Lancet 2012: 380(9859):2224-60

[149] Aaron Lerner, Patricia Jeremias, Torsten Matthias 'The World Incidence and Prevalence of Autoimmune Diseases is Increasing' International Journal of Celiac Disease ' Volume 3: Number 4 2015 pp 151-155. doi: 10.12691

[150] T Umasunthar J Leonardi B 'Incidence of fatal food anaphylaxis in people with food allergy: a Systemic Review and Meta-analysis' Clin Exp Allergy Dec 2013 43(12):1333-1341

[151] Ibid

[152] Gwen Smith 'Why so many allergies now?' Food Allergy, November 20 2010

[153] Ramyani Gupta, Aziz Sheikh, David P Strachan 'Time trends in allergic disorders in the UK' Thorax 62 (1): 91-96, 2007

[154] Lerner A et al 'Changes in intestinal tight junction permeability associated with industrial food additives explain the rising incidence of autoimmune disease.'Autoimmunity Review Jun:14(6): 479-89: 2015

[155] ibid

[156] Devaraj S, Wang Polagrunto 'High fat, energy dense fast foods style breakfasts result in an increase in oxidative stress in the metabolic system' Metabolism 2008: 57: 867-70

[157] NIH Human 'Microbiome project defines normal bacterial makeup of the body' US National Library of Medicine, 2015

[158] Elaine O Petrof 'Probiotics and Gastrointestinal Disease: Clinical Evidence and Basic Science' Antiinflamm Antiallergic Ahents Med Chem 2009 Sept 1;8(3): 260-269

159 Erica and Justin Sonnenburg 'Starving our microbial self: The deleterious consequences of a diet deficient in microbiota accessible carbohydrates' Cell Metab 20 No 5 Nov 4, 2014:779-86

160 Dr David Perlmutter 'Brain Maker- The Power of Gut Microbes to Heal and Protect Your Brain' p33 2015

161 Josef Neu 'Cesarean versus vaginal delivery: Long term infant outcomes and the Hygiene Hypothesis' Clin Perinatol 2011 June : 38(2): 321-331

162 M G Domigeuz Bello 'Delivery mode shapes the Acquisition and Structure of the Initial Microbiota across multiple body habitats in Newborns' Proc Natl Acad Sci USA 107, No 26: 11971-75 Epub June 21 2010

163 Josef Neu "cesarean versus vaginal delivery: Long term infant outcomes and the Hygiene Hypothesis' Clin Perinatol 2011 June: 38(2): 321-331

164 Joel Fuhrman 'The End of Diabetes' pp8 2013

165 B Hone Kei Yip et al 'Casearean section and risk of autism across gestational age: A multi-national cohort study of 5 million births' Int J of Epidemiology 2017 April 46(2) 429-439

166 V K Ridaura et al 'Gut microbiota from twins discordant for obesity modulate metabolism in mice' Science 341 no 6150 (Sept 6 2013)

167 Dethlefsen et al 'An Ecological and Evolutionary perspective on human micro biome mutualism and diseases' Nature 449: 811-818:10:1038 2007

168 David Kessler 'Antibiotics and the Meat We Eat' New York Times, March 27 2013

169 'Early antibiotics exposure leads to lifelong metabolic disturbance in mice' News Release NUY Lagone Medical Centre August 14 2014

170 H D Holscher et al 'Fibre supplementation influences phylogenetic structure and functional capacity of the human intestinal microbiome: follow up of a Randomised Controlled Trial' Am Journal Clin Nutr 101 no 1 Jan 2015: 55-64

171 Fukui H 'Decreased Barrier Function Does it Really Influence the Risk of Inflammation?' Inflamm Intest Dis 2016: 1: 135-145

172 Sonoda N, Furuse M et al 'Chlostridium perfringens enterotoxin fragment removes specific claudins from tight junction strands: Evidence for direct involvement of cloudiness in tight junction barrier' J Cell Biol 1999147 195-204 Pub Med

173 M C Arrieta, L Bistritz, J B Meddings 'Alterations in intestinal permeability' Gut 2006 Oct: 55(10) 1512-1520

174 Obrenovich MEM 'Leaky Gut Leaky Brain?' Microorganisms 2018 Oct 18: 6(4)

175 Jessica M Yano, Kristie Yu et al 'Indigenous Bacteria from the gut microbiota regulate host serotonin biosynthesis' Cell 2015 April 9:161(2):264-276

[176] John R Kelly, Paul J Kennedy 'Breaking down the barriers: The gut micro biome, intestinal permeability and stress related psychiatric disorders' Front Cell Neurosci 2015: 9: 392

[177] C Zhang et al 'Structural Modulation of Gut Microbiota in Life-long Calorie Restricted Mice' Nat Commun 4: 2013: 2163

[178] Kristin Schmidt, Phillip Cowen et al 'Prebiotic intake reduces waking cortisol response and alters emotional bias in healthy volunteers' Psychopharmacology 2015:232(10):1793-1801

[179] Kirsten Tillisch, Emeran Mayer et al 'Consumption of fermented milk product with probiotic modulates brain activity' Gastroenterology 2013 June: 144(7): 10:1053

[180] Adam Brickman, Usman Khan 'Enhancing dentate gyrus function with dietary flavanols improves cognition in older adults' Nat Neuroscience 2014 Dec:17(12):1798-1803

[181] F Cardona et al 'Benefits of polyphenols on gut microbiota and implications in human health' J Nutr Biochem 24 No 8 August 2013

[182] R J T Mocking 'Meta-analysis and meta-regression of Omega 3 polyunsaturated fatty acid supplementation for major depressive disorder' Transl Psychiatry 2016 March:6(3): e756

[183] Robertson RC 'Omega 3 polyunsaturated fatty acids critically regulate behaviour and gut microbiota development in adolescence and adulthood'Brain Behave Immune 2017 Jan: 59: 21-37

[184] Tufts Centre for the Study of Drug Development.

[185] https://www.telegraph.co.uk/news/health/news/8267876/Statins-the-drug-firms-goldmine.html

[186] Irving Kirsh 'Antidepressants and the placebo effect' Zeitschrift Fur Psychologie 222.3 (2014): 128-34

[187] Dr Peter Gotzsche 'Deadly Psychiatry and Organised Denial'

[188] Franz MJ, Van Wormer 'Weight loss outcomes: a systematic review and meta analysis of weight loss clinical trials with minimum 1 year follow up' J Am Diet Assoc 2007:107:(10): 1755-1767

[189] Weight Loss and weight Management Market 2017

[190] Fast Food Market Report - Global Newswire 2017

[191] Federal Trade Commission Report, 'Marketing Food to Children and Adolescents: A Review of Industry Expenditures, Activities and Self-Regulation' 2006

[192] Ebiquity 2016

[193] L Sharp, D Donnelly, A Hegarty 'Risk of several cancer is higher in urban areas after adjusting for socioeconomic status. Results from a two country population based study of 18 Common Cancers' Journal of Urban Health: Bulletin of the New York Academy of Medicine 91 no 3 (jan 2014): 510-25

[194] S J D O'Keefe, J V Li, L Lahti et al 'Fat, fibre and cancer risk in African Americans and rural Africans' Nature Communications 6 April 2015:6342

[195] Y Fan, X Jin, C Man, Z Goa, X Wang 'Meta-analysis of the association between the inflammatory potential of the diet and colorectal cancer risk' Oncotarget 8 no 35 (August 2017):59592-600

[196] Martinez Gonzalez MA PREDIMED 'A ProVegetarian food pattern and reduction in total mortality in the Prevention with Medieteranean Diet' American Journal of Clinical Nutrition 2014: 100: 320s-28s

[197] Keleme LE Kushi LH 'Associations of dietary protein with disease mortality in a prospective study of postmenopausal women' American Journal of Epidemiology 2005 161(3) 239- 49

[198] Morgan E Levine 'Low protein intake is associated with major reduction in IGF-1, cancer and overall mortality in the 65 and younger but not older population' Cell Metabolism 19.3 March 2014:407-17

[199] Min Zhang et al 'Dietary intakes of mushrooms and green tea combine to reduce the risk of breast cancer in Chinese women' International Journal of Cancer 124.6 March 2008 1404-8

[200] Dean Ornish Foreword to John Robbins 'The Food Revolution' 10th Edition

[201] M Suzuki, D C Wilcox 'Okinawa Centenarian Study: Investigating Healthy Aging Among the World's Longest Lived People' Encyclopaedia of Geropsychology ed Nancy Pachana Singapore 2017

[202] Dan Buettner 'The Blue Zones: Lessons for Living longer from the people who've lived the longest' 21 April 2009

[203] American Association of Endocrine Surgeons Presidential address 'Beyond Surgery' Caldwell Esselte, San Jose California, April 15, 1991

[204] Singh PN et al 'Dietary risk factors for Colon Cancer in a Low Risk Population' American Journal of Epidemiology 148 (1998): 761-74

[205] Singh PN et al 'Dietary risk factors for Colon Cancer in a Low Risk Population' American Journal of Epidemiology 148 (1998): 761-74

[206] Ibid

[207] Hiryama T 'Diet & Cancer' Nutriton and Cancer 1 1979:67-81

[208] www.ncbi.clm.nih.gov/m/pubmed/23169929

[209] Pisani P et al 'Carrots, Green Vegetables and Lung Cancer: A Case-Control Study.' Int J Epidemiol 1986 Dec;15(4):463-8.

[210] X Xu, Cheng Y et al 'Dietary carrot consumption and the risk of prostate cancer.' Eur J of Nutr 2014 Dec: 53(8):1615-23. doi: 10.1007/s00394-014-0667-2. Epub 2014 Feb 12.

[211] Health professionals Follow Up Study 'Dairy Products Linked to Prostate Cancer' Associated Press April 2000

[212] Giovannucci E 'Tomatoes, tomatoe based products and lycopene and cancer: Review of the Epidemiological Literature' Journal of the National Cancer Institute 91 (1999): 317-31

[213] 'Vegetables Lower Prostate Cancer Risk' Journal of the National Cancer Institute 92 (2000): 61-8

[214] Decarli A et al 'Macronutrients, Energy Intake and Breast Cancer Risk' Epidemiology 8(1997): 425-28

[215] Hirayama T 'Epidemiology of Breast Cancer with Special Reference to the Role of Diet' Preventative Medicine 7 (1978) 173-95

[216] Dagfinn Aune et al 'Fruit and Vegetable Intake and the Risk of Cardiovascular Disease, Total Cancer and All Cause Mortality - A Systemic Review and Dose Response Meta-analysis of Prospective Studies' International Journal of Epidemiology 46.3 Jun 2017: 1029-56

[217] Brown MJ, Ferruzzi MG et al 'Carotenoid bioavailability is higher from salads ingested with full fat than with fat reduced salad dressings as measured with electrochemical detection' Am J Clin Nutr 2004:80(2):396-403

[218] Kim SY, Yoon S, Kwon SM 'Kale juice improves coronary artery disease risk factors in hyperchoesterolemic men' Biomed Environ Sci 2008 April 21(2):91-7

[219] Victoria Kirsh et al 'Prospective study on fruit and vegetable intake and risk of prostate cancer' Journal of the National Cancer Institute August 2007: 1200-1209

[220] Cai Xia Zhang et al 'Greater vegetable and fruit intake is associated with a lower risk of breast cancer among Chinese women' International Journal of Cancer 125.1 July 2009:181-188

[221] Folkard DL et al 'Effect of Sulforaphane on NOD2 via NF-kB: Implications for Chrons Disease' J Inflame (London) 2015

[222] Hawng JH, Lim SB 'Antioxidant activity and anti-inflammatory actives of broccoli florets in LPS-stimulated RAW 264.7 cells' Prev Nutr Food Sci 2014

[223] Zhang X, Shu XO et al 'Cruciferous vegetable consumption is associated with reduced risk of total and cardiovascular disease mortality' Am J Clin Nutr 2011:94(1): 240-6

[224] Carcinogenesis. 2005 Feb;26(2):387-93.

[225] Elena Jovanovski et al 'Effect of Spinach, a High Dietary Nitrate Source, on Arterial Stiffness and Related Hemodynamic Measures: A Randomized, Controlled Trial in Healthy Adults' Clin Nutr Res 2015 Jul; 4(3): 160–167.

[226] Yang Y et al 'Carotenoid analysis of several dark-green leafy vegetables associated with a lower risk of cancers.' Biomed Environ Science 1996 Dec: 9(4):386-92.

227 Nat Rev Neurosci. 2008 Jul; 9(7): 568–578.

228 Shishu, Kaur IP 'Inhibition of mutagenicity of food-derived heterocyclic amines by sulforaphane--a constituent of broccoli' Indian J Exp Biol. 2003 Mar;41(3):216-9.

229 Zimmer AR et al 'Antioixdant and anti-inflammatory properties of capsicum baccatum: from traditional use to scientific approach' J Ethnopahrmacol 2012

230 Schwartz B et al 'Possible mechanisms of action of mushroom derived gluons on inflammatory bowel diseases and associated cancer' Ann Transl Med 2014

231 Elsayed EA et al 'Mushrooms: A potential natural source of anti-inflammatory compounds for medical applications' Mediators Inflamm 2014

232 Min Zhang et al 'Dietary Intakes of Mushrooms and Green Tea Combine to Reduce the Risk of Breast Cancer in Chinese Women' International Journal of Cancer 124.6 March 2008: 1404-8

233 'The anti-proliferative and antioxidant activities of common vegetables: a Comparative study Food Chemistry January 2009

234 Ashraf K et al 'Effects of Allium sativum (garlic) on systolic and diastolic blood pressure in patients with essential hypertension'. Pak J Pharm Sci. 2013 Sep: 26(5):859-63

235 Borek C 'Garlic reduces dementia and heart-disease risk' J Nutr. 2006 Mar;136(3 Suppl):810S-812S. doi: 10.1093/jn/136.3.810S.

236 Kianoush S et al 'Comparison of therapeutic effects of garlic and d-Penicillamine in patients with chronic occupational lead poisoning'. Basic Clin Pharmacol 2012 May;110(5):476-81. doi: 10.1111/j.1742-7843.2011.00841.x. Epub 2011 Dec 29.

237 World Cancer Research Fund / American Institute for Cancer Research. 'Food, Nutrition, Physical Activity and the Prevention of Cancer: a Global Perspective Washington DC AICR 2007

238 Yashin YI, Nemzet BV 'Creation of a databank for content of antioxidants in food products by amperometric method' Molecules 2010:15:(10): 7450-66

239 Luu HN,Blot WJ, Xiang YB et al 'Prospective evaluation of the association of nut/peanut consumption with total and cause specific mortality' JAMA Inter Med 2015:175(5):755-66

240 Fraser GE, Shavlik 'Ten years of Life : is it a matter of choice?' Arch Int Medicine 2001:161: (13): 1645-52

241 Eustruch R, Ros E et al 'Primary prevention of cardiovascular disease with a mediterranean diet' N Engl J Med 2013: 368(14):1279-90

242 Guasch Ferre M, Bullo M et al 'Frequency of nut consumption and mortality risk in the PREDIMED nutrition intervention trial' BMC Med 2013:11:164

[243] J Agric Food Chem. 2008 Jun 25;56(12):4444-9.

[244] J. Agric. Food Chem., 2006, 54 (14), pp 5027–5033

[245] Priyanka Kajla 'Flaxseed - a potential functional food source' J Food Sci Technol April 2015: 52(4): 1857-1871

[246] Thompson LU. Chen JM et al 'Dietary flaxseed laters tumour biological markers in post menopausal breast cancer. Clin cancer Res 2005: 11(10): 3828-35

[247] Mohammadi-Sartang M et al 'Flaxseed supplementation on glucose control and insulin sensitivity: a systematic review and meta-analysis of 2 5 randomised, placebo controlled trials' Nutr Rev Feb 2018 1:76(2): 125-139

[248] Rodrigues Leyva D, Weighell W, Edel AL 'Potent anti-hypertensive action of dietary flaxseed in hypertensive patients' Hypertension 2013:62(6):1081-9

[249] Lowcock EC, Cotterchio M 'Consumption of Flaxseeds - a rich source of lignans is associated with reduced breast cancer risk' Cancer Causes Control April 2013 : 24(4): 813-6

[250] Pan A, Chen M et al 'ALA and heart disease - a systematic review and meta-analysis' Am Jour Clinic Nutr Dec 2012: 96(6): 1262-73

[251] ' Changes in 2-hydroxyestrone and 16alpha-hydroxyestrone metabolism with flaxseed consumption: modification by COMT and CYP1B1 genotype' Cancer Epidem Biomarkers Prev 2007 Feb : 16(2): 256-62

[252] Flax Council of Canada

[253] Vuksan V, Jenkins AL et al 'Salba-chia in the treatment of overweight and obese patients with type 2 diabetes: A double-blind randomized controlled trial'. 2017 Feb:27(2):138-146. Nutr Metab Cardiovasc Dis. doi: 10.1016/j.numecd.2016.11.124. Epub 2016 Dec 9.

[254] Tome-Carniero J et al 'Grape reservatrol increases serum adiponectin and downregulates inflammatory genes in the peripheral blood mononuclear cells: a triple blind placebo controlled one year clinical trial in patents with stable coronary artery disease' Cardiovasc Drugs Ther 2013

[255] Kelley DS et al 'Sweet bing cherries lower circulating concentrations of markers for chronic inflammatory diseases in healthy humans' J Nutr 2013

[256] Aviram M, Rosenblat M, Dornfield L et al 'Pomegranate juice consumption reduces oxidative stress, atherogenic modifications to LDL and platelet aggregation: studies in humans & in atherosclerotic apolioprotein e deficient mice' AmJ Clin Nutr 2000: 71(5):1062-76

[257] Aedin Cassidy, Kenneth Mukamal, Lynda Liu 'High anthocyanin intake is associated with a reduced risk of myocardial infarction in young to middle aged women' Circulation: Journal of American Heart Association, 2013: 127:188-196

[258] McAnulty LS, Collier SR, Landram MJ 'Six weeks daily ingestion of whole blueberry powder increases natural killer cell counts and reduces arterial stiffness in sedentary males and females' Nutr Res 2014 July: 34(7): 577-84

[259] Ibid

[260] https://www.ncbi.nlm.gov/pmc/articles/PMC3813433/ 'Dietary flavonoid fisetin: A novel dual inhibitor of PI3K/Akt and mTOR for prostate cancer management'

[261] Clin Cancer Res. 2011 February 1;17(3):598-610

[262] David B. Haytowitz and Seema Bhagwat 'USDA Database for the Oxygen Radical Absorbance Capacity (ORAC) of Selected Foods' Release 2

[263] Dias MM et al 'Pro-apoptotic activities of polyphenolics from açai (Euterpe oleracea Martius) in human SW-480 colon cancer cells' Nutr Cancer. 2014;66(8):1394-405. doi: 10.1080/01635581.2014.956252. Epub 2014 Oct 20.

[264] Fragoso MF et al 'Inhibition of mouse urinary bladder carcinogenesis by açai fruit (Euterpe oleraceae Martius) intake' Plant Foods Hum Nutr. 2012 Sep;67(3):235-41.

[265] Silva DF et al 'Cytotoxic effects of Euterpe oleracea Mart. in malignant cell lines' BMC Complement Altern Med. 2014 May 29;14:175. doi: 10.1186/1472-6882-14-175.

[266] Shibu Poulose, Donna F Bielinski, and Barbara Shukitt-Hale 'Neuronal housekeeping via activation of autophagy by blueberry, strawberry, acai berry and walnut extracts'. FASBE Journal

[267] Huffington Post September 9, 2013

[268] Biomolecular and Clinical Aspects of Chinese Wolfberry CRC Press/Taylor & Francis 2011

[269] Beatty S, Murray IJ, Hensob DB et al 'Macular pigment and risk for age related macular degeneration in subjects from a Northern European Population' Invest Opthalmol Vis Sci 2001:42(2):439-46

[270] 'Monounsaturated fatty acid (avocado) rich diet for mild hypercholesterolemia' Lopez Ledesma et al Arch Med Res 1996 27(4): 519-23

[271] 'Effects of a vegetarian diet vs a vegetarian diet enriched with avocado in hypercholesterolemic patients' RCT Carranza-Madrigal et al Arch Med Res 1997 28(4):537-41

[272] 'Avocado consumption is associated with better diet quality and nutrient intake and lower metabolic syndrome risk in US adults - results from the National Health and Nutrition Examination Survey' (NHANES) 2001-2008

[273] 'Carotenoid absorption from salad and salsa by humans is enhanced by the addition of avocado or avocado oil' Unle NZ, Bohn T, Clinton SK, Schwartz SJ Journal Nutr 2005 March 135(3):431-1

[274] 'Antioxidant and prebiotic activity of five peonidin-based anthocyanin extracted from purple sweet potato' Sun H et al Sci Rep 2018

[275] Anand P, Kunnumakkara AB et al 'Bioavailability of Curcumin; problems and promises' Mol Pharm 2007 4(6):807-8

[276] Shoba G et al 'Influence of pipeline on the pharmacokinetics of cur cumin in animals and human volunteers' Planta Med 1998: 64(4); 353-6

[277] Jurenka JS 'Anti-inflammatory properties of curcumin, a major constituent of Curcuma longa: a review of preclinical and clinical research' Altern Med Rev. 2009 Jun;14(2):141-53.

[278] Menon VP 'Antioxidant and anti-inflammatory properties of curcumin' Adv Exp Med Biol. 2007;595:105-25.

[279] Suzhen Dong et al 'Curcumin Enhances Neurogenesis and Cognition in Aged Rats: Implications for Transcriptional Interactions Related to Growth and Synaptic Plasticity' PLoS One. 2012; 7(2): e31211

[280] Carroll RE 'Phase IIa clinical trial of curcumin for the prevention of colorectal neoplasia' Cancer Prev Res (Phila). 2011 Mar;4(3):354-64. doi: 10.1158/1940-6207.CAPR-10-0098.

[281] Tayyen RF 'Curcumin content of turmeric and curry powders' Nutr Cancer. 2006;55(2):126-31.

[282] Savini I 'Origanum vulgare induces apoptosis in human colon cancer caco2 cell' Nutr Cancer 2009:61(3):381-9. doi: 10.1080/01635580802582769.

[283] 'Carvacrol inhibits proliferation and induces apoptosis in human colon cancer cells' Anticancer Drugs. 2015 Sep;26(8):813-23. doi: 10.1097/CAD.0000000000000263.

[284] EE Mazokopakis, IK Starakis et al 'The hypolipidaemic effects of Spirulina (Arthrospira platensis) supplementation in a Cretan population: a prospective study' J Sci Food Agric. 2014 Feb; 94(3):432-7. doi: 10.1002/jsfa.6261. Epub 2013 Jul 10.

[285] Mohamed Ismail et al 'Chemoprevention of rat liver toxicity and carcinogenesis by Spirulina' Int J Biol Science 2009; 5(4): 377–387.

[286] Akao Y et al 'Enhancement of anti-tumor natural killer cell activation by orally administered Spirulina extract in mice'. Cancer Sci. 2009 Aug;100(8):1494-501. doi: 10.1111/j.1349-7006.2009.01188.x. Epub 2009 May 6.

[287] B Matthew, Nair PP et al 'Evaluation of Chemoprevention of oral cancer with Spirulina Fusiformis' Nutr Cancer. 1995;24(2):197-202

[288] Matsubara et al. "Radioprotective effect of metallo-thionine," presented at Radial Rays Conference, Tokyo Japan 1985

[289] Nutrients. 2017 Jul 6;9(7). pii: E708. doi: 10.3390/nu9070708

[290] J Nutr Sci Vitaminol (Tokyo). 2003 Oct;49(5):334-9

[291] Obes Res Clin Pract. 2013 Mar-Apr;7(2):e95-e105. doi: 10.1016/j.orcp.2013.01.002.

[292] Neuroscience Letters, Volume 464, Issue 3, 30 October 2009, Pages 193-198

[293] Int Immunopharmacol. 2003 Jun;3(6):889-900

[294] J Toxicol Sci. 2011 Jan; 36(1):121-6

[295] Stephen Crozier et al 'Cacao seeds are a 'Super Fruit': A comparative analysis of various fruit powders and products' Chemistry Central Journal2011 5:5

[296] T Schewe, Y Steffen 'How do dietary flavanols improve vascular function?' <u>Arch Biochem Biophys.</u> 2008 Aug 15;476(2):102-6. doi: 10.1016/j.abb.2008.03.004. Epub 2008 Mar 10.

[297] Wienreb O 'Neurological mechanisms of green tea polyphenols in Alzheimers and Parkinsons diseases' J Nutr Biochem 2004

[298] Tipoe GL et al 'Green tea polyphenols as an antioxidant and anti-inflammatory agent for cardiovascular protection' Cardiovasc Hematol Disocrd Drug Targets 2007

[299] Molina N et al 'Green polyphenols change the profile of inflammatory cytokine release from lymphocytes of obese and lean rats and protect against oxidative damage' Int Immnopharmacol 2015

[300] Tipoe GL et al 'Green tea polyphenols as an antioxidant and anti-inflammatory agent for cardiovascular protection' Cardiovas Hematol Disocrd Drug Targets 2007

[301] Anthony Samsel, Stephanie Seneff 'Glyphosate's suppression of Cytochrome P450 and Amino Acid Biosynthesis by the Gut Microbiome: pathways to Modern Diseases' Entropy 2013: 15(4): 1416-1463

[302] Agency for Research on Cancer 2015 and IARC Report

[303] Defra Committee on Pesticide Residues in Food (PRiF)

[304] Sheah JY 'Consumption of Red Meat but not cooking oils high in polyunsaturated fat is associated with higher arachidonic acid status in Singapore Chinese Adults' Nutrients 2017

[305] Allen NE 'The associations of diet with serum insulin like Growth Factor 1and its main binding proteins in 292 women meat eaters, vegetarians and vegans' Cancer Epidemiol Biomarkers Prev 2002 Nov : 11(11): 1441-8

[306] Tang WH 'Intestinal microbial metabolism of phosphatidylcholine and cardiovascular risk' N Engl J Med 2013 April 25:368(17): 1575-84

[307] David Perlmutter

[308] http://foodrevolution.org

[309] US Council of Environmental Quality

[310] R D Morris 'Drinking water and cancer' Environ Health Perspect 1995 Nov: 103 (Suppl 8): 225-231

[311] 'Sustainable Medicine' Dr Sarah Myhill Chapter 3 pp151

[312] Bertram LA, Stefanick ML, Saquib N, et al: Physical activity, additional breast cancer events, and mortality among early-stage breast cancer survivors: findings from the WHEL Study. Cancer Causes Control 2011;22:427-435.

[313] Irwin ML, Smith AW, McTiernan A, et al: Influence of pre- and postdiagnosis physical activity on mortality in breast cancer survivors: the health, eating, activity, and lifestyle study. J Clin Oncol 2008;26:3958-3964.

[314] Y Yamanaka, K Honma, S Hashimoto 'Effects of physical exercise on human circadian rhythmns' Sleep and Biological Rhythms 4, No 3, Sept 2006:199-206

[315] S A Tabish 'Is diabetes becoming the biggest epidemic of the twenty first century?' International Journal of Health Sciences 1, No 2, July 2007:v-viii

[316] National Heart, Lung and Blood Institute 'Coronary heart disease risk factors' 2016

[317] S C Moore, I M Lee, E Weiderpass et al 'Association of leisure time physical activity with risk of 26 types of cancer in 1.44 million adults' Journal of American Medical Association Internal Medicine 176 no 6 June 2016:816-25

[318] P A Sheridan, H A Paich, J Handy 'Obesity is associated with impaired immune response to influenza vaccination in humans' International Journal of Obesity 2005:36,No 8, August 2012:1072-77

[319] F S Luppino, LM de Wit et al 'Overweight obesity and depression: a systematic review and met-analysis of longitudinal studies' Archives of General Psychiatry' 67, No 3, March 2010:220-29

[320] S A Shapses, L C Pop 'Obesity is a concern for bone health with ageing' Nutrition Research 39 March 2017:1-13

[321] J C Nguyen, A S Killcross, T A Jenkins 'Obesity and Cognitive Decline: Role of inflammation and vascular changes' Frontiers in Neuroscience 8 December 2014:375

[322] T Tchkonia, D E Morbeck, T Von Zglinicki 'Fat tissue, ageing and cellular senescence' Aging Cell 9 No 5 May 2010: 667-84

[323] IM Lee 'Physical Activity and Cancer Prevention Data from Epidemiological Studies' Med Sci Sports Exerc Nov 2003 35 (11) 1823-1827

[324] MJM Magbanua 'Physical activity and prostate gene expression in men with lours prostate cancer.' Cancer causes & control 25 no 4 (Feb 2014):515-23

[325] K A Ashcraft, R M Peace et al 'Efficacy and mechanisms of aerobic exercise on cancer initiation, progression and metastasis: a critical systematic review of in vivo preclinical data' Cancer Research 76 No 14 (July 2016): 4032-50

[326] K M Mustian, LK Sprod et al 'Exercise recommendations for cancer related fatigue, cognitive impairment, sleep problems, depression, pain, anxiety and physical dysfunction; a review' Oncology Haematology Review 8, No 2 (January 2012): 81-88

[327] K M Mustian, L Peppone, TV Darling et al 'A 4 week home based aerobic and resistance exercise program during radiation therapy' a pilot randomised clinical trial' Journal of Supportive Oncology 7, No 5, Sept-Oct 2009: 158-67

328 Hutnick NA, Williams NI, Kraemer WJ, et al: Exercise and lymphocyte activation following chemotherapy for breast cancer. Med Sci Sports Exerc 2005;37:1827-1835.

329 'Multi-centre randomised control trial of yoga for sleep quality among cancer survivors' Journal of Clinical Oncology 31, No 26 (September 2013): 3233-41

330 B Oh, P N Butow, B Mullan et al 'Effect of medical Qigong on cognitive function, quality of life and a biomarker of inflammation in cancer patients: A randomised control trial' Supportive Care in Cancer 20 No 6 (June 2012): 1235-42

331 K M Mustian, CM Alfano 'Comparison of pharmaceutical, psychological and exercise treatments for cancer related fatigue: A meta-anaylsis' Journal of American Medical Association Oncology 3 No 7 (July 2017):961-68

332 Ghose A, Kundu R, Toumeh A, et al. A review of obesity, insulin resistance, and the role of exercise in breast cancer patients. *Nutr Cancer* 2015;**67**:197–202.

333 Goodwin PJ. Obesity, insulin resistance and breast cancer outcomes. *Breast* 2015; 24(Suppl 2):S56–9.

334 BHF Physical Activity Statistics 2015 pg 13

335 S W Cole, A S Nagaraja 'Sympathetic nervous system regulation of the tumour microenvironment ' Nature Reviews: Cancer 15 No 9 (Sept 2015):563-72

336 Blix E, Perski A et al 'Long term occupational stress is associated with regional reduction in brain tissue volumes' PLOS One 2013:8(6)

337 Black P H 'Stress and the Inflammatory response: a review of neurogenic inflammation' Brain Behav Immun 2002 Dec 16 (6): 622-53

338 P H Thacker, L Y Han et al 'Chronic stress promotes tumour growth and angiogenesis in a mouse model of ovarian carcinoma' Nature Medicine 12 no 8 (August 2006): 939-944

339 Y Childa, M Hamer, J Wardle et al 'Does stress related psychosocial factors contribute to cancer incidence and survival?' Nature Clinical Practice Oncology 5, No 8 2008

340 K Lillberg, PK Verkasalo, J Capri et al 'Stressful life events and risk of breast cancer in 10,808 women: a short study' American Journal of Epidemiology 157, 2003:415-23

341 M A Price, CC Tennant, PN Butow et al 'The role of physiological factors in the development of breast carcinoma: Part 2. Life event stressors, social support, defence style and emotional control and their interactions' Cancer 91(4):2001:686-97

342 M A Rosenkrantz, R J Davidson 'A comparison of mindfulness based stress reduction and an active control in modulation of neurogenic inflammation' Brain Behaviour and Immunity 27, No 1 (January 2013): 174-84

343 F Zedan, A L Adler-Neal 'Mindfulness meditation based pain relief is not mediated by endogenous opioids' Journal of Neuroscience 36 No 11 March 2016:3391-97

[344] Willougby Britton, Nathaniel E and Jonathan Gould 'A Randomised Controlled Pilot trial of Classroom Based Mindfulness Meditation compared to an Active Control Condition in 6th Grade Children' J Sch Psychol 2014 June(3): 263-278

[345] ibid

[346] NHS Digital Data 2016

[347] S Dworkis 'Recovery Yoga - A practical guide for chronically ill, injured and post-operative people' Three Rivers New York Press 1997

[348] D Gebhardt and C E Crump 'Employee fitness and wellness programs in the workplace' American Psychologist 45 (1990) 262-272

[349] J Lasater 'Yoga for Repetitive Strain Injury' OneBody Inc August 7 2001

[350] L Payne 'The Business of Teaching Yoga' Los Angeles Samata International Multi-media 2000

[351] D McDowell 'Harried Internet Execs are finding relaxation and inner peace through yoga' Yoga Journal Jan/Feb 2001 76-80

[352] S Taylor 'Introducing a yoga group in an acute inpatient psychiatric facility' OT Practice 6 (2000) 22-23

[353] K M Mustian, L K Sprod et al 'Mutlicantre Randomised Control Trial of Yoga for sleep quality among cancer survivors' Journal of Clinical Oncology 31, no 26, September 2013:3233-41

[354] K D Chandwani, G Perkins, HR Nagendra at el 'Randomised Control Trial of yoga in women with breast cancer undergoing radiotherapy' Journal of Clinical Oncology 32, no 10 (April 2014):1058-65

[355] Matthew Walker Business Insider

[356] Prof Maiken Nedergaard NIH 'How Sleep Clears the Brain' October 28th 2013

[357] Anand ST, MH Ebell 'Circadian disrupting exposures and breast cancer risk: A meta-analysis' Int Arch Occup Environ Health 2015 July:88(5):533-47

[358] K L Weihs, S J Simmonds, J Mizrahi 'Dependable social relationships predict overall survival in stages 2 & 3 breast carcinoma patients' Journal of Psychosomatic Research 59 No 5 November 2005:299-306

[359] S Hughes 'Social support predicts inflammation, pain and depressive symptoms: longitudinal relationships among breast cancer survivors' Psychoendocrinology 42 April 2014:38-44

[360] M Karin, F R Greten 'NF KappaB: Linking inflammation and immunity to cancer development and progression' Nature Reviews: Immunology 5 no 10 October 2005: 749-59

[361] C Kroenke, Y L Michael, EM Poole et al 'Post-diagnosis social networks and breast cancer mortality in the after breast cancer pooling project' Cancer 123, no 7 (April 2017): 1228-37

[362] Gustavsson J, Cederberg C, Sonnesson U et al 'Global food losses and food waste: Extent, causes and prevention' Rome, Food and Agriculture Organisation 2011

[363] FAO Food Wastage Footprint: Full Cost Accounting. www.fa.org/3/a-i3991e.pdf October 27 2014 Rome: Food and Agriculture Organisation 2014

[364] ibid

[365] https://timeforchange.org

[366] https://www.ourworldindata.org

[367] ibid

[368] https://ourworldindata.org

[369] ibid

[370] United Nations Report

[371] ibid

[372] ibid

[373] https://www.wri.org

[374] NRDC Report 2005-2014 World Resources Institute

[375] Gideon Eshel and Pamela Martin 'Diet, Energy & Global Warming' Earth Interactions Vol 10 2006

[376] Peter Scarbourogh, Paul Appleby, Anja Mizdrak 'Dietary greenhouse gas emissions meat eaters, fish eaters, vegetarians and vegans in the UK' Climatic Change July 2014, Volume 125 Issue 2, pp179-192

[377] Professor G David Tilman 'Nature' November 12

[378] Ibid

[379] New Scientist Magazine 18 July 2007, pp 15

[380] The Telegraph - https://www.independent.co.uk/life-style/food-and-drink/vegans-uk-rise-popularity-plant-based-diets-veganism-figures-survey-compare-the-market-a8286471.html

[381] 2018 Compare the Market Cars Against Humanity Survey - https://www.comparethemarket.com/car-insurance/content/cars-against-humanity

[382] Reducing foods environmental impacts through producers and cosumers J Poore, T Nemecek Science 01 June 2018 Voume 360 Issue 6392 pp 987-992 doi:10.1126/science.aaq0216

[383] Proceedings of the National Academy of Sciences March 26, 2018

[384] Hoekstra AY 'The water footprint of animal products in the meat crisis: Developing more sustainable production and consumption' Earthscan 2010: 22-33

[385] 'New Zealand Salmon Research Halted' Associated Press, Feb 26th 2000

[386] Allsopp et al. State of the World's Oceans, 2009, Springer

[387] Consumer Lab 2013, Covaci 2010, Foran 2003, Levine 2005

[388] Consumer Lab 2013

[389] Bao Y, Han J. Hu FB et al 'Association of nut consumption with total and cause specific mortality' N Eng J ed 2013:369(21):2001-11

[390] Nurk E, Refsum H et al 'US per capita food supply trends; more calories, refined carbohydrates and fats' Food Review 2002:25:2-15

Lightning Source UK Ltd.
Milton Keynes UK
UKHW051839200819
348291UK00001B/1/P